Decision Making in Pain Management

Decision Making in Pain Management

Second Edition

Somayaji Ramamurthy, MD
Professor, Department of Anesthesiology
University of Texas Health Sciences Center at San Antonio
San Antonio, Texas

Euleche Alanmanou, MD
Assistant Professor of Anesthesiology
University of Texas Medical Branch at Galveston
Medical Staff, Driscoll Children's Hospital
Corpus Christi, Texas

James N. Rogers, MD
Professor, Department of Anesthesiology
University of Texas Health Sciences Center at San Antonio
San Antonio, Texas

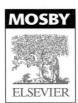

MOSBY

ELSEVIER

MOSBY
ELSEVIER

Four Penn Center, Suite 1800
1600 John F. Kennedy Boulevard
Philadelphia, Pennsylvania 19103

Notice

Knowledge and best practice in this field are constantly changing. As new research and experience
broaden our knowledge, changes in practice, treatment, and drug therapy may become necessary or
appropriate. Readers are advised to check the most current information provided (i) on procedures
featured or (ii) by the manufacturer of each product to be administered, to verify the recommended
dose or formula, the method and duration of administration, and contraindications. It is the
responsibility of the practitioner, relying on their own experience and knowledge of the patient,
to determine diagnoses, to determine dosages and the best treatment for each individual patient, and
to take all appropriate safety precautions. To the fullest extent of the law, neither the Publisher nor
the Editors assume any liability for any injury and/or damage to persons or property arising out or
related to any use of the material contained in this book.

THE PUBLISHER

First Edition 1993.

Library of Congress Cataloging-in-Publication Data
Decision making in pain management / [edited by] Somayaji Ramamurthy, James N.
    Rogers, Euleche Alanmanou.—2nd ed.
        p. ; cm.
    Includes bibliographical references and index.
    ISBN-13: 978-0-323-01974-3   ISBN-10: 0-323-01974-9
    1. Pain–Treatment–Decision making. 2. Analgesia–Decision making.
3. Anesthesia–Decision making. I. Ramamurthy, Somayaji. II. Rogers, James N. (James
Norman) III. Alanmanou, Euleche.
    [DNLM: 1. Pain–diagnosis. 2. Decision Trees. 3. Pain–therapy. 4. Palliative Care. WL
704 D294 2005]
    RB127.D43 2005
    616′.0472–dc22   2004044994

ISBN-13: 978-0-323-01974-3
ISBN-10: 0-323-01974-9

Publisher: Natasha Andjelkovic
Editorial Assistant: Katie Davenport
Senior Project Manager: Mary B. Stermel
Marketing Manager: Emily M. Christie

Printed in United States of America

Last digit is the print number: 9 8 7 6 5 4 3 2

To

Alon P. Winnie, M.D.,

A great teacher and friend,

In appreciation of his achievements and

his tireless efforts to reduce human suffering

LIST OF CONTRIBUTORS

Euleche Alanmanou, MD
Assistant Professor of Anesthesiology,
    University of Texas Medical Branch at Galveston;
    Medical Staff, Driscoll Children's Hospital,
    Corpus Christi, Texas

Sergio Alvarado, MD
Assistant Professor, Department of Anesthesiology,
    University of Texas Health Sciences Center at San
    Antonio, San Antonio, Texas

Douglas M. Anderson, MD
Associate Professor, Department of Anesthesiology,
    University of Texas Health Sciences Center at
    San Antonio, San Antonio, Texas

Michele L. Arnold, MD
Scottsbluff Physiatry Associates, Scottsbluff,
    Nebraska

Renee Bailey, MD
Department of Medicine (Neurology), University of
    Texas Health Sciences Center at San Antonio,
    San Antonio, Texas

Richard Barohn, MD
Professor and Chairman, Department of Neurology,
    University of Kansas Medical Center, Kansas City,
    Kansas

Nikesh Batra, MD
Private Practice, Columbus, Ohio

Jerry A. Beyer, MD
Director, Cardiothoracic Anesthesia Services, Wilford
    Hall Medical Center, Lackland AFB, Texas

Bert Blackwell, MD
Medical Director, Pain Clinic, East Jefferson Hospital,
    Metairie, Louisiana

Nikolai Bogduk, MD
Director, Department of Clinical Research, Royal
    Newcastle Hospital, Newcastle, New South Wales,
    Australia

Gordon Bosker, MEd, CPO
Department of Rehabilitation Medicine, University of
    Texas Health Sciences Center at San Antonio,
    San Antonio, Texas

Octavio Calvillo, MD, PhD
Attending Anesthesiologist, The Methodist Hospital,
    Houston, Texas

Javier Canon, MD
Addiction Psychiatrist, University Center for Pain
    Medicine, Department of Anesthesiology, University
    of Texas Health Sciences Center at San Antonio,
    San Antonio, Texas

Stephen W. Dinger, DO
Department of Rehabilitation Medicine, University of
    Texas Health Sciences Center at San Antonio,
    San Antonio, Texas

Susan J. Dreyer, MD
Associate Professor of Orthopaedics, Emory University,
    Emory Orthopaedics and Spine Center, Atlanta,
    Georgia

Thomas A. Edell, MD
Assistant Professor of Anesthesiology, Director,
    Pain Medicine, Wilford Hall Medical Center,
    Lackland AFB, Texas

Jay Ellis, MD
Clinical Professor, Department of Anesthesiology,
    University of Texas Health Sciences Center at
    San Antonio, San Antonio, Texas

Mirelle Foster, MD
Medical Director of Acute Rehabilitation Unit, Sid
    Peterson Memorial Hospital, Kerrville, Texas

Ted Gingrich, MD
Anesthesia Consultants of Fresno, Fresno,
    California

Andrew Gitter, MD
Department of Rehabilitation Medicine, University of
    Texas Health Sciences Center at San Antonio,
    San Antonio, Texas

Kenneth R. Goldschneider, MD
Director, Division of Pain Management,
    Cincinnati Children's Hospital Medical Center,
    Cincinnati, Ohio

James G. Griffin, PT, ATC
Clinical Assistant Professor, Department of
    Anesthesiology, University of Texas Health Sciences
    Center at San Antonio, San Antonio, Texas

Catherine Hoerster, PhD
Transplant Psychologist, Texas Transplant Institute for
    Methodist Healthcare Systems, San Antonio, Texas

Stuart W. Hough, MD
Pain Management Specialists, PC, Rockville, Maryland

Paul T. Ingmundson, PhD
Staff Psychologist, Audie L. Murphy Memorial Veterans Hospital; Staff Polysomnographer, Sleep Disorders Laboratory, Neurodiagnostic Center, University Hospital of San Antonio, San Antonio, Texas

John C. King, MD
Professor, Department of Rehabilitation Medicine, University of Texas Health Sciences Center at San Antonio; Director of Reeves Rehabilitation Center, University Health System, Department of Physical Medicine, Audie L. Murphy Memorial Veterans Hospital, San Antonio, Texas

Qassem Kishawi, MD
Assistant Clinical Professor, Department of Anesthesiology, University of Connecticut School of Medicine, Assistant Attending, St. Francis Hospital and Medical Center, Hartford, Connecticut

Kelly Gordon Knape, MD
Clinical Professor, Department of Anesthesiology, University of Texas Health Sciences Center at San Antonio, San Antonio, Texas

Erik M. Kussro, DO
Alaska Rehabilitation Medicine, Anchorage, Alaska

Ellen Leonard, MD
South Texas PM&R Group, Inc., San Antonio, Texas

Jonathan P. Lester, MD
Concentra Medical Centers – New Jersey, Bellmawr, New Jersey

Aaron Malakoff, MD
Medical Director, Hope Hospice, New Braunfels, Texas

Magaly V. Marrero, PhD
Health Support Psychology, San Antonio, Texas

Stephen B. Milam, DDS, PhD
Professor and Hugh B. Tilson Endowed Chair, Department of Oral and Maxillofacial Surgery, University of Texas Health Sciences Center at San Antonio, San Antonio, Texas

Susan Noorily, MD
Clinical Professor, Department of Anesthesiology, University of Texas Health Sciences Center at San Antonio, San Antonio, Texas

Somayaji Ramamurthy, MD
Professor, Department of Anesthesiology, University of Texas Health Sciences Center at San Antonio, San Antonio, Texas

T.R. Christian Reutter, DO
Private Practice, San Francisco, California

John R. Roberts, MD
Tennessee Valley Pain Consultants, Huntsville, Alabama

James N. Rogers, MD
Professor, Department of Anesthesiology, University of Texas Health Sciences Center at San Antonio, San Antonio, Texas

Mark E. Romanoff, MD
Medical Director, Southeast Pain Care, Charlotte, North Carolina

I. Jon Russell, MD, PhD
Associate Professor of Medicine, Director, University Clinical Research Center, University of Texas Health Sciences Center at San Antonio, San Antonio, Texas

Lawrence S. Schoenfeld, PhD, ABPP
Professor and Director of Clinical Psychology Residency and Fellow Programs, University of Texas Health Sciences Center at San Antonio, San Antonio, Texas

Ioannis Sharibas, MD
Clinical Assistant Professor, Department of Anesthesiology, Baylor College of Medicine, Houston, Texas

Erik Shaw, DO
Department of Rehabilitation Medicine, University of Texas Health Sciences Center at San Antonio, San Antonio, Texas

Maurice G. Sholas, MD, PhD
Assistant Professor and Director, Pediatric Rehabilitation Program, Louisiana State University Health Sciences Center, New Orleans, Louisiana

Tracy Sloan, PhD
Private Practice, San Antonio, Texas

Dale Solomon, MD
Tejas Anesthesia, P.A., San Antonio, Texas

Robert Sprague, MD
Chief of Anesthesia Operative Services, Heywood Hospital, Gardner, Massachusetts

Suzette M. Stoks, PhD
Assistant Professor, South Texas Addiction Research and Technology (START) Center, University of Texas Health Sciences Center at San Antonio, San Antonio, Texas

William E. Strong, MD
Staff Anesthesiologist, Central Utah Surgical Center, Orem, Utah

Jeffrey T. Summers, MD
Clinical Assistant Professor, Department of Anesthesiology, University of Mississippi Medical Center, Jackson, Mississippi

Ley L. Taylor-Jones, DO
Private Practice, Plano, Texas

Linda Tingle, MD
Clinical Associate Professor, Department
of Anesthesiology, University of Texas Health
Sciences Center at San Antonio, San Antonio,
Texas

Renee Van Stavern, MD
Assistant Professor of Neurology, Wayne State
University Comprehensive Stroke Program, Detroit,
Michigan

Anna M. Varughese, MD
Associate Professor of Clinical Anesthesia and
Pediatrics, Cincinnati Children's Hospital Medical
Center, Cincinnati, Ohio

Norbert J. Weidner, MD
Associate Professor of Clinical Anesthesia and
Pediatrics, Cincinnati Children's Hospital Medical
Center, Cincinnati, Ohio

Lynda Wells, MD, DABPM
Associate Professor, Department of Anesthesiology,
University of Virginia Health System, Charlottesville,
Virginia

Roger Wesley, MD
Staff Anesthesiologist, Lewis-Gale Medical Center,
Salem, Virginia

Marcos A. Zuazu, MD
Associate Professor, Department of Anesthesiology,
University of Texas Health Sciences Center at
San Antonio, San Antonio, Texas

PREFACE TO THE SECOND EDITION

Many clinicians, especially pain management physicians, have reiterated the usefulness of the algorithmic approach to the evaluation and treatment of pain, which was outlined in the first edition of *Decision Making in Pain Management.*

There have been great advances in the concepts, approaches, treatment options, and technology in pain medicine, which necessitate significant revision in order to make the book more relevant to the present day practitioner.

This book is not meant to replace in-depth, highly referenced textbooks in pain medicine. It may, nevertheless, be a valuable supplement, providing pain clinicians with a logical, concise, step-wise approach to the identification, diagnosis, and management of various acute or chronic painful conditions or syndromes.

We have maintained the multidisciplinary approach with inputs from various specialties. While many chapters have been added to reflect the advances in the field of pain medicine, several other chapters, including the descriptions of nerve block techniques, have been deleted in this edition because the actual techniques are better explained in regional anesthsia textbooks, rather than in an algorithmic approach. Also, outlines were provided for *select* chapters that we felt benefited from that format. In areas of controversies, the chapters may reflect the preferences of the individual author.

We would like to thank all our many contributors, whose efforts will make this book unique, useful, and give it a multidisciplinary character. We would also like to thank Natasha Andjelkovic, PhD, of Elsevier for her perseverance.

A note of thanks to Ashley Alanmanou, DDS, whose help, patience and devotion in preparing this manuscript were truly amazing.

We offer special thanks to Ms. Linda Shimerda, for her tireless effort in coordinating the activities of multiple editors and authors. Without her, this book would not have been possible.

Somayaji Ramamurthy, MD
Euleche Alanmanou, MD
James N. Rogers, MD

CONTENTS

EVALUATION

INITIAL MANAGEMENT OF ACUTE PAIN

EVALUATION OF THE CHRONIC PAIN PATIENT

EVALUATION OF PAIN IN CHILDREN

EVALUATION OF THE GERIATRIC PAIN PATIENT

ASSESSMENT OF SUBSTANCE ABUSE POTENTIAL

PSYCHOLOGICAL EVALUATION

SLEEP DISTURBANCES AND CHRONIC PAIN

DISABILITY AND QUALITY OF LIFE

POSTTRAUMATIC STRESS DISORDER

PAIN MEASUREMENT

IMAGING STUDIES

DISCOGRAPHY

ELECTROMYOGRAPHY AND NERVE CONDUCTION STUDIES (UPPER/LOWER)

THERMOGRAPHY

EXAMINATION UNDER SEDATION

TESTING AND TREATMENT WITH INTRAVENOUS LOCAL ANESTHETICS AND OTHER DRUGS

DIFFERENTIAL EPIDURAL/SPINAL BLOCKADE

DIAGNOSTIC NEURAL BLOCKS

Initial Management of Acute Pain

JAY ELLIS

A. First things first. Pain is a complex sensory and emotional experience because of tissue injury or as described in terms of tissue injury. Assess for reversible, treatable causes of tissue injury that threaten life, limb, or organ function such as compartment syndrome, ischemic pain, or compressive neuropathy.

B. History and physical examination. Assess pain for intensity, location, quality, radiation, aggravating and alleviating factors, and temporal relationships (timing).
   1. Intensity. Use an age-appropriate pain rating scale. Assess pain level at rest and with activity to identify incident pain or pain associated only with certain movements or activities.
      a. Children 0 to 2 years of age: Assess level of irritability, vital signs, activity.
      b. Children 3 to 12 years of age: Faces Scale, picture board with faces from happy and smiling to extremely sad and crying, representing graded increases in pain from none to extreme
      c. Adults and older children: Verbal pain score, on a scale from 0 to 10, with zero indicating no pain and 10 the worst possible pain imaginable
   2. Location. Pain that is precisely located to site of injury/surgical incision often (but not always) indicates local tissue injury and nociception. Vague, poorly localized pain often (but not always) represents visceral organ pain
   3. Quality. Certain sensations suggest certain types of problems. "Pins and needles," burning, tingling, and numbness suggest possible ischemia or nerve compression. Cramping, colicky pain suggests obstruction of a hollow viscus.
   4. Radiation. Does the pain travel? Radiation in characteristic patterns suggests a specific site, for example, L4–5 disk herniation causing posterior thigh and calf pain.
   5. Aggravating and alleviating factors. Does rest relieve pain or does activity increase it? Which activities? Does heat or cold make it better or worse? These provide clues to cause and suggest treatment.
   6. Temporal relationships. Is the pain constant, intermittent, getting better, staying the same, or getting worse? Pain that comes and goes suggests smooth or skeletal muscle contraction/spasm as an element of the pain.

C. Diagnostic tests. Dictated by disease state.

D. General management principles. Classification of pain into mild (1 to 4/10 on Verbal Pain Score), moderate (5 to 7/10 on Verbal Pain Score), and severe (8 to 10/10 on Verbal Pain Score), helps determine initial therapy.

   1. Mild pain: Treat with physical modalities as appropriate. Use ice to reduce swelling and heat to promote edema resolution. Massage relieves muscle aches and spasm. Holding a pillow against a surgical incision splints the incision during pulmonary therapy.
      a. Analgesics: oral acetaminophen 325 to 1000 mg every 4 to 6 hours up to 4 g every 24 hours. Reduce dose for patients with a history of liver insufficiency or history of regular alcohol ingestion of more than three drinks per day.
      b. Oral nonsteroidal antiinflammatory drugs (NSAIDs). Suggested doses are ibuprofen 400 to 800 mg orally tid up to 3200 mg every 24 hours or naproxen 250 to 500 mg bid. There is no evidence to suggest that one NSAID is more effective than another for acute pain management. The most rational method of choosing an NSAID is cost. Side effect profiles are remarkably similar for all NSAIDs for acute, short-term management. Indomethacin has the most prominent antiinflammatory effects of common NSAIDs and may be less advisable for use in patients at risk for renal injury. All NSAIDs except COX-2 (cyclooxygenase 2) inhibitors affect platelet function and hemostasis and are contraindicated in patients with coagulopathy or where bleeding could be catastrophic (postoperative neurosurgical patients). All NSAIDs cause gastrointestinal symptoms and increase the risk of gastrointestinal bleeding. NSAIDs should be avoided in patients at high risk for gastrointestinal bleeding. COX-2 inhibitors have fewer antiplatelet effects and may be more advantageous for postoperative pain control and in patients on other anticoagulants. The increased risks of cardiac and vascular events in patients with COX-2 inhibitors deserve attention.
      c. Ketoralac. The initial dose for single treatment is 60 mg IM or 30 mg IV. Reduce dose by half for patients who weigh less than 50 kg, have renal impairment, or are older than 65 years of age.

   If mild pain persists despite use of physical modalites and simple analgesics go to methods for treating:

   2. Moderate pain. Use physical modalities and a mild analgesic as indicated, but moderate pain usually requires administration of an opioid medication for effective treatment. Less potent opioids are usually sufficient. Oral combinations of acetaminophen–codeine, acetaminophen–hydrocodone, or acetaminophen–oxycodone are usually effective

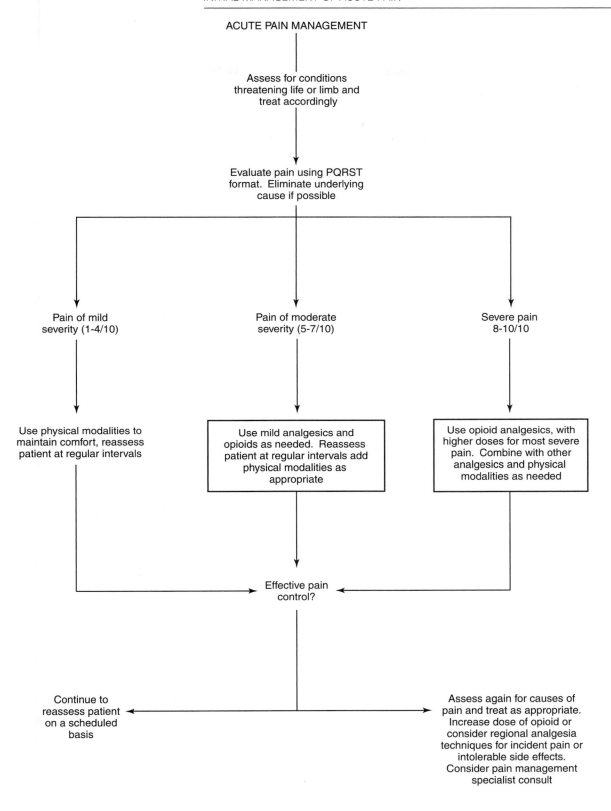

in doses of one or two tablets orally every 4 to 6 hours. The maximum dose of combination medications is limited by the amount of acetaminophen in the tablet. The maximum dose of acetaminophen is 4 g every 24 hours and should be reduced by at least 30% for those with a history of liver disease or regular alcohol ingestion of three drinks or more each day. If moderate pain fails to respond to oral therapy with less potent opioids or oral therapy is contraindicated, go to treatment for:

3. Severe pain. Severe pain usually requires prompt treatment with a potent opioid. While the oral route may be effective, the delay in onset of 30 to 60 minutes makes initial treatment with parenteral therapy more desirable. Interindividual variation in opioid requirement is large, making initial dosage recommendations only a starting point for most patients. Some patients need 10 times the initial recommended dose to achieve pain relief. Patients with higher pain scores require larger initial doses of opioid to control pain. Common starting doses of parenteral opioids are as follows: morphine at a dose of 2 to 5 mg IV, with onset of relief in 5 to 8 minutes and duration of 3 to 4 hours; meperidine at a dose of 20 to 50 mg IV, with onset of relief in 3 to 5 minutes and duration of 3 to 4 hours; hydromorphone at a dose of 2 to 5 mg IV, with onset of relief in 3 to 5 minutes and duration of 2 to 3 hours; fentanyl at a dose of 1 to 2 mcg/kg IV, with onset of relief in 1 to 2 minutes and duration of 1 to 2 hours.

The end point of opioid administration is pain relief (verbal pain score of 3 or less) or development of intolerable side effects.

All opioids cause nausea, vomiting, constipation, miosis, dose-dependent sedation, and respiratory depression. Nausea and vomiting can be managed by switching to another opioid or by administering an antiemetic such as promethazine 12.5 to 25 mg IV or IM every 6 hours as needed. Constipation is best treated with the use of a colonic motility agent such as oral or rectal bisacodyl or senna extract. Morphine and meperidine cause histamine release.

E. Specific treatment. Patient-controlled analgesia (PCA) is an effective way to administer opioid medication with pain relief equal or superior to that of as-needed administration and higher patient satisfaction ratings. Side effects are equal to or reduced when compared to as-needed administration.
1. Patient requirements are sufficient mental capacity to understand the treatment technique and physical ability to push the infusion button
2. Recommended settings are as follows: morphine, loading dose of 4 to 20 mg IV, demand dose 1 mg every 10 minutes, 4-hour lockout of 16 mg. A word about basal infusion rates: Basal infusion rates increase the risk of respiratory complications with PCA without necessarily increasing effectiveness of analgesia. Basal infusions may be necessary for patients with a high opioid requirement resulting from chronic opioid use (cancer pain patients, substance abuse).

Patients on mechanical ventilation who are not at risk for apnea may benefit from a basal infusion
3. Pain refractory to opioids. Pain poorly responsive to opioids may be due to compartment syndrome/ischemia; in this case, treat the underlying problem. Pain due to neural injury requires adjuvant analgesics such as tricyclic antidepressants (amitriptyline), anticonvulsants (gabapentin), or regional anesthesia for pain control. Incident pain—pain due to activity or movement, with little pain at rest—is difficult to control with opioids. Doses necessary to control incident pain cause excessive sedation at rest. Consider regional anesthesia (nerve blocks, epidural analgesia) and stabilization of fractures to control pain.
4. Interindividual variation for opioid requirement. Doses of opioids required for pain control vary by a factor of 10 between individuals. For example, the average dose of morphine for open cholecystectomy pain is 5 mg IV, but doses range from 2 to 20 mg IV.
5. Epidural analgesia. Small amounts of opioids given in epidural or intrathecal space provide profound analgesia with less sedation than parenteral administration. Combined with dilute solutions of local anesthetics via constant infusion or patient-controlled epidural analgesia, epidural analgesia is very effective for incident and neuropathic pain.
6. Regional anesthesia. Nerve blocks can provide analgesia anesthesia of regions of the body. Intercostal nerve blocks for rib fractures, femoral nerve block for femur fracture, and brachial plexus block for upper extremity pain are just a few useful examples.

F. Ongoing assessment. Assess patients for pain at regular intervals, making pain score the "fifth vital sign." Monitor for side effects and complications and treat aggressively.

G. Complications and side effects.
1. NSAIDs: bleeding, platelet dysfunction, gastrointestinal distress/hemorrhage, renal injury
2. Opioids: constipation, nausea/vomiting, sedation, pruritis, respiratory depression
3. PCA: Overdose of opioid from misprogramming of pump
4. Epidural/intrathecal analgesia: same as for opioids plus urinary retention and delayed respiratory depression (up to 24 hours) with epidural/intrathecal morphine.

REFERENCES

Loeser JD: *Bonica's Management of Pain*, 3rd ed. Philadelphia, Lippincott Williams & Wilkins, 2001.

Practice guidelines for acute pain management in the perioperative setting: an updated report by the American Society of Anesthesiologists Task Force on Acute Pain Management. *Anesthesiology* 2004; 100:1573–1581.

Evaluation of the Chronic Pain Patient

SOMAYAJI RAMAMURTHY

The evaluation should take into consideration the multidimensional nature of chronic pain, consisting of nociceptive input, changes in the peripheral central nervous system, referred pain from visceral and somatic structures, multiple therapeutic procedures, and medication use that results in side effects, disability, and deconditioning. The associated psychological factors including depression and behavioral changes, as well as social and economic consequences secondary to unemployment and financial problems, are further complicating factors.

A. Review of medical records. The patient's medical records and the history of previous therapeutic modalities, with their results and complications, should be reviewed thoroughly before the evaluation. A questionnaire is useful to obtain information regarding the patient's pain level; pain descriptors; previous medical procedures and medications; current pharmacotherapy, especially the use of anticoagulants and herbal and over-the-counter medications; sleep; mood; activity; and exercises. Information regarding legal claims related to work injury and automobile or other accidents is very relevant. A pain diagram is extremely useful in determining the location and radiation of the pain, and in addition characterizes the pain, such as burning, shooting, or with associated numbness. The pain diagram is used not only to determine the details about the pain but it may also provide insight into the psychological factors. We find routine use of the Beck depression inventory very informative. Reviewing the details provided by the patient's questionnaire makes the interview and history-taking much better directed and thorough, saves time, and reassures the patient that the physician is well informed of his or her condition.

B. History. A thorough history is taken including the review of systems followed by questions directed specifically toward the pain, related to its origin; type; character (such as burning, stabbing, and so forth), radiation; and aggravating and relieving factors. The relevant information obtained from the questionnaire is extremely useful in directing the questions to determine whether the type of pain is likely to be nociceptive, neuropathic, or referred. Details regarding the results of the previous therapeutic modalities, complications, allergies are helpful in planning the management.

C. Physical examination. The physical examination starts as soon as the clinician enters the patient's room. The patient's mood, expression, range of motion of the painful body part when the patient is concentrating on giving the history, and interaction with family members in the examination room provide important insight. A general neurologic examination may reveal neurologic changes including sensory, motor, reflex changes, and nerve tension signs, which can assist in the diagnosis of radicular pain, complex regional pain syndrome, and neuropathic pain. Evaluation of the gait and range of motion of the joints together with particular tests to delineate specific pathology of hip, knee, facet, sacroiliac, and other joints, as well as examination of the muscular trigger points, are necessary to determine the source of pain. Maneuvers that reproduce the patient's exact pain are very informative. Signs of nonorganic pain include nondermatomal, inconsistent decrease in sensation to pinprick; significant discrepancy in range of motion with distraction; and significant pain behavior with range of motion and palpation during examination that was not observed in the patient during the history taking.

D. Investigation. After the history and physical examination and review of the previous studies including imaging, further tests may be needed. Most of the chronic pain patients are likely to have had significant imaging studies before an evaluation by a pain specialist. Imaging is useful to rule out fractures, tumors, or other pathology. But it is very important to be aware that tests such as magnetic resonance imaging (MRI) can reveal significant anatomic abnormalities even in asymptomatic individuals; thus it is very important to correlate the findings with the results of a thorough history and physical examination to avoid unnecessary invasive procedures. Electromyography (EMG) and nerve conduction studies if positive are very helpful to confirm change in the physiologic function of the muscles and nerves even though a negative EMG nerve conduction may not rule out pathology. Drug screening tests may be necessary to evaluate a patient's consumption of prescription and illicit drugs.

E. Neural blockade and intravenous testing. Differential nerve blocks have been utilized in the diagnosis and to plan the treatment of pain syndromes. Diagnostic injections such as medial branch blocks, sacroiliac joint injections, and discography and nerve root blocks are very valuable in the diagnosis of pain originating from the spine. Even when there is pain relief, the important role of placebo should be taken into consideration before planning invasive procedures. The lack of pain relief following a nerve block helps to avoid unnecessary neurodestructive procedures.

Intravenous testing using a placebo, lidocaine, opioid agonists and antagonists, benzodiazepines, and pentothal are extremely useful in the differential diagnosis of nonperipheral pain. Unfortunately these tests are not frequently employed because of the significant time required and lack of financial reimbursement.

F. Psychological and functional testing. The initial evaluation of the patient may indicate a need for further psychological testing and evaluation of functional ability and impairments and need for orthotics and assist devices.

REFERENCES

Godwin J, Zahid Bajwa Z: Evaluating the patient with chronic pain. In: Warfield CA, Godwin J, Bajwa Z (eds) *Principles and Practice of Pain Medicine*, 2nd ed. New York, McGraw-Hill, 2004, pp. 55–60.

Loeser JD (ed): *Bonica's Management of Pain,* 3rd ed., Philadelphia, Lippincott Williams & Wilkins, 2001.

EVALUATION OF THE CHRONIC PAIN PATIENT

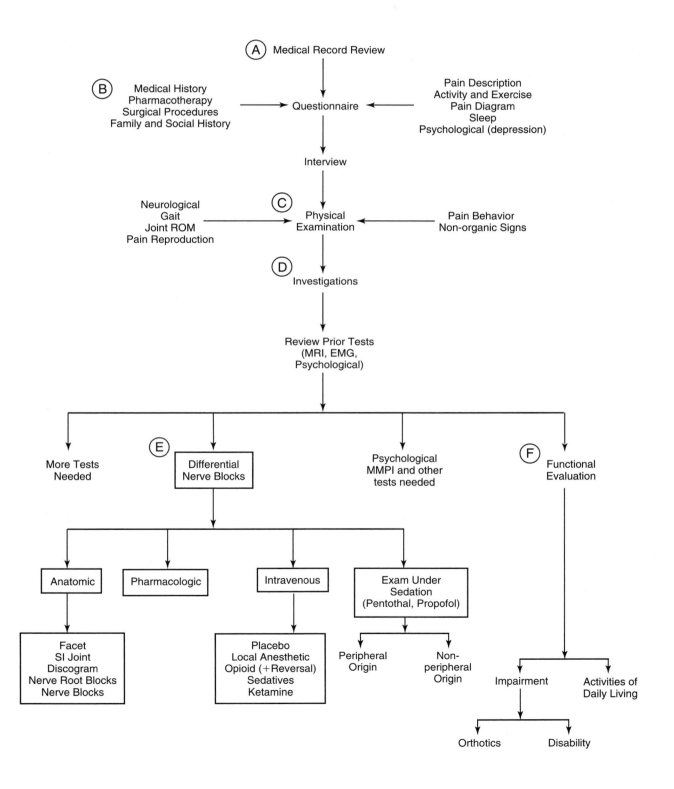

Evaluation of Pain in Children

ANNA M. VARUGHESE, NORBERT J. WEIDNER,
AND KENNETH R. GOLDSCHNEIDER

Pain in neonates and children has historically been underreported, misunderstood, and undertreated. Although the subject of pediatric pain has been in the spotlight during the past decade, recent investigations show limited improvement in prevailing practices in the field despite efforts to change the practice of clinicians.

A. The universal objectives of pain assessment are at least threefold: (1) to detect the presence of pain; (2) to estimate the potential impact of pain on the patient, which then influences the decision-making process or methods of intervention; and (3) to reassess pain at frequent intervals and determine the effectiveness of these interventions. The evaluation should include a review of the patient's history and physical examination. Patients should be assessed using developmentally and clinically appropriate tools. Although multiple tools exist to measure and assess pain in children, many are not well validated and not applicable to all age groups, and none has been universally accepted. Generally, pain assessment instruments in children can be categorized as observational, self-reported, and the results of physiological instruments. In children 5 years of age and older, assessment is facilitated by the self-report, which is accompanied by observational descriptors. In younger children and children with cognitive disabilities, physiological parameters (e.g., changes in heart rate and blood pressure, palmar sweating, changes in transcutaneous oxygen tension) and observational descriptors (e.g., crying, facial expression, leg position, touch, behavior) have been used to assess pain.

   1. Some age-appropriate tools are the Neonatal Infant Pain Scale (NIPS) (0–14 years), the Children's Hospital Eastern Ontario Pain Scale (CHEOPS) (1–5 years), OUCHER (a pain scale for children) (>5 years), the Visual Analog Scale (VAS) (>8 years), and the COMFORT scale for unconscious patients; moreover, the Noncommunicating Children's Pain Checklist (NCCPC) and more recently the NCCPC-PV (postoperative version) have been validated for use in children with intellectual disabilities.
   2. Investigations are limited to those that help with the plan for pain management (e.g., coagulation studies to rule out a coagulopathy before regional analgesia, renal profile to determine the opioid of choice). Morphine is avoided in patients with impaired renal function due to the accumulation of the active metabolite morphine 6-glucuronide.

B. The options available for managing acute pain are systemic treatment with analgesics such as opioids or nonsteroidal antiinflammatory drugs (NSAIDs), regional analgesia (central or peripheral nerve blocks), or a combination of the above. The choice is made after considering many factors (i.e., the etiology, location, and intensity of pain; the impact of pain on the patient, the presence of contraindications). Regional analgesia is not the preferred option in the presence of abnormal coagulation, febrile bacteremia, ongoing neurologic defects, or parent/patient refusal.

C. Systemic treatment with analgesics is useful for the following groups of pediatric pain patients.

   1. Surgical and trauma patients in whom regional anesthesia is not appropriate because of the surgical site or surgical intensity or in whom it is contraindicated
   2. Cancer patients with pain caused by the disease process or chemotherapy; those with pain associated with procedures
   3. Hematologic patient with sickle cell disease and pain from vasoocclusive crises not amenable to regional anesthesia
   4. General medical patients with acute pain (e.g., due to cystic fibrosis, pancreatitis, lupus, or juvenile rheumatoid arthritis)

D. Regional techniques often offer better analgesia with fewer side effects. Major complications (e.g., permanent neuronal injury) are decidedly uncommon. More serious complications involve a local anesthetic toxicity or narcotic-induced respiratory depression. Less serious but bothersome side effects (e.g., pruritus, nausea and vomiting, urinary retention) are related to centrally administered narcotics.

E. Systemic analgesia with opioids can be provided orally, parenterally, and transcutaneously. Patient-controlled analgesia is suitable for developmentally normal children 6 years of age or more. For younger children and children with cognitive disabilities, nurse/caregiver- or parent-controlled analgesia is an option. In the absence of allergies, morphine is often the first drug of choice. If side effects occur or pain control is inadequate with increasing doses, hydromorphone and fentanyl are alternatives. Supplementation with NSAIDs and acetaminophen improves the quality of analgesia and the patient's ability to ambulate after surgery. Ketorolac has few side effects and provides excellent supplemental analgesia; it should be avoided, however, in the presence of continued bleeding, hypovolemia, or decreased urinary output. The intramuscular route is avoided if possible.

F. Central blocks are performed much more commonly than peripheral nerve blocks in children. Continuous epidural analgesia and single-shot caudal analgesia is the most frequently performed block. The puncture site and location of the tip of the catheter determine the drug used. The issue of placing the epidural catheter in awake versus asleep children has been debated.

In children 8 years of age and older, placing the catheter while the child is awake or lightly sedated is encouraged. Thoracic puncture in sleeping younger patients is reserved for cases where the benefits outweigh the risks; and it should be performed by experienced practitioners. The addition of butorphanol to the epidural infusion can reduce the severity of itching. The use of an α_2–adrenergic drug may prolong the analgesia for single-shot caudal application with an acceptable side effect profile.

REFERENCES

Berde CB: Acute postoperative pain management in children. *ASA Refresher Course Lect* 1995;225:1–7.

Breau LM, Finley GA, McGrath PJ, Camfield CS: Validation of noncommunicating children's pain checklist-postoperative version. *Anesthesiology* 2002;96:528–535.

Mathews JR, McGrath PJ, Pigeon H: Assessment and measurement of pain in children. In: Schecter NL, Berde CB, Yaster M (eds) *Pain in Infants and Children and Adolescents.* Baltimore, Williams & Wilkins, 1993, pp 96–111.

EVALUATION OF PAIN IN CHILDREN

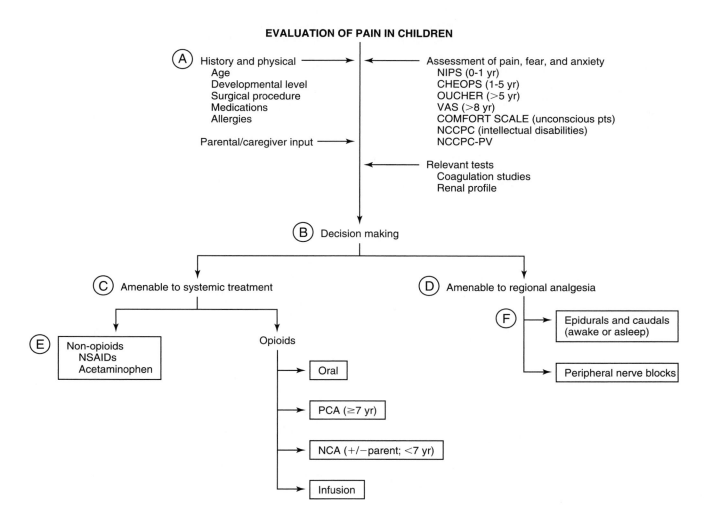

Evaluation of the Geriatric Pain Patient

SOMAYAJI RAMAMURTHY

Pain complaints are twice as common in the population older than 60 years than in the younger population. However, pain in the elderly is undertreated because of misconceptions such as that the elderly are expected to have pain or they are too ill and too sensitive to medications and cannot be safely treated. This is further compounded by the patient's not wanting to bother the family with their pain complaints and a decreasing ability to express themselves clearly secondary to short-term memory problems, the onset of dementia, and the debilitating effects of numerous medications being taken for various systemic illnesses.

A. A thorough history and complete review of the medical records, including all medications the patient is taking and has previously tried is important because elderly patients have significant concurrent illnesses requiring numerous medications. Because of the debility, short-term memory problems, and associated dementia, it is essential to obtain complete information. This frequently requires obtaining the information from the caregivers regarding the medications, activities of daily living, history of falls, and pain behavior. Frequently, patients are not aware of anticoagulant and antiplatelet medications they are taking. This can lead to serious problems, secondary to drug interactions or following invasive procedures.

B. The pain evaluation can be extremely difficult because of poor eyesight, impaired hearing, debility, memory problems, and dementia. The Verbal Descriptive Scale (VDS) appears to be the easiest test to complete and the most informative. However, a combination of the Visual Analogue Scale (VAS), Numerical Rating Scale (NRS), and the VDS is likely to yield information that is more complete. Questions requiring short yes or no answers are more likely to be understood. Pain diaries may be critical to document reliably the responses to medications and procedures. In patients with significant dementia, observation of the pain behavior and information gathered from the caregivers is essential when evaluating the patient's pain.

C. In addition to a thorough neurologic examination, it is essential to evaluate for significant deconditioning, decreased joint motion, and muscle tightness. A multidisciplinary examination is useful for evaluating gait ("get up and go test"), mobility, and the need for assistance (cane, walker, wheelchair), the activities of daily living, and pain behavior. Significant anxiety and depression are common and require thorough evaluation and treatment to control pain adequately.

REFERENCES

Ferrell BA: Pain management in the elderly people. *J Am Geriatr Soc* 1991;39:64.

Ferrell BA, Ferrell BR, Rivera L: Pain in the cognitively impaired nursing home patients. *J Pain Symptom Manage* 1995;10:591.

Sorkin B, Turk D: Pain management in the elderly. In: Roy R (ed) *Chronic Pain in Old Age.* Toronto, University of Toronto Press, 1995, pp 156–180.

EVALUATION OF THE GERIATRIC PATIENT

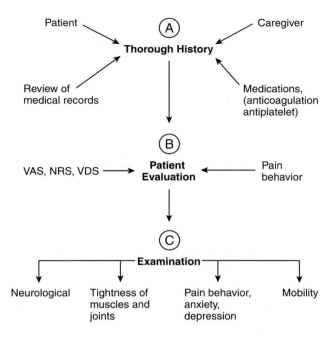

Assessment of Substance Abuse Potential

MAGALY V. MARRERO

Opiates are commonly used to treat chronic, nonmalignant pain. Much controversy remains regarding the use of traditional definitions of abuse and dependence when treating pain patients. The emphasis on tolerance and withdrawal in these traditional definitions [*Diagnostic and Statistical Manual, 4th Edition* (DSM-IV)] make them inappropriate when diagnosing pain patients prescribed opiates. Our perception of low back pain patients misusing their opioid medication may be colored by our mental image of the stereotypic illicit drug user or addict, but these individuals are quite different.

Traditional psychological tests assist in determining co-morbidity but do not provide effective predictive value unless patients are already concerned about addiction. Inherent difficulties are present when diagnosing addictive disease in chronic pain patients maintained on opioid analgesics. At this time, assessment of substance abuse potential relies on the use of a comprehensive approach based on a biopsychosocial model, addiction literature, and studies attempting to develop quick, cost-efficient screening questionnaires to predict risk for developing problematic opioid behaviors. A multidisciplinary approach that involves the use of contingency opioid contracts, patient education, and involvement of psychiatrists, psychologists, or addiction specialists is recommended when treating chronic nonmalignant pain with opiates.

A. A history of polysubstance abuse and positive biogenetics may be risk factors for addiction. The risk appears to decrease when (1) a previous abuse problem is related to alcohol or cocaine abuse only, (2) when the history of polydrug abuse is remote, or (3) there is continued support through a stable family, Alcoholics Anonymous, or a similar support group.

B. Co-morbidity of a mental health disorder(s) is frequently found in individuals with an addictive disorder. Their presence does not necessarily indicate that an addiction disorder is present. Further evaluation and follow-up with a mental health professional is recommended.

C. Mental status examinations are an important part of obtaining a baseline of function that can later be used to determine if noncompliance is due to mental confusion or sedation.

D. The predictive value of "drug-seeking" behaviors must be balanced by findings in chronic pain patients. About 20% of nonaddicted patients report the same behaviors. A small sample of patients have reported indicators that are denied by all pain patients who do not have an addictive disease.

REFERENCES

Chabal C, Erjavek MK, Jacobson L, et al: Prescription opiate abuse in chronic pain patients: clinical criteria, incidence, and predictors. *Clin J Pain* 1997;13:150–155.

Compton P, Durakjjan J, Miotto K: Screening for addiction in patients with chronic pain and "problematic" substance use: evaluation of a pilot assessment tool. *J Pain Symptom Manage* 1998;16: 355–363.

Fishman SM, Wilsey B, Yang J, et al: Adherence monitoring and drug surveillance in chronic opoid therapy. *J Pain Symptom Manage* 2000;20:293–307.

Robinson RC, Gatchel RJ, Polatin P, et al: Screening for problematic prescription opioid use. *Clin J Pain* 2001;17:220–228.

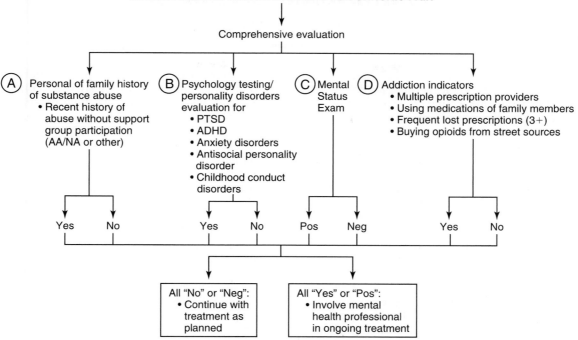

OPIATE PRESCRIPTION CONSIDERED FOR CHRONIC PAIN

Comprehensive evaluation

(A) Personal of family history of substance abuse
• Recent history of abuse without support group participation (AA/NA or other)

Yes   No

(B) Psychology testing/ personality disorders evaluation for
• PTSD
• ADHD
• Anxiety disorders
• Antisocial personality disorder
• Childhood conduct disorders

Yes   No

(C) Mental Status Exam

Pos   Neg

(D) Addiction indicators
• Multiple prescription providers
• Using medications of family members
• Frequent lost prescriptions (3+)
• Buying opioids from street sources

Yes   No

All "No" or "Neg":
• Continue with treatment as planned

All "Yes" or "Pos":
• Involve mental health professional in ongoing treatment

Psychological Evaluation

MAGALY V. MARRERO

Chronic pain is a complex, individual, multidimensional, subjective experience. The chronic pain model consists of sensory, affective, and cognitive components. The value of the psychological evaluation lies not only in determining the presence of psychopathology but in identifying a patient's perceived relationship to their illness or injury, degree of suffering, and level of disability. In chronic pain patients, psychological evaluation may identify individual strengths and weaknesses that may assist with successful medical management. Evaluation may identify specific treatments that would minimize psychological distress, provide clues about patient response to specific modalities, and identify clinical problems that may need to be addressed prior to proceeding with invasive procedures.

A. Referral for psychological evaluation is usually recommended when physical findings cannot explain symptom reports of severity, functional impairment, or disability. Patients who exhibit pronounced emotional distress and fail to respond to treatment or who use health care services, medications, or alcohol excessively (or any or all of these behaviors) are also candidates for psychological evaluation.

B. Comprehensive psychological evaluation in the chronic pain population requires a skilled clinician with specialized training in chronic pain. Familiarization with recent chronic pain literature assists in the gathering of biopsychosocial information and cognitive patterns that may affect a patient's perception and response to pain.

C. Sensory measurement scales help patients and clinicians develop a common language about pain intensity, changes in intensity, degree of analgesia achieved, affective components of pain, and other dimensions.

D. Psychometric testing allows an evaluation of mood, personality, perceptions about medical care, motivation, perceived disability, pain beliefs, psychosocial context, illness behavior, and coping mechanisms.

E. No "chronic pain" personality has been identified. Personality tests have long been used to evaluate pain patients to help identify the context in which the pain problem exists. The most commonly used of these are the Minnesota Multiphasic Personality Inventory (MMPI) and the MMPI-2. A number of empirically based typologies have been developed using these tests to enhance the clinical understanding and treatment of pain patients.

REFERENCES

Gatchel RJ, Turk DC: *Psychosocial Factors in Pain: Clinical Perspectives.* New York, Guilford Press, 1999.
Greene RL: *The MMPI-2/MMPI: An Interpretive Manual.* Boston, Allyn & Bacon, 1991.
Turk DC, Melzack R: *Handbook of Pain Assessment.* New York, Guilford Press, 1992.

PSYCHOLOGICAL EVALUATION

A useful criteria for referral of chronic pain patient

- ○ Inconsistent reports of
  Severity, functional impairment, or disability.
- ○ Non-organic findings
- ○ Pronounced emotional distress
- ○ Failure to respond to several treatment modalities
- ○ Pain behavior enabled by family members
- ○ Possible secondary gains
- ○ Excessive use of
  Health care services, medications, and/or alcohol

Comprehensive psychological evaluation

Interview
  Pain history
    Location
    Sensation
    Severity
    Frequency
    Modulating factors
    Previous treatment
    Efficacy of treatment
    Associated signs and symptoms
    Medications
  Daily activity
  Present functioning
    Physical
    Social
    Occupational
  Social history
  Medical history
    General
    Psychiatric
    Addictive
  Mental Status Exam

Frequently used psychometric
instruments
    Verbal rating scales (VIRS)
    Numerical rating scales
    Visual analog scales
    McGill pain Questionnaire
    Medical outcomes survey (SF-36)
    Pain beliefs questionnaire
    Millon behavioral health inventory
    Millon behavioral medicine
    Survey of pain attitudes
    Multidimensional pain inventory
    Minnesota multiphasic
    Personality inventory-2 (MMPI-2)

Sleep Disturbances and Chronic Pain

PAUL T. INGMUNDSON

Sleep disturbances are common among chronic pain patients; complaints of poor sleep occur in up to 70% in some reported series. A variety of sleep disorders are associated with complaints of pain.

A. The basis for the diagnosis of any sleep disorder is a history of the sleep complaint, including a review of the medical and psychiatric history and use of medications. A collateral history from the bed partner, including information about the frequency and types of movements, arousals, and any respiratory abnormalities, is often critical in arriving at a tentative diagnosis. A sleep log, documenting hours spent in bed, time asleep, and daytime naps, also may yield useful data for the initial assessment.

B. A variety of extrinsic factors need to be assessed in evaluating a sleep compaint. Noisy sleep environment; inappropriate use of alcohol, stimulants, or sedative hypnotic medications; poor sleep hygiene; jet lag; and shift work are all examples of extrinsic factors that may contribute to a complaint of poor sleep.

C. Disorders of excessive daytime sleepiness are sometimes termed hypersomnias. A complaint of hypersomnia accompanied by loud, irregular snoring raises the suspicion of obstructive sleep apnea, which must be confirmed in an overnight laboratory study (nocturnal polysomnography). Associated features may include hypertension, obesity, and morning headaches.

D. Disorders associated with repetitive movement during sleep may be associated with complaints of pain and fatigue on awakening. Restless legs syndrome (RLS) consists of creeping, painful sensations in the lower extremities that can be relieved only by movement and may be associated with difficulties in initiating sleep. Periodic limb movements during sleep (PLMS) are stereotyped, repetitive movements of the extremities that occur during sleep. Virtually all patients with RLS have PLMS, although the converse is not true. The incidence of PLMS increases with age and may occur without an associated complaint of disturbed sleep. Clonazepam, 0.5 mg to 2.0 mg, or temazepam, 30 mg, has been reported to be effective. Reports of successful treatment with bromocriptine and L-dopa may implicate dopaminergic mechanisms in the etiology of the disorder.

E. Nocturnal bruxism, or tooth grinding, is frequently associated with complaints of facial pain and may involve destruction of dental and joint tissue. The cause is unknown, although psychosocial stressors are frequently implicated as trigger factors. Treatment generally consists of an occlusive splint, or nightguard. Biofeedback or relaxation training may be helpful in some cases, although the clinical efficacy of these for bruxism remains to be established.

F. Psychiatric conditions, particularly anxiety and depression, are often associated with disturbed sleep, although the presence of psychiatric symptoms should not preclude investigation of other possible etiologies.

G. Chronic musculoskeletal pain, in the absence of specific laboratory findings, or evidence of connective tissue or metabolic disease, has been labeled fibrositis, fibromyalgia, or myofascial pain. The disorder is frequently associated with complaints of nonrestorative sleep. Nocturnal polysomnography in such patients often demonstrates alpha-frequency (8 to 11.5 Hz) intrusions in the EEG, or nonrapid eye movement sleep. The alpha EEG finding is also observed during febrile illness and postviral syndromes, but is generally absent in insomnia or depressive disorders. Treatment generally consists of a sedating tricyclic (e.g., amitriptyline) in conjunction with nonsteroidal antiinflammatory analgesics. The use of short half-life benzodiazepines such as triazolam is generally discouraged, although benzodiazepines with intermediate range half-lives (e.g., nitrazepam) have proved useful in some cases. Behavioral approaches to treatment may often be helpful.

H. Idiopathic insomnia is a childhood-onset disorder of initiating or maintaining sleep that cannot be attributed to other psychiatric or medical factors. Psychophysiologic, or "learned," insomnia usually has an adult onset and is associated with agitation and somatized tension. Patients in both groups are frequently prescribed benzodiazepines, although the chronic nature of the complaint may lead to problems with tolerance or dependence. Ultimate resolution of the disturbance often requires some form of behavioral intervention.

I. Chronic pain patients typically report spending much time in bed or at rest, although they also describe their sleep as disturbed and frequently unrestorative. Behavioral approaches to sleep disturbances focus on modifying maladaptive sleep behaviors. The stimulus control method focuses on altering cues in the sleep environment that may be associated with arousal rather than sleep. The sleep restriction method titrates the amount of time spent in bed to the patient's sleep efficiency, a ratio of sleep time to the amount of time spent in bed. Both approaches, or combinations thereof, may help consolidate the sleep phase and improve the subjective quality of sleep.

REFERENCES

American Sleep Disorders Association: *The international classification of Sleep Disorders* Lawrence, KS, Allen Press, 1990.

Moldofsky H: Sleep and fibrositis syndrome. *Rheum Dis Clin North Am* 1989;15:91–103.

Montplaisir J, Godbout R: Restless legs syndrome and periodic movements during sleep. In: Kryger MH, Roth T, Dement WC, (eds). *Principles and Practice of Sleep Medicine.* Philadelphia, WB Saunders, 1989.

Morin CM, Kowatch RA, Wade JB: Behavioral management of sleep disturbances secondary to chronic pain. *J Behav Ther Exp Psychiatry* 1989;20:295.

Pilowksky I, Crettendon I, Townley M: Sleep disturbance in pain clinic patients. *Pain* 1985;23:27.

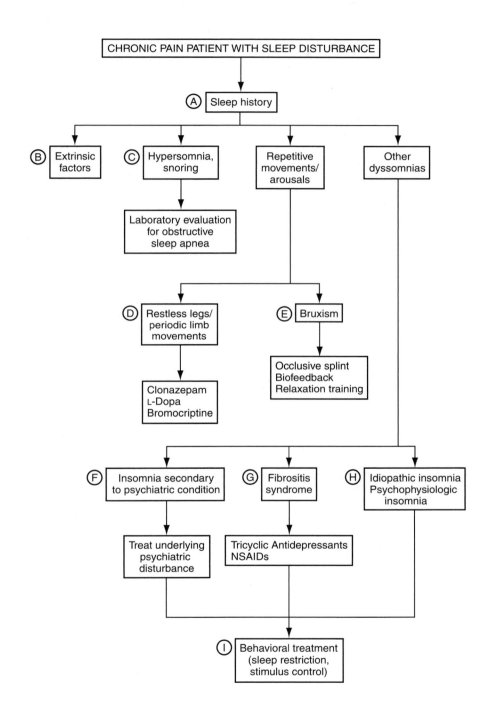

Disability and Quality of Life

ERIK SHAW

When chronic pain is discussed, disability and quality of life are interrelated concepts. Many studies have attempted to address this and even examine the role of certain factors on each separately and together. The roles of clinical problems, psychological factors, and social stressors are all important. The question of what elements contribute to shifting acute pain into the chronic challenge it can be are also addressed in this chapter.

A. The World Health Organization (WHO) originally defined impairment, disability, and handicap as classifications for dysfunction. Briefly stated, *impairment* is any loss or abnormality of psychological, physiologic, or anatomic structure or function (AMA guidelines are very useful in assessing the impairment of human organ systems); *disability* is any restriction or lack of ability to perform an activity in the manner or within the range considered normal for a human being; and *handicap* is a disadvantage for a given individual resulting from impairment or disability that limits or prevents the fulfillment of a role that is normal (depending on age, sex, and social and cultural factors) for that individual. In the new International Classification of Functioning, Disability and Health (ICF), the World Health Assembly has attempted to classify functions, structures, activities, and participation. This framework can help provide the fundamental basis from which to focus on disability.

B. Several questionnaires have attempted to evaluate various parameters of disability. Among the most frequently used is the Roland-Morris Disability Questionnaire (RDQ), which determines disability due to low back pain, and was derived from the Sickness Impact Profile (SIP), a broader health status query. The RDQ has good reliability and face validity, although it does not measure important factors such as psychological and social difficulties. The Oswestry Disability Index (ODI) also examines patients with chronic low back pain, and is a good predictor of return to work.

C. Quality of life (QOL) is defined by WHO as "the individuals' perceptions of their position in life, in the context of the cultural and value system in which they live and in relation to their goals, expectations, standards and concerns." Measures for QOL should have an appropriate scope, be understood and completed by patients, and be statistically validated. Popular measures include the SIP and Medical Outcomes Study Short-Form 36 (SF-36).

D. Psychological factors can also play an important role in disability and QOL. If problems are detected early, specific interventions can be initiated that may help to limit disability and improve QOL. In general, it can be difficult to differentiate between psychological distress, depressive symptoms, and depressive mood. A significant predictor of unfavorable outcome is psychological distress. Somatization can also point to unfavorable scores for disability. Further, psychological distress and somatization may predict chronic disability and poor QOL. Evidence suggests, however, that addressing fear avoidance behavior can have a beneficial effect on clinical outcomes.

The concepts of disability and QOL are broad, interrelated topics. Discussed briefly here, they have great clinical importance in the practice of pain management.

REFERENCES

Cieza A, Stucki G: New approaches to understanding the impact of musculoskeletal conditions. *Best Pract Res Clin Rheumatol* 2004;18:141–154.

Guidelines to the Evaluation of Permanent Impairment, 4th ed. Chicago, American Medical Association, 1995.

Pincus T: A systematic review of psychological factors as predictors of chronicity/disability in prospective cohorts of low back pain. *Spine* 2002;27:E109–120.

Roland M, Fairbank J: The Roland–Morris Disability Questionnaire and the Oswestry Disability Questionnaire. *Spine* 2000;25: 3115-3124.

Scott DL, Garwood T: Quality of life measures: use and abuse. *Bailliere's Clin Rheumatol.* 2000;14:663–687.

World Health Organization: *International classification of impairments, disabilities, and handicaps.* Geneva, WHO, 1980.

DISABILITY AND QUALITY OF LIFE

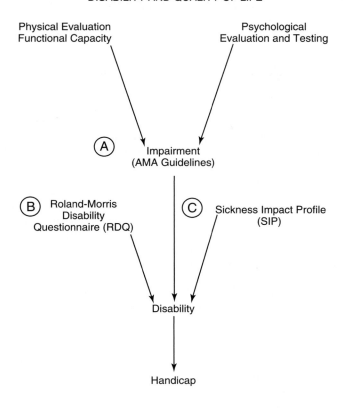

Posttraumatic Stress Disorder

SUZETTE M. STOKS AND LAWRENCE S. SCHOENFELD

Posttraumatic stress disorder (PTSD) is an anxiety disorder characterized by the development of chronic symptoms following exposure to a highly traumatic stressor. As many as 80% of persons meeting the criteria for PTSD also have co-morbid diagnoses, most commonly depression, another anxiety disorder, or a substance abuse disorder. Increasing attention has been drawn to the co-occurrence of psychological trauma and physical symptoms. The lifetime prevalence of PTSD has been estimated to range from 1% to 14% and has been found to be twice as high in women (10.4%) as in men (5%). Recent studies have suggested a high prevalence of PTSD symptoms among chronic pain patients; and in one study as many as 80% of combat veterans with PTSD also reported chronic pain. Individuals with both physical symptoms and PTSD report higher levels of pain, lower quality of life, greater functional impairment, and more psychological distress than their counterparts with either symptom alone. Additionally, compared to nontraumatized individuals, trauma survivors report more medical symptoms and use more medical services. PTSD symptoms often go undetected in patients presenting with pain complaints, yet such symptoms often complicate the clinical picture and adversely affect treatment outcome if not addressed. Consequently, increasing attention is being given to the importance of recognizing and treating PTSD in pain patients.

A. To qualify for a diagnosis of PTSD, a person first must have been exposed to a traumatic event in which he or she experienced, witnessed, or was confronted with an event or events that involved actual or threatened death or serious injury or a threat to the physical integrity of self or others; the person's response must have involved intense fear, helplessness, or horror. A similar response to a less severe stressor should be evaluated for the possibility of an adjustment disorder.

B. The traumatic event is then persistently reexperienced through intrusive, distressing recollections of the event, distressing dreams of the event, acting or feeling as if the event were recurring (e.g., flashbacks), intense psychological distress or physiological reactivity upon exposure to cues associated with the trauma.

C. Persistent avoidance of stimuli (e.g., thoughts, people, places) associated with the trauma and numbing of the individual's general responsiveness (e.g., feeling emotionally numb or detached from other people) also occur.

D. Increased symptoms of arousal must be present manifested by at least two of the following: difficulty falling or staying asleep, irritability or anger outbursts, difficulty concentrating, hypervigilance, or an exaggerated startle response.

E. The symptoms must persist for more than 1 month. A delayed-onset subtype is seen less frequent and occurs when symptoms do not appear until at least 6 months after the trauma. Similar symptom presentations with shorter duration should be evaluated for the possibility of acute stress disorder.

F. Once a diagnosis of PTSD is established, treatment should be provided by a qualified clinician. Treatment selection should take into account the expected efficacy against PTSD, the patient's treatment goals (e.g., symptom reduction versus improving the capacity for human relatedness), possible difficulties or side effects, and patient motivation and willingness to engage in the proposed treatment as well as treatment length, cost, and the patient's availability of resources.

G. Cognitive-behavioral therapy (CBT)-based approaches have been the most widely studied interventions for PTSD. They encompass a variety of techniques, including exposure therapy, systematic desensitization, stress inoculation training, cognitive therapy, assertiveness training, biofeedback, and relaxation. CBT has been shown to be effective in reducing symptoms of PTSD; however, not all patients benefit from CBT, and it is not yet clear what factors predict success with this treatment approach.

H. Eye movement desensitization and reprocessing (EMDR) appears to be more effective than wait-list control, but there is a lack of methodologically sound research in this area. During EMDR patients are asked to keep in mind a disturbing image, negative cognition, and bodily sensations associated with the trauma while tracking the clinician's moving finger in the patient's visual field. This is repeated until the distressing aspects of the trauma are reduced and more adaptive cognitions about the trauma emerge.

I. Group psychotherapy has been associated with a positive treatment outcome regardless of whether the intervention directly addresses the trauma. Group therapy can provide a unique opportunity for patients to normalize their distress and receive social support.

J. Psychodynamic therapy for the treatment of PTSD has been the subject of little empirically based efficacy research, in part due to the fact that treatment goals tend to be more diffuse than mere symptom reduction and are not easily measured by available assessment methods. This approach seeks to mobilize the patient's adaptive functioning by exploring the unconscious, and it may include addressing wishes, fantasies, fears, and defenses relating to the traumatic event. This mode of treatment is highly effective for some patients, but it may be prolonged and expensive.

K. Pharmacotherapy is also used to treat PTSD. Selective serotonin reuptake inhibitors (SSRIs) are currently recommended as first-line pharmacotherapy for PTSD. In general, pharmacotherapy has been shown to reduce symptoms effectively, but it does not have a clear effect on the course of the disorder and therefore may be most effective as an adjunct to psychological and social treatments.

L. Other approaches, such as hypnosis, psychosocial rehabilitation, marital and family therapy, and creative arts therapies, show promise in the treatment of PTSD. They are often effective during impasses that other treatment approaches fail to work through. However, more research is needed to establish these approaches as effective techniques.

REFERENCES

American Psychiatric Association: *Diagnostic and Statistical Manual of Mental Disorders: Fourth Edition.* Washington, DC, American Psychiatric Association, 1994.

Beckham JC, Crawford AL, Feldman ME, *et al:* Chronic posttraumatic stress disorder and chronic pain in Vietnam combat veterans. *J Psychosom Res* 1997;43:379–389.

Foa EB, Keane TM, Friedman MJ (eds) *Effective Treatments for PTSD: Practice Guidelines from the International Society for Traumatic Stress Studies.* New York, Guilford Press, 2000.

Geisser ME, Roth RS, Bachman JE, Eckert TA: The relation-ship between symptoms of post-traumatic stress disorder and pain, affective disturbance and disability among patients with accident and non-accident related pain. *Pain* 1996;66:207–214.

Samson AY, Bensen S, Beck A, *et al:* Posttraumatic stress disorder in primary care. *J Family Pract* 1999;48:222–227.

Sharp TJ, Harvey AG: Chronic pain and post traumatic stress disorder: mutual maintenance? *Clin Psychol Rev* 2001; 21:857–877.

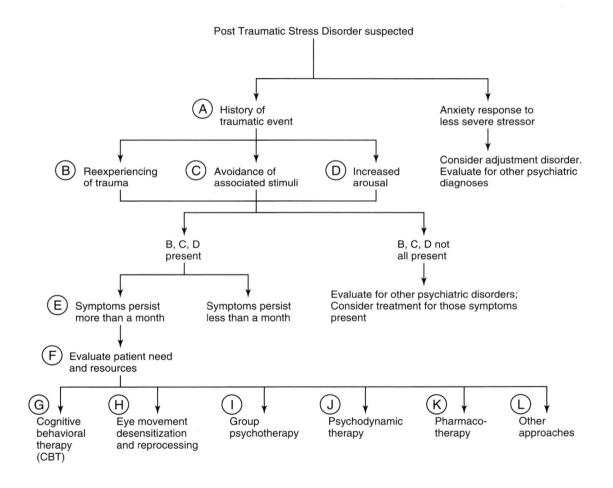

Pain Measurement

EULECHE ALANMANOU

Patient care is improved by monitoring the severity and duration of pain. It is now widely accepted that pain is a complex experience involving sensory, emotional, psychological, and sociologic factors. The subjective nature of pain explains the difficulty with its measurement. The same standard cannot be used to measure pain in all circumstances.

A. Pain could be measured using single dimensional or multidimensional self-assessment tools. If the patient's self-assessment of pain is not consistent with physical findings, a behavioral assessment is recommended. The most commonly used pain evaluation tools are of a single dimension and include the following (see Appendix 3): Verbal Descriptor Scale, Visual Analogue Scale, Numerical Rating Scale, and Pain Relief Scale. They are quick and easy to use but risk oversimplifying the patient's pain.

B. The multidimensional self-assessment tools take into account the motivational and affective dimension of the pain. The verbal descriptors of these tools and the precise description of the location of the pain may be useful for differentiating the etiologies of pain (somatic or visceral pain versus neuropathic pain). One of the most supported assessment tools is the McGill Pain Questionnaire (MPQ), developed by Melzack and colleagues in 1975 (see Appendix 3). An abbreviated version of the MPQ was introduced by Melzack in 1987. The MPQ has been designed to assess the three dimensions of pain: sensory, affective, evaluative. Other multidimensional pain scales include the Brief Pain Inventory (BPI), the Dartmouth Pain Questionnaire, the Minnesota Multiphasic Personality Inventory (MMPI), the West Haven-Yale Multidimensional Pain Inventory (WHYMPI), and the Quebec Back Pain Disability Scale (QBPDS).

C. Measurement of pain behavior used in conjunction with other, previous measurements can help quantify diverse pain problems. The behavior assessment methods include direct observation by the clinician, monitoring pain medication use, a pain diary, and pain drawing on a body diagram.

D. The appropriate use of pain measurement tools depend on the goals established. For initial assessment and follow-up after therapeutic intervention, a single-dimensional measurement method can be used. As part of the diagnostic workup of chronic pain, single-dimensional, multidimensional, psychological, and behavioral methods are recommended.

E. Addressing the specific impairment may help a clinician face the challenge of pain assessment in cognitively impaired patients.

F. Please refer to Chapter 3, page 8, for assessment of pain in children. In general, multidimensional methods are applied starting at 12 to 14 years of age.

REFERENCES

Chapman CR, Syrjala KL: Measurement of pain. In: Bonica JJ (ed) *The Management of Pain*, 2nd ed. Philadelphia, Lea & Febiger, 1990.

McGrath PA: Evaluating a child's pain. *J Pain Symptom Manage* 1989;4:198.

Melzak R: The McGill Pain Questionnaire: major properties and scoring methods. *Pain* 1975;1:277.

Melzak R: The short-form McGill Pain Questionnaire. *Pain* 1987;30:191.

Turk DC, Melzack R: *Handbook of Pain Assessment*. New York, Guilford Press, 1992.

Valley MA: Pain measurement. In: Raj PP (ed) *Pain Medicine: A Comprehensive Review*, 2nd ed. St. Louis, Mosby, 2003.

PAIN MEASUREMENT

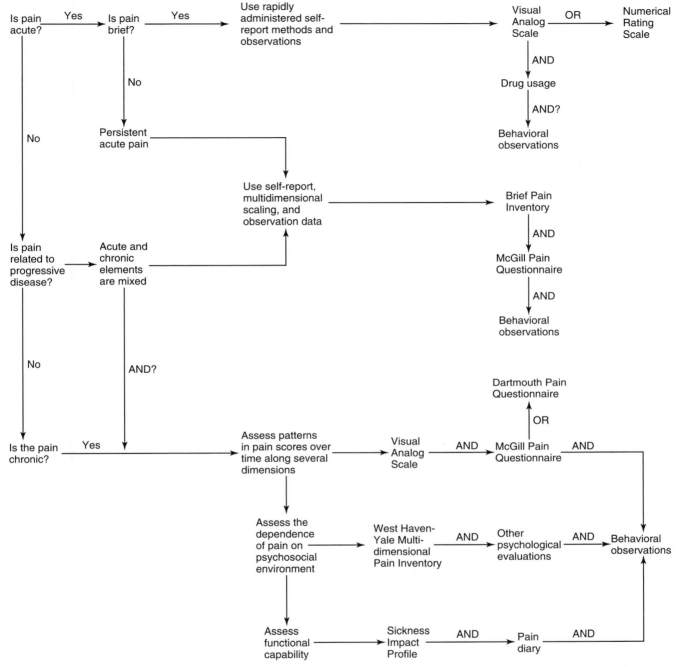

Modified from Chapman CR, Syrjala KL: Measurement of pain. In: Loeser JD (ed) *Bonica's Management of Pain,* 3rd ed. Philadelphia, Lippincott Williams & Wilkins, 2001, with permission.

Imaging Studies

SOMAYAJI RAMAMURTHY AND SERGIO ALVARADO

Radiologic imaging is a useful tool not only in diagnosis of pain syndromes, but also in management and therapy of chronic pain. Communication between the radiologist and the consulting physician is essential to optimizing the benefit of imaging studies including choice of the most appropriate modality. Most importantly, imaging is a supplement to, not a substitute for a thorough history and physical examination.

A. Most patients with acute pain will not need diagnostic imaging studies. If suspicion is raised during history and physical examination, then proceeding with imaging is warranted. Elements of a patient's evaluation that should trigger consideration of diagnostic studies include history of trauma that may have resulted in a fracture. A history of cancer; constitutional symptoms such as fever, chills, and unexplained weight loss; recent bacterial infection; intravenous drug use; immunosuppression; and extremes of age may raise suspicion of a neoplastic or infectious process causing pain. Any significant neurologic findings on examination may warrant imaging studies, especially in the case of severe or progressive neurologic deficit in the lower extremities, recent onset of bladder dysfunction, or saddle anesthesia, which might suggest a cauda equina syndrome. Acute pain that persists beyond 6 weeks despite conservative care should be investigated with diagnostic imaging, usually plain radiography.

B. Plain radiography is often a useful initial study to obtain, especially in the case of musculoskeletal disorders including trauma. It is the most widely available, least expensive modality and its reliability, rapidness, and portability make it an effective screening tool.

C. Computed tomography (CT) is used as an adjunct to plain radiography for further investigating musculoskeletal processes, especially in regard to joint spaces where the anatomic features are complex and obscured by overlying structures. It is the study of choice for intrathoracic and intraabdominal processes. In the setting of spine imaging, it has largely been replaced by magnetic resonance imaging (MRI). It remains useful for guidance in percutaneous procedures, especially when needle placement is in areas where there are high risks of complications if adjacent structures are compromised such as in celiac plexus blocks, cervical spine injection, and cranial nerve blocks.

D. MRI has become the modality of choice for definitively imaging many areas especially intracranial, spine, and musculoskeletal. The contraindications to MRI are presence of ferromagnetic implants, cardiac pacemakers, intracranial clips, or claustrophobia. Most implantable intrathecal infusion devices in use today are MRI compatible, although that should be verified with the particular manufacturer. Spinal cord stimulators at the present time are not considered to be compatible. As with other techniques, MRI can reveal abnormalities in asymptomatic patients. In one series, 63% of asymptomatic persons had disc protrusion, and 13% had disc extrusion, emphasizing the importance of clinical correlation with imaging findings to avoid inappropriate therapy. Contrast enhancement with gadolinium may help identify early inflammatory and infectious processes such as postprocedural discitis and is the modality of choice for evaluation of a suspected intrathecal catheter tip granuloma. Gadolinium does not contain iodine and is safe in patients with iodine allergy.

E. Myelography is a method of visualizing the spinal canal and thecal sac. It involves injection of a small amount of nonionic contrast into the thecal sac via a dural puncture followed by imaging in multiple projections, allowing the contrast to delineate the subarachnoid space, spinal cord, and the nerve root sleeves. It can be combined with CT, and is especially valuable in evaluating arachnoiditis and extradural abscess. MRI has largely replaced myelography. Although myelography is useful when patients have a contraindication to MRI, or when abnormalities on MRI do not correlate with clinical findings, MRI has largely replaced myelography.

F. Nuclear medicine scanning, most commonly bone scintigraphy with technetium (Tc)-99m phosphate indicates bone turnover, which is a common occurrence in bone metastases, primary spine tumors, fracture, infarction, infection, and other disorders involving bone metabolism.

G. Arthrography involves injection of contrast into a joint space to further evaluate the joint. It can be combined with CT and MRI, although for the most part it has been replaced with MRI.

H. Discography can be useful diagnostically in conjunction with CT or MRI to localize a disc herniation or characterize the extent of disc degeneration, as well as confirm the source of symptoms. A volume of contrast media is injected into the disc space to determine the integrity of the intervertebral disc. It is often followed by CT to enhance structural imaging of the disc. The injectate pressurizes the disc and the patient is able to confirm whether or not there is pain and if it is concordant. Proprietary systems available for documenting opening and maximum pressures of injection into the disc may help distinguish chemical from mechanical sources of back pain. Findings should be interpreted cautiously, as there is a possibility of false-positive results. Discography is invasive and has risk of infection and neural injury

IMAGING STUDIES

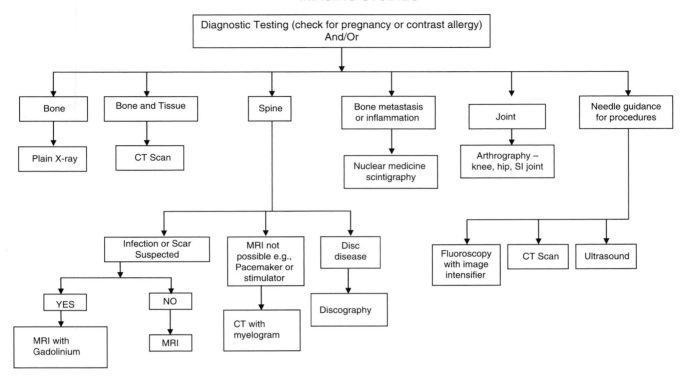

and should be reserved as a confirmatory test, not an initial diagnostic tool.

I. The advent of fluoroscopy, especially portable C-arm fluoroscopic units, has had a great impact on the performance of interventional pain management techniques. Needle placement percutaneously under fluoroscopic guidance with administration of contrast to confirm placement as well as absence of intra-vascular or intrathecal injection has greatly improved the accuracy and safety of these procedures and has evolved into a standard of care for many of them.

J. Ultrasound is an excellent tool for body imaging and visualization of soft tissue and relatively superficial vascular structures. Recently, much interest has been generated in performing ultrasound guided regional techniques for both acute and chronic pain. It appears that as the technology continues to evolve, greater utilization of this modality for treatment will ensue.

Choice of a particular modality is usually based on tissue type and likely diagnosis. For headache and facial pain, CT is best for severe, sudden headaches, trauma, and presumed sinusitis. MRI is a better choice for chronic headache and temporomandibular dysfunction. In chest and abdominal pain, plain radiography is a good initial choice with a lack of finding leading to consideration of echocardiography, ECG, CT, ultrasound, or gas-trointestinal contrast examinations for further evalua-tion. For neck and upper extremity complaints, plain radiographs are a good start, followed by CT in the presence of acute trauma, and MRI if the problems are chronic. In low back pain for which imaging is indicated, plain films are the initial choice followed by MRI for most situations. An exception may be bony impingement of neural structures, which is better evaluated by CT. MRI without and with gadolinium enhancement is the modality of choice for failed back surgery syndrome.

REFERENCES

Eckard VR, Batnitzky S, Abrams BM, et al: Radiology and the diagnosis and management of pain. In: Raj PP (ed) *Practical Management of Pain,* 3rd ed. St. Louis, Mosby, 2000.

Greher M, Kirchmair L, Enna B, et al: Ultrasound-guided lumbar facet nerve block: accuracy of a new technique confirmed by computed tomography. *Anesthesiology* 2004;101:1195–1200.

Humphreys SC, Eck JC, Hodges SD: Neuroimaging in low back pain. *Am Fam Physician* 2002;65:2299–2306.

Discography

QASSEM KISHAWI

Disc abnormalities are responsible for half the cases of back pain. Aging replaces water and polysaccharides with collagen, and the disc loses its elastic properties. This makes the disc unable to handle axial forces, resulting in fissures and cracks in the disc and making the disc susceptible to pain. Although degenerated discs typically lose their height, there is no correlation between disc height and symptoms. For that reason and because regular imaging [radiography, computed tomography (CT), magnetic resonance imaging (MRI)] gives a good idea of the shape of each disc, discography is the only method to confirm whether a disc is intrinsically painful. Discography is an invasive diagnostic tool designed to stimulate the disc by increasing the intervertebral pressure and reproducing the patient's pain. It can be done anywhere in the cervical, thoracic, or lumbar discs, with the latter being the most common.

Discogenic pain is typically a deep, dull midline aching in the low back that might radiate to the gluteal areas but is rarely experienced below the knees or legs. It usually worsens with axial loading and may present acutely after sudden bending or twisting. Indications for discography include evaluating suspected discs before performing surgical discectomy or spinal fusion, axial pain with a negative myelogram, spinal stenosis with single root symptoms, and failed back syndrome when conservative measures have failed. On the other hand, patients who are not candidates for definitive management of discogenic pain (surgery, intradiscal electrothermal therapy) are not candidates for discography. Other contraindications include the existence of sensory or motor loss, discitis, local skin infection, coagulopathies, allergy to contrast material, and the inability of the patient to cooperate during the procedure due to his or her mental condition or a language barrier. Relative contraindications include pregnancy, disc herniation with signs of acute radiculopathy, and unresolved psychological issues.

A. Preparations include obtaining patient's consent after the procedure and risks/benefits are fully explained. Patient is given nothing orally and has an accompanying adult. Full physical and neurologic examinations are performed before and after the procedure, and previous diagnostics are reviewed. An intravenous infusion is started, and broad-spectrum antibiotics are given before the procedure. The patient is placed prone with standard American Society of Anesthesiologists (ASA) monitors on. Light sedation is provided as needed to keep the patient comfortable but still able to cooperate with the procedure.

B. Usually one disc above and one below the suspected level are also injected as control levels, and the suspected level is injected last. The approach is from the side opposite the patient's pain. The following parameters are noted: resistance on entry to the annulus, compliance of the nucleus on injection, pain provocation on injection, and distribution of dye inside and outside the disc. Antibiotics and local anesthetics are injected before withdrawing the needle at each level. Anteroposterior and lateral discographic images are then obtained as well as a postprocedure CT scan within 2 hours to highlight the features of internal disc disruption.

C. Postprocedure instructions include watching for complications, limiting the patient's activity, and providing back support and oral analgesics. A next-day phone call and a follow-up visit are standard. Complications include discitis (septic and aseptic), epidural abscess, rupture of the disc, nerve root injury, dural puncture, headache, and pneumothorax. The patient should be evaluated immediately if any of the above is suspected. Diagnostic tests include a complete blood count, erythrocyte sedimentation rate, C-reactive protein assay, blood cultures, and MRI. When infection is suspected, broad-spectrum antibiotics should be started; and, if indicated, an abscess is drained.

REFERENCES

Cleveland Clinic Pain Management and Regional Anesthesia Symposium, Key West, FL 2002.

Cousins MJ, Bridenbaugh PO (eds): *Neural Blockade in Clinical Anesthesia and Management of Pain*, 3rd ed. Philadelphia, Lippincott-Raven, 1998.

Raj PP, Lou L, Erdine S, et al: *Radiographic Imaging for Regional Anesthesia and Pain Management*. New York, Churchill Livingstone, 2003.

Tollison CD, Satterthwaite JR, Tollison JW (eds): *Practical Pain Management*, 3rd ed. Philadelphia, Lippincott Williams & Wilkins, 2001.

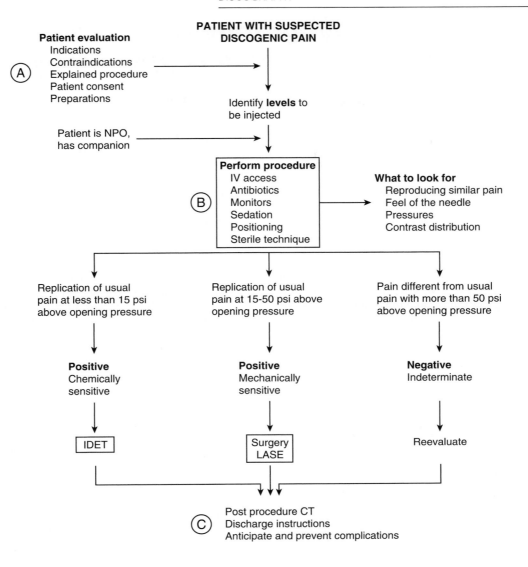

PATIENT WITH SUSPECTED DISCOGENIC PAIN

Patient evaluation
Indications
Contraindications
Explained procedure
Patient consent
Preparations

(A)

Identify **levels** to be injected

Patient is NPO, has companion

Perform procedure
IV access
Antibiotics
Monitors
Sedation
Positioning
Sterile technique

(B)

What to look for
Reproducing similar pain
Feel of the needle
Pressures
Contrast distribution

Replication of usual pain at less than 15 psi above opening pressure

Replication of usual pain at 15-50 psi above opening pressure

Pain different from usual pain with more than 50 psi above opening pressure

Positive
Chemically sensitive

Positive
Mechanically sensitive

Negative
Indeterminate

IDET

Surgery
LASE

Reevaluate

Post procedure CT
Discharge instructions
Anticipate and prevent complications

(C)

Electromyography and Nerve Conduction Studies (Upper/Lower)

ERIK SHAW

As with most diagnoses in medicine, electrodiagnosis (EDX) begins with a thorough history and physical exam. If a patient has neurologic or muscular symptoms such as shooting or burning pain, numbness, or weakness, electromyography (EMG) and nerve conduction studies (NCSs) can be useful in the evaluation and treatment. Many lesions of the peripheral nervous system (dorsal root ganglion and distal) can be assessed with EDX. NCSs typically involve external stimulation of the peripheral nervous system via a surface stimulator and recording electrodes. NCS gathers information regarding the function of motor and sensory nerves. This information can point to aberrations in either the myelin or axon. Needle EMG directly examines muscle and may yield findings in the presence of myopathies, neuropathies, plexopathies, and radiculopathies. The tests are complementary and both should be performed in most circumstances. Comparison studies in unaffected regions or extremities may help to elucidate nerve function more fully.

A. In the case of suspected neuropathy, EDX studies may show the type, whether axonal or demyelinating; the severity; as well as any muscle involvement that may be present as a result of denervation of the muscle. Severe neuropathies may cause weakness. By studying other regions that may be clinically silent, such as the other lower extremity or an upper extremity, the disease process may be graded more accurately and a more precise depiction of the clinical process given. For example, many cases of carpal tunnel syndrome may be bilateral, with only one hand clinically involved. Using this example further, by examining a lower extremity, the examiner may more precisely say that it is carpal tunnel syndrome rather than a generalized neuropathy involving upper and lower extremities. For suspected neuropathies, EMG needle exam is generally recommended. Severe neuropathies may show denervation.

B. Radiculopathies pose their own diagnostic challenge. For EDX, both NCS and EMG are appropriate. While the NCS may be normal, in severe cases in which many axons (>80%) are damaged, NCS changes may be noted. Needle EMG will be the most telling, however. Knowledge of anatomy and anatomic variations, distributions, and order of innervation are critical to completing a thorough and accurate EMG evaluation. In cases in which radiculopathy is strongly clinically suspected and EMG is negative, a diagnosis of radiculopathy may still be made. Irritation of the nerve root may not cause permanent axonal injury or may not have damaged enough axons to show denervation.

C. Temperature of the extremity will significantly alter the NCS and may cause disease to be missed or found in its absence. Electrical interference is ubiquitous, and proper techniques should be employed to minimize this. Time duration after a significant injury requires 7 to 21 days for demyelination to be seen with EMG. Other less severe compression or ischemic neuropathies may be clinically apparent before they may be assessed electrodiagnostically.

D. Laboratory results may be abnormal, such as those seen in myopathic processes, or radiologic imaging studies may be suspected abnormal. For some neuromuscular diseases, such as myasthenia gravis, antibody assays are available that may be helpful in completing the clinical picture.

E. It is important to realize that while EDX can be helpful in locating the lesion, it will not delineate the etiology. It can differentiate axonal lesions from demyelinating lesions and establish a pattern (unilateral, symmetric, asymmetric, sensory or motor or both), but responsibility for the final diagnosis is with the clinician. Motor and sensory NCSs are well suited for identifying demyelination and axonal loss. As disease progresses and more nerves become involved, differentiation between the two becomes increasingly difficult.

F. Needle EMG is of benefit when determining severity of the lesion and axonal loss. At rest, muscle is normally electrically silent. With disease, the muscle membrane can become unstable and depolarize spontaneously; "positive sharp waves and fibrillations" can be reflective of degeneration of the axon and signify that a disease process is an active one. They may be seen in acute or chronic lesions, although they often regress with time and reinnervation. Evidence of reinnervation from collateral sprouting may also be evident on EMG and may herald eventual recovery.

G. Lastly, it is important to inform the patient about the testing he or she will undergo. Testing requires the patient to be cooperative and willing, but it can be uncomfortable for some individuals. There are a few contraindications to EDX. First is patient refusal. In addition, needle EMG may be avoided when coagulopathies, lymphedema, or anasarca is present and should not be performed in muscles soon to be biopsied.

REFERENCE

Dumitru D, Amato AA, Zwaats MJ, et al: *Electrodiagnostic Medicine*, 2nd ed. Philadelphia, Hanley and Belfus, 2002.

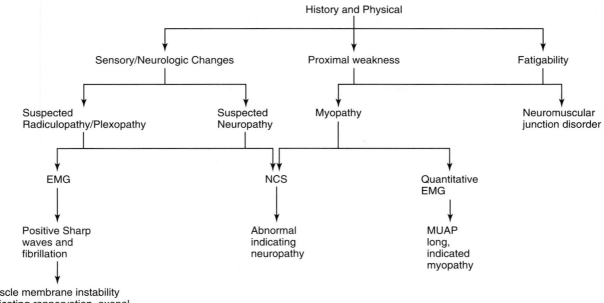

History and Physical

Sensory/Neurologic Changes | Proximal weakness | Fatigability

Suspected Radiculopathy/Plexopathy | Suspected Neuropathy | Myopathy | Neuromuscular junction disorder

EMG | NCS | Quantitative EMG

Positive Sharp waves and fibrillation | Abnormal indicating neuropathy | MUAP long, indicated myopathy

Muscle membrane instability indicating rennervation, axonal loss and sprouting

Thermography

JOHN R. ROBERTS

Although thermography has been used in the evaluation of many disorders, from headache to vascular pathology, its use as a primary diagnostic tool to differentiate specific disease processes has not been reported in the literature. It is usually considered a confirmatory test in lieu of other, more traditional diagnostic studies such as radiologic imaging or electromyography/nerve conduction velocity (EMG/NCV) tests. This chapter describes the use of thermography in a more novel role: as a method to differentiate causes of extremity pain.

Painful disorders of the extremities often present a diagnostic dilemma because of the high concentration of innervation and multiple sites for potential injury, from the spine to more distal structures. There is presently no test to measure the subjective painful process uniformly or objectively from one patient to another. However, the delicate sympathetic nerves are often also damaged along with larger fibers. Dysfunction in these nerves can be objectively measured using thermography. Regional changes in skin temperature as a reflection of altered blood flow can be helpful for supporting the diagnosis of sympathetic nerve dysfunction.

Unlike conventional imaging techniques, such as magnetic resonance imaging (MRI) or radiographs that show structural or anatomic abnormalities, thermography details dynamic physiologic changes that reflect the underlying pathology. An increase in sympathetic activity causes vasoconstriction and a resultant decrease in skin temperature. Decreased sympathetic flow causes increased regional blood flow and increased skin temperature. Documentation of these changes can be useful for diagnosing the abnormality and following the disease process.

Traditionally, small temperature probes have been used to compare temperature changes in the involved extremity compared with those in the corresponding contralateral area. A discrepancy of at least 1°C in matched areas is considered abnormal under controlled circumstances. However, these small probes measure the skin temperature only directly underneath the probe. Multiple measurements are required to delineate a pattern of abnormality in an extremity. Thermographic images display temperature differentials in the entire area scanned. These images reflect alterations in blood flow superficially, or up to 27 mm deep. These characteristics make thermography a sensitive, unique tool for evaluating areas of suspected pathology instead of using the traditional spot checks. The pattern of temperature change can be useful for differentiating causes of pain such as peripheral nerve injury, spinal root pathology, and complex regional pain syndrome. Nondermatomal, circumferential temperature changes found in areas not specific to vascular distributions are suspicious for a complex regional pain syndrome. If changes are noted in the distribution of a peripheral nerve, the more proximal nerve root is unlikely to be the source. If a dermatomal pattern is observed, focusing the evaluation on the spinal root is warranted.

There are two common methods for producing thermographic images. Both methods are noninvasive, painless, and relatively easy to use. Infrared thermography instruments scan a field of view in two directions simultaneously to produce an image. The qualitative data obtained reflect quantitative temperature differentials with a precision of 0.1°C. Liquid crystal thermography utilizes contact screens impregnated with a methyl ester derivative that changes color when exposed to different temperatures. This method is subject to more error, however, and is inherently less precise. This chapter assumes the use of infrared thermography as the standard.

Because thermography is a relatively new diagnostic modality and provides highly sensitive qualitative data, it is vulnerable to error from multiple variables. Care must be taken when collecting the data to obtain useful information in a reproducible fashion. A standardized approach to testing is suggested here. The examination room must have a stable ambient temperature of 20° to 21°C. Fluorescent lighting, a carpeted floor, and an examination table in the center of the room reduce exogenous heat error. The patient should wear loose clothing and not have recently exercised, smoked, or ingested vasoactive chemicals. Color changes are valid, corresponding to a range of 24° to 34°C. Colder temperatures are reflected as blue-to-black hues, and warmer temperatures are pink to red. The difference in temperature provides the important diagnostic information.

REFERENCES

Bruehl S, Lubenow TR, Nath H, et al: Validation of thermography in the diagnosis of reflex sympathetic dystrophy. *Clin J Pain* 1996;12:316–325.

Dotson RM: Clinical neurophysiology laboratory tests to assess the nociceptive system in humans. *J Clin Neurophysiol* 1997;14:32–45.

Green J: Neurothermography. *Semin Neurol* 1987;7:313–316.

Park ES, Park CI, Jun-KI, et al: Comparison of sympathetic skin response and digital infrared thermographic imaging in peripheral neuropathy. *Yonsei Med J* 1994;35:429–437.

Takahashi Y, Takahashi K, Moriya H: Thermal deficit in lumbar radiculopathy: correlations with pain and neurologic signs and its value for assessing symptomatic severity. *Spine* 1994;19:2443–2450.

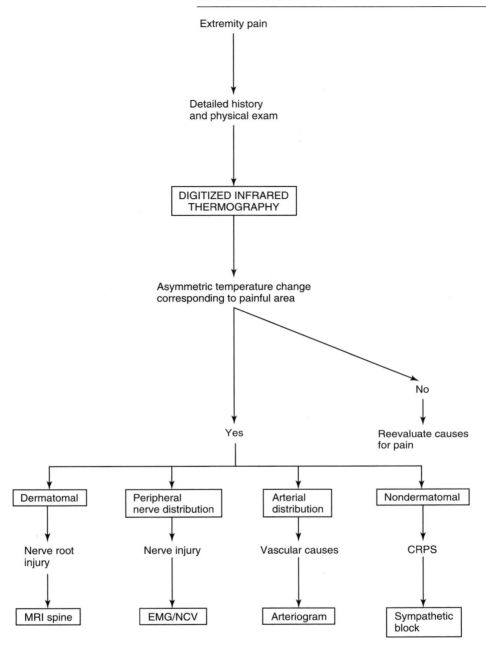

Examination Under Sedation

ROGER WESLEY AND SOMAYAJI RAMAMURTHY

Frequently we encounter "complex pain" patients who present diagnostic or therapeutic dilemmas. These patients may have pain of multifactorial, uncertain, or unknown etiology with a confusing or inconsistent course; the pain may not respond to conventional therapy; and there may be symptoms more pronounced than the organic etiology would predict. This may be related to psychosocial overlay, since pain is a subjective experience, sometimes influenced heavily by cultural learning, psychological and social variables, and secondary gain. Before subjecting these patients to expensive or invasive diagnostic tests, intensive or risky treatment regimens, or surgical intervention, it is desirable to identify those in whom a psychological etiology prevails, so as to minimize risk to the patient, conserve medical resources, and provide more appropriate therapy. Pentothal testing is a useful diagnostic aid for these patients.

A. Traditionally, psychological testing such as the Minnesota Multiphasic Personality Inventory (MMPI) or Eysenck personality inventory has been used to identify those patients who may be predisposed to a nonorganic etiology for their pain. Similarly, diagnostic neural blockade has been used to assess the relative influence of organic and psychosocial factors in chronic pain patients.

B. Pentothal testing is a modification of the sodium amytal interview, initially developed in 1961 and subsequently described in detail by Soichet (1978), in which a detailed psychological and physical examination is performed during increasing levels of sedation. It is believed that barbiturate sedation may eliminate the influence of malingering or psychosocial overlay on the examination. Pentothal testing involves assessment of a previously painful physical maneuver under sodium pentothal sedation. The basis of the test is the fact that while a patient is under light sedation, he or she is capable of demonstrating a primitive reaction to pain and is unable to demonstrate a supratentorial response.

C. The patient fasts overnight, and informed consent is obtained. After IV cannulation, monitors are applied, including continuous ECG, pulse oximetry (SpO_2), and blood pressure cuff. Equipment for airway resuscitation, including positive pressure ventilation, and resuscitative drugs are kept close at hand.

D. The response to a previously painful maneuver is assessed. For example, a grimace or withdrawal in response to a straight leg raise test is documented.

E. Sodium pentothal is administered in 50-mg increments until loss of voice response and lash reflex is attained. (In place of sodium pentothal, 10 to 20 mg increments of propofol can be substituted.)

F. A stimulus known to be painful (Achilles heel pinch or 50-Hz ministimulus tetanus) is applied, and any grimace or withdrawal response is documented.

G. The previously painful maneuver is repeated, and a response or lack of one is recorded. The presence of a response is considered confirmation of peripheral pathology, and further conventional treatment, neurolytic block, or surgery if applicable, may be instituted. Lack of a painful response suggests a nonperipheral etiology, indicating that the patient may have central or psychogenic pain or may be malingering, and that invasive, neurolytic block or surgical treatment is unlikely to benefit the patient. Psychological therapy may be helpful.

REFERENCES

Krempen JF, Silver RA, Hadley J: An analysis of differential epidural spinal anesthesia and pentothal pain study in the differential diagnosis of back pain. *Spine* 1979;4:452.

Soichet RP: Sodium amytal in the diagnosis of chronic pain. *Can Psychiatr Assoc J* 1978;23:219.

Waters A: Psychogenic regional pain alias hysterical pain. *Brain* 1961;84:1.

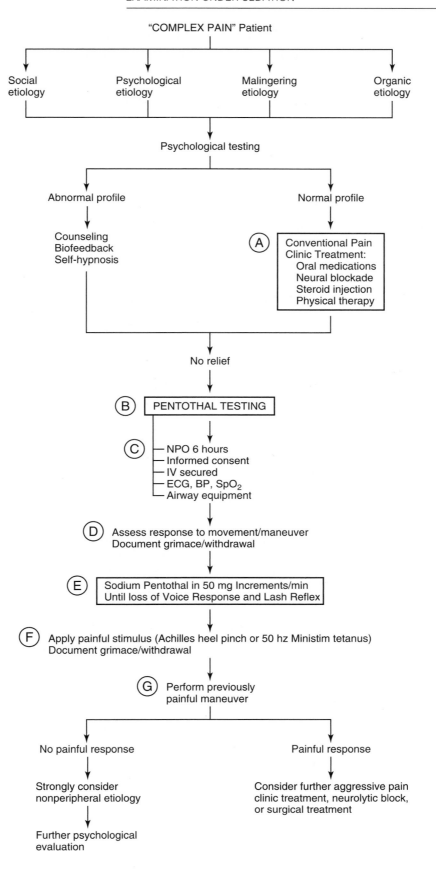

Testing and Treatment with Intravenous Local Anesthetics and Other Drugs

SERGIO ALVARADO

Chronic pain syndromes are often difficult to treat because of their multifactorial etiologies and the complex interaction of physical and psychosocial components. Identifying useful therapies in a particular patient can consume a great deal of time and resources. The administration of various intravenous (IV) agents may not only be effective treatments, but also aid in predicting the usefulness of certain classes of drugs.

A. Infusion of lidocaine intravenously has been studied by many investigators as a treatment for various neuropathic pain syndromes and as a useful test to predict the efficacy of treating chronic pain syndromes with sodium channel blocking agents such as mexiletine, carbamazepine, and topiramate. Infusion protocols for treatment vary widely, with boluses ranging from 2 to 5 mg/kg over a minimum of 3 minutes with or without an infusion afterward. Alternatively, the dose is infused over 30 to 60 minutes. Intervals between treatments vary based on patient response and duration of effect. In the author's practice a 5 mg/kg bolus is given as a slow IV push, with interruption of the infusion if the patient develops central nervous system (CNS) side effects such as perioral numbness, auditory disturbances, dizziness, or lightheadedness. Administration is resumed when the adverse effects subside. Standard hemodynamic monitoring including heart rate, ECG, blood pressure, and pulse oximetry is mandatory with full resuscitation equipment readily available. Testing regimens vary from a fixed 100 mg per patient to 5 mg/kg body weight. The authors use a series of bolus injections with the patient blinded. Two of the injections are placebo (normal saline), and the others are 50-mg boluses of lidocaine for a total of 5 mg/kg, maximum 200 mg per patient, with temporary interruption of injection if CNS effects occur.

B. Similarly, infusion of opioids may be useful in treating refractory pain or pain flares, and in predicting efficacy of treatment with chronic oral opioids. Morphine is used most often for treatment, although any of the parenterally available agents may be used. For testing purposes, an agent of rapid onset and brief duration such as fentanyl or alfentanil is a more practical choice, although a technique using patient-controlled analgesia with morphine has been described, with lack of dosing constraints touted as an advantage. A positive response to the opioid can be verified by administering naloxone and observing an immediate reversal of analgesic effect. Presence of euphoric effects without reduction of pain is considered a negative response.

C. If there appears to be a significant anxiety component to a patient's pain behavior, intravenous administration of anxiolytic agents such as the benzodiazepines midazolam and diazepam may be useful diagnostically. To further confirm the anxiolytic's effect, the benzodiazepine antagonist flumazenil may be administered. The patient may then benefit from behavioral and pharmacologic therapies to relieve anxiety.

D. In the case of sympathetically maintained pain, administration of the α-adrenergic antagonist phentolamine has been shown to be useful diagnostically. Raja also showed that administering phentolamine intravenously resulted in analgesia that was similar to local anesthetic blockade of the sympathetic ganglion. The protocol involves blinding of the patient and administration of two placebo injections with the phentolamine administered as 1 mg/kg over 10 minutes with standard hemodynamic monitoring.

E. Recently, a ketamine infusion protocol has been described to predict potential responsiveness to oral dextromethorphan for neuropathic pain. With the patient blinded, ketamine 0.1 mg/kg is administered in addition to a placebo control. Using greater than or equal to 67% reduction in pain as the criterion for a positive response, the test had a positive predictive value of 90%, negative predictive value of 80%, with specificity of 92%.

Given the difficulty in treating many chronic pain syndromes, careful administration of intravenous agents may provide a useful therapeutic option. When using these agents for diagnostic and prognostic purposes, caution must be used in interpreting patient response.

REFERENCES

Cohen SP, Chang AS, Larkin T, Mao J: The intravenous ketamine test: a predictive response tool for oral dextromethorphan treatment in neuropathic pain. *Anesth Analg* 2004;99:1753–1759.

Mao J, Chen LL: Systemic lidocaine for neuropathic pain relief. *Pain* 2000;87:7–17.

O'Gorman DA, Raja SN: In: Raj PP (ed) *Practical Management of Pain*, 3rd ed. St. Louis, Mosby, 2000, pp. 723–729.

TESTING AND TREATMENT WITH INTRAVENOUS AGENTS

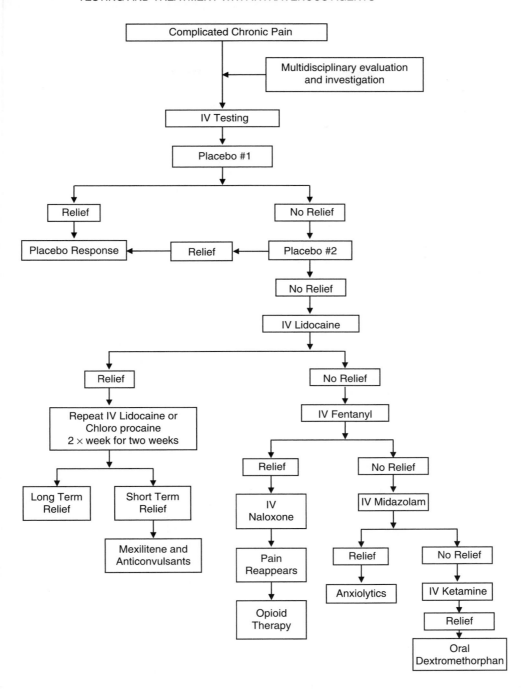

Differential Epidural/Spinal Blockade

WILLIAM E. STRONG AND SOMAYAJI RAMAMURTHY

Many patients are referred to the pain clinic with chronic pain problems of unknown etiology despite extensive evaluation. A differential epidural/spinal block can help identify the mechanism of pain. Its usefulness is based on the differential sensitivity of nerve fibers to local anesthetic agents (Table 1). This procedure is most useful for patients with pain in the lower extremities, lower abdomen, pelvis, or low back. The epidural form can be used for thoracic pain. The purpose of the block is to define the mechanism of pain, whether sympathetic, somatic, or central in origin. The procedure is useful in diagnosis and prognosis and can be therapeutic. Differential spinal block was first described by Sarnoff and Arrowood (1946) and was modified by Raj and Ramamurthy (1988) to include differential epidural blocks. A modified retrograde spinal block has been described.

A. A thorough history and physical examination is required in the initial evaluation of all patients at the pain clinic. Additional studies such as imaging and electromyography (EMG)/nerve conduction are performed as indicated, although in most cases the studies have already been completed. Psychological testing completes the initial evaluation, and this point in diagnosis can usually be as certain and treatment begun. If the etiology is still unclear a differential block is an appropriate next step.

B. The differential block can be performed as a progressive spinal or retrograde (modified) spinal, continuous spinal, or continuous epidural block. An advantage of the continuous technique is that patients do not have to lie on their side with a needle in their back for the duration of the entire procedure. Disadvantages of the epidural technique are slower onset and less clear endpoints. Since these patients are receiving a central neuraxial block, the usual monitoring, IV access, and airway resuscitation equipment should be immediately available.

C. Perform the spinal or epidural block in the usual manner. For the spinal technique (noncontinuous), patients must remain on their side with the needle in the subarachnoid space during the entire procedure. All injections should be made with syringes that have the same volume and appearance so that the patient will be unaware of the solution that is being used. The sensation is tested with pinprick and sympathetic function with the cutaneous temperature probe or sympathogalvanic response before and 5 minutes after each injection. Whether an epidural or spinal technique is chosen, the initial injection should be with 0.9% saline as a placebo. Pain relief following this injection is considered a placebo response. A placebo response does not rule out organic etiology because 30% to 35% of patients whose pain is of an organic etiology can obtain significant pain relief with a placebo.

D. If the patient receives no pain relief with the placebo, inject a low concentration of local anesthetic (0.25% procaine or spinal or 0.5% for epidural) to produce a sympathetic block. If the pain is relieved with a confirmed sympathetic block and with intact sensation, the pain is most likely sympathetically mediated. This patient's pain may respond to a series of sympathetic block. Misdiagnosis can occur if presence of sympathetic block and absence of sensory block is not verified.

E. If the patient continues to have pain, inject a higher concentration of local anesthetic (0.5% procaine for spinal, 1% lidocaine for epidural). If pain is relieved after loss of sensation to pinprick, a somatic etiology is likely and the patient may be a candidate for further peripheral nerve blocks or surgery.

F. If the pain is not relieved with a sensory nerve block, inject a concentration of local anesthetic (1% or higher concentration of procaine for spinal, 2% lidocaine for

---

TABLE 1
Classification of Nerve Fibers on the Basis of Fiber Size (Relating Fiber Size to Fiber Function and Sensitivity to Local Anesthetics)

Group	Fiber	Conduction	Modality	Sensitivity to Local Anesthetics (Subarachnoid Procaine)
A (Myelinated) Alpha	20 μm	100 mps	Large motor, proprioception (reflex activity)	1%
Beta	20 μm	100 mps	Small motor, touch, and pressure	1%
Gamma	20 μm	100 mps	Muscle spindle fibers (muscle tone)	1%
Delta	4 μm	5 mps	Temperature and sharp pain Possibly touch	0.5%
B (myelinated)	3 μm	3–14 mps	Preganglionic autonomic fibers	0.25%
C (unmyelinated)	0.5–1 μm	1.2 mps	Dull pain, temperature, touch (like delta, but slower)	0.5%

mps, meters per second.
From Ramamurthy S, Winnie AP: Regional anesthetic techniques for pain relief. *Semin Anesth* 1985;4:237; with permission.

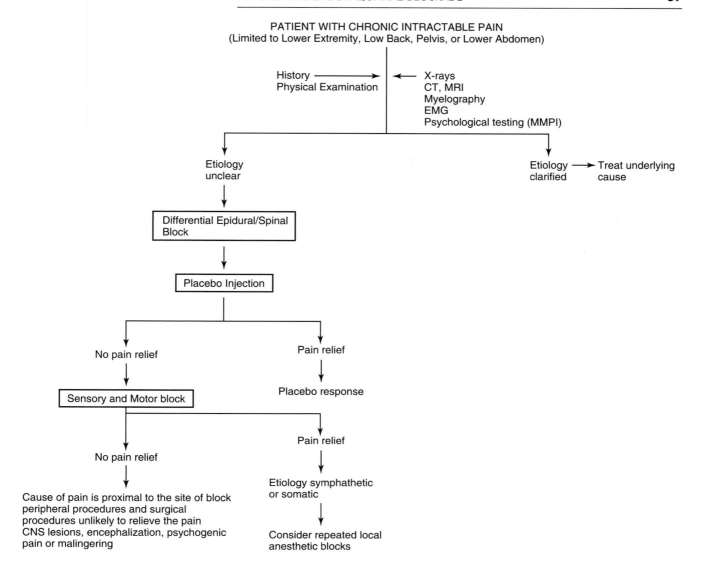

PATIENT WITH CHRONIC INTRACTABLE PAIN
(Limited to Lower Extremity, Low Back, Pelvis, or Lower Abdomen)

History ⟶ ← X-rays
Physical Examination   CT, MRI
Myelography
EMG
Psychological testing (MMPI)

Etiology   Etiology ⟶ Treat underlying
unclear   clarified   cause

Differential Epidural/Spinal
Block

Placebo Injection

No pain relief   Pain relief

Sensory and Motor block   Placebo response

No pain relief   Pain relief

Cause of pain is proximal to the site of block   Etiology symphathetic
peripheral procedures and surgical   or somatic
procedures unlikely to relieve the pain
CNS lesions, encephalization, psychogenic   Consider repeated local
pain or malingering   anesthetic blocks

epidural) to more completely block sensory and motor fibers. If the pain is relieved, a somatic etiology is likely and peripheral nerve blocks or surgery may be helpful. If the patient obtains no pain relief with complete somatic nerve block, the etiology of the pain is proximal to the site of the block and neither peripheral blocks nor surgical procedures will be of benefit. No pain relief with this procedure can occur in the case of central nervous system (CNS) lesions, encephalization, malingering, or psychogenic pain.

Complications of the differential epidural/spinal block procedure are the same as those associated with other spinal or epidural procedures. These include hypotension secondary to sympathetic block, postdural puncture headache, backache, bleeding, and hematoma.

DIFFERENTIAL BLOCK—MODIFIED TECHNIQUE

With this technique, the indications and the patient preparation are similar to that of the standard differential epidural and spinal technique. After injection of the placebo, if the pain persists, a high concentration of local anesthetic such as 5% procaine for spinal or 2% lidocaine for epidural is injected to ensure good sensory and motor block. The spinal needle is removed and the patient is turned to the supine position. If the patient has no pain relief despite having a significant sensory and motor block in the painful area then the etiology is proximal to the site of block. This patient is not likely to benefit from procedures such as injections or surgery. Proximal etiology such as CNS lesions, encephalization, malingering, or psychogenic pain is to be considered.

If the patient has pain relief, then the etiology would be either sympathetic or somatic. The patient is observed for return of pain and the sensory and sympathetic blocks are simultaneously monitored. If the pain relief is present only for the duration of sensory block then a somatic etiology is likely. If the pain relief persists even after recovery from the sensory block this patient has a pain condition in which long-term pain relief follows temporary interruption of sympathetic and somatic pathways. This patient could have sympathetically mediated pain or a condition that may be relieved by repeated local anesthetic blocks.

This technique has several advantages. Patients do not have to lie on their side after injection of the local anesthetic. This is comfortable for the patient and also facilitates examination of the patient to evaluate the effectiveness of the local anesthetic block while attempting to reproduce the painful maneuvers. The time required to perform this technique is much shorter than that for the classical technique, especially when the pain is not likely to be relieved despite significant sensitive motor block. Endpoints are also much better defined than in the classical technique.

REFERENCES

Gasser HS, Erlanger J: Role of fiber size in establishment of nerve block by pressure or cocaine. *Am J Physiol* 1929;88:581

Raj PP, Ramamurthy S: Differential nerve block studies. In: Raj P (ed) *Practical Management of Pain*. Chicago, Year Book, 1988, p. 173.

Sarnoff SJ, Arrowood JG: Differential spinal block. *Surgery* 1946; 20:150.

Diagnostic Neural Blocks

EULECHE ALANMANOU

The use of nerve block as a diagnostic tool has gained a popularity that is not always backed by the critical review of the available data. In patients with acute pain, the stimulus creates impulses in nociceptors and the conduction of these signals can be blocked by local anesthetics before they are perceived in the central nervous system (CNS). With chronic pain, the site of generation and the mechanism of maintenance of nociceptor activity are not always clear. There is a complex interplay of peripheral and central mechanisms involving nociceptor activity, sympathetic contribution, spinal processing, plasticity, and convergent input. The issues that compound the complexity of a patient's pain include cultural, environmental, psychological, and disuse factors.

Nerve blocks with local anesthetics in high concentration interrupt both afferent and efferent neural conduction; in contrast, with low concentrations of local anesthetics this interruption might become selective. Thus neural conduction in small fibers (A-δ) and nonmyelinated nerve fibers (C fibers) may be interrupted, whereas there is only a modest effect on large myelinated fibers, which are predominantly motor or proprioceptive agents.

The limitations of a diagnostic nerve block should be kept in mind because these blocks are simply useful additions to the available diagnostic and prognostic tools. Full evaluation of the patient and the pain problem is warranted for determining if a nerve block is appropriate. A review of the available investigations is performed, and new studies are ordered if necessary. A psychological or psychiatric evaluation can provide additional insight.

The decision to block a specific site depends on the painful body part (Table 1). Performance of the regional anesthesia technique requires, in addition to technical excellence, knowledge of anatomic and physiologic foundations and limitations of the procedure. The physician should be prepared to deal with potential side effects and complications. The patient should sign an informed consent that details the risks of the procedure.

A. Before the block is performed, a pain measurement (i.e., the Visual Analog Scale) is applied, any motor or sensory deficit is determined, and the temperature over the affected area is recorded. These indicators are then compared to those on the contralateral site and documented.

B. Once a nerve block is performed, it is essential to confirm that the targeted nerve has been reached. It is also useful to know if an undesired blockade has occurred, such as blockage of an adjacent nerve. The postblock examination includes assessment of temperature, sweating, and the sympathogalvanic response to evaluate the sympathetic response. Any sensory and motor change should be documented and a new pain measurement undertaken.

C. Because treatment often depends on an accurate diagnosis, cautious interpretation of diagnostic nerve blocks is warranted. The sensitivity of such blocks can be enhanced during their performance by fluoroscopic, sonographic, or computed tomographic guidance. The specificity of blocks is more difficult to control. Some of the factors that decrease the specificity of diagnostic blocks include placebo effects and expectation bias.

D. In practice, pain relief of more than 50% after a confirmed block requires a repeat block when the pain returns.

E. If the relief can be consistently reproduced, consider a block at regular intervals, continuous infusion of analgesic, injection of steroids, or a neuroablative procedure. Keep in mind that relief obtained with a nerve block may help predict the response to neural decompression but its value for predicting the response to neuroablation is unproved. Moreover, the available studies raise doubt as to whether analgesia after sympathetic blockade necessarily indicates a sympathetic contribution to pain.

F. If there is no pain relief after a confirmed block, consider that the origin of pain might be proximal to the site of the block. The etiologies might include a CNS lesion, a psychogenic process, malingering, or encephalization.

TABLE 1
Site of Block

Site of Pain	Sympathetic	Somatic
Head	Stellate ganglion block	C2 block; trigeminal block (or branches)
Neck	Stellate ganglion block	Cervical plexus block (or individual nerve)
Arm	Stellate ganglion block	Brachial plexus block (or individual nerve)
Thorax	Thoracic epidural; paravertebral block; intercostal block	Thoracic epidural; paravertebral block; intercostal block
Abdomen	Celiac plexus block; splanchnic	Paravertebral block; intercostal block
Pelvis	Superior hypogastric block	Caudal, epidural, saddle, sacral root block
Leg	Lumbar paravertebral sympathetic block	Lumbar paravertebral somatic block

Modified from Ramamurthy S, Winnie AP: Regional anesthetic techniques for pain relief. *Semin Anesth* 1985;4:237, with permission.

REFERENCES

Buckley FP: Regional anesthesia with local anesthetic. In: Loeser JD (ed) *Bonica's Management of Pain*, 3rd ed. Philadelphia, Lippincott Williams & Wilkins, 2001.

Hogan QH, Abram SE: Neural blockade for diagnosis and prognosis: a review. *Anesthesiology* 1997;86:216.

Raja SN: Nerve blocks in the evaluation of chronic pain: a plea for caution in their use and interpretation. *Anesthesiology* 1997;86:4.

Ramamurthy S, Winnie AP: Regional anesthetic techniques for pain relief. *Semin Anesth* 1985;4:237.

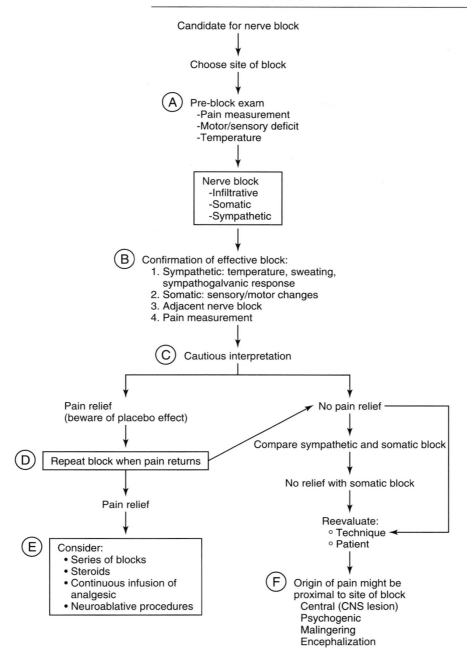

Candidate for nerve block

↓

Choose site of block

↓

(A) Pre-block exam
-Pain measurement
-Motor/sensory deficit
-Temperature

↓

Nerve block
-Infiltrative
-Somatic
-Sympathetic

↓

(B) Confirmation of effective block:
1. Sympathetic: temperature, sweating, sympathogalvanic response
2. Somatic: sensory/motor changes
3. Adjacent nerve block
4. Pain measurement

↓

(C) Cautious interpretation

Pain relief (beware of placebo effect)

No pain relief

↓

Compare sympathetic and somatic block

↓

No relief with somatic block

↓

(D) Repeat block when pain returns

↓

Pain relief

Reevaluate:
○ Technique
○ Patient

↓

(E) Consider:
• Series of blocks
• Steroids
• Continuous infusion of analgesic
• Neuroablative procedures

(F) Origin of pain might be proximal to site of block
Central (CNS lesion)
Psychogenic
Malingering
Encephalization

ACUTE PAIN

Patient-Controlled Analgesia
Acute Herpes Zoster
Acute Upper Extremity Pain
Acute Lower Extremity Pain
Acute Thoracic Pain
Acute Vertebral Pain
Acute Abdominal Pain
Acute Pancreatic Pain
Obstetric Pain

Patient-Controlled Analgesia

JAY ELLIS

Patient-controlled analgesia (PCA) is an effective form of acute pain control that allows patients to regulate their own analgesic medication delivery with mechanical safeguards in place to prevent overdose. Studies comparing PCA to traditional intramuscular opioid dosing on an "as-needed" (PRN) basis found PCA to be as good or better than PRN dosing for controlling pain without an increase in complications (Etches 1999; Lehmann 1999). One study questioned the economic cost of PCA, stating that scheduled intramuscular dosing provided equivalent analgesia and outcomes at lower cost (Keita et al. 2003). The primary criticism of this conclusion is that outcomes for PRN administration or scheduled administration of medication on a busy nursing unit may not reach the precision and reproducibility found in an ongoing clinical trial. PCA is a nursing-force expander.

The PCA device consists of a programmable infusion pump that delivers a predetermined dose of analgesic medication (the demand dose) when the patient activates a button. The patient cannot receive another dose of medication during a predetermined period of time, called the "lockout interval," no matter how many times he or she pushes the button. The usual lockout interval is 5 to 15 minutes. In addition, 1-hour and 4-hour lockout intervals specify the maximum amount of medication a patient can receive during a 1-hour or a 4-hour period. This serves as an additional safeguard against overdose. There is also the capacity to generate a constant infusion with or without the demand dose. Most commercially available devices come equipped with locks and user password codes to prevent tampering with the device.

A. Patient-controlled analgesia has been used successfully in patients of all ages, from school-age children to the elderly (Lavand'Homme and De Kock 1998; Trentadue et al. 1998). A patient who is a candidate for PCA must have sufficient mental capacity to understand the purpose of the machine, be physically able to press the button, and be willing to take responsibility for administering the pain medication. Ideally, this education takes place before the patient is in excruciating pain or mentally compromised by large doses of sedative-hypnotic agents. Family and friends should not be allowed to use the device except under strict protocols, which change the therapy from patient-controlled to parent- or spouse-controlled analgesia. Patients need to understand that the machine has limits to prevent them from overdosing and that they should press the button as often as they feel the need. Patient requests for medication during the lockout interval are a useful measure of the effectiveness, or ineffectiveness, of therapy.

B. Morphine is the most commonly used medication for PCA, although meperidine, hydromorphone, and several others have been described (Camu et al. 1998; Pang et al. 1999; Plummer et al. 1997;

Rapp et al. 1996). There is no evidence that any of the medications is sufficiently better than morphine to warrant replacing morphine as the most commonly used medication in the general patient population. Individual patients may have special needs (allergic reactions, severe side effects) that make one of the other medications a more attractive option. The biggest advantage of morphine is that it comes in readily available commercially prepared containers for easy use.

C. Side effects and complications from PCA are less than or equal to those found with other forms of opioid administration. Nausea occurs in 30% to 50% of patients receiving PCA morphine and vomiting in 14% to 30%, rates similar to those found in other acute opioid administration studies (Tramer and Walder 1999; Tsui et al. 1996). Respiratory depression requiring treatment occurs in 0.5% to 1.6% of patients depending on the setting and method of administration. Studies looking at risk factors for respiratory depression identified demand doses of morphine higher than 1.5 mg, age over 65 years, abdominal surgery, and a background constant infusion of morphine as risk factors for respiratory depression (Sidebotham et al. 1997). Some practitioners think a background infusion improves analgesia and improves sleep in patients receiving PCA for postoperative pain control. Studies dispute this belief and show that analgesia appears similar for at least certain types of postsurgical patients, making the routine use of background infusions a questionable practice (Lavand'Homme and De Kock 1998; Smythe et al. 1996). Exceptions to this rule include patients with severe pain requiring high doses of opioids (e.g., severe cancer pain) to control pain. A background infusion could help avoid the extreme peaks and valleys of large-dose bolus opioid use or the problem of the patient having to hit the button every 5 minutes, day and night. In addition, patients who use large doses of opioids chronically for pain may benefit from a background infusion to substitute for their daily medication until they can resume oral therapy.

D. Initiation of opioid therapy usually requires a loading dose of medication to get the patient's pain under control so small incremental doses of opioid can maintain the analgesia. The loading dose varies widely from patient to patient and reaches doses equivalent to 10 to 15 mg of morphine or more in some individuals. Failure to achieve reasonable control of the pain with the loading dose causes the patient and the facility staff quickly to lose faith in the technique, as the patient repeatedly hits the button to no apparent benefit. Next the patient should receive a demand dose of 1 to 1.5 mg of morphine, or an equivalent amount of another opioid, every 5 to 15 minutes.

PATIENT-CONTROLLED ANALGESIA

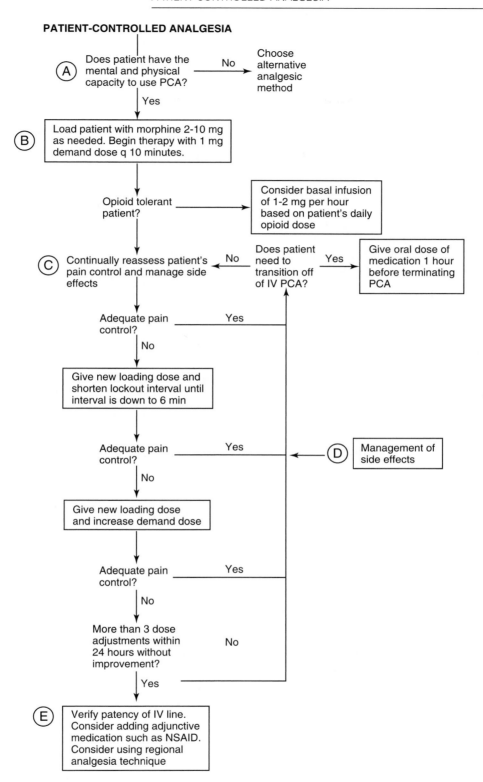

Ⓐ Does patient have the mental and physical capacity to use PCA?

No → Choose alternative analgesic method

Yes

Ⓑ Load patient with morphine 2-10 mg as needed. Begin therapy with 1 mg demand dose q 10 minutes.

Opioid tolerant patient? → Consider basal infusion of 1-2 mg per hour based on patient's daily opioid dose

Ⓒ Continually reassess patient's pain control and manage side effects

No ← Does patient need to transition off of IV PCA? → Yes → Give oral dose of medication 1 hour before terminating PCA

Adequate pain control? — Yes

No

Give new loading dose and shorten lockout interval until interval is down to 6 min

Adequate pain control? — Yes ← Ⓓ Management of side effects

No

Give new loading dose and increase demand dose

Adequate pain control? — Yes

No

More than 3 dose adjustments within 24 hours without improvement? — No

Yes

Ⓔ Verify patency of IV line. Consider adding adjunctive medication such as NSAID. Consider using regional analgesia technique

The clinical onset of morphine analgesia averages 6 minutes, so more frequent dosing is not recommended (Upton et al. 1997). The smaller doses and longer intervals are recommended for individuals most susceptible to opioid side effects, such as the elderly. The 1-hour and 4-hour lockouts should reflect the maximum dose allowable for the demand dose and the corresponding lockout interval. For example, a patient receiving 1 mg demand dose with a 6-minute lockout and no background infusion should not have a 1-hour lockout limit of more than 10 mg.

E. Patients require regular reassessment to gauge the effectiveness of therapy and address the problem of side effects. Patients with poor pain control after the demand dose need a larger demand dose. Patients with good, though transient, pain control need a shorter lockout interval. Patients who state that the "machine isn't working" need the patency of their intravenous line confirmed; and if the intravenous infusion is working, the patient needs a repeat loading dose, a higher demand dose, and possibly a shorter lockout interval.

F. Management of side effects is an important component of effective PCA therapy. Several studies have looked at prophylactic antiemetic therapy given separately or as a part of the demand dose (Dresner et al. 1998; Tramer and Walder 1999). Droperidol is effective in treating PCA-induced nausea and vomiting, but the recent warnings regarding droperidol and prolonged-QT syndrome has discouraged its use. 5-Hydroxytrypamine-3 (5HT-3) receptor antagonists and the older antidopaminergic agents such as prochlorperazine or promethazine are effective as well. Alternatively, another opioid may be tried (e.g., switching from morphine to hydromorphone). Patients may not be as nauseated with another opioid. Another option is to add an adjunctive analgesic medication such as ketoralac to reduce the dose of opioid needed. Nausea is a dose-related side effect.

G. Patient-controlled analgesia is not a "set and forget" therapy. Both physician and nursing staff need to understand the effective elements of therapy, management of side effects, and prevention of complications. One study looking at PCA managed by an acute-pain service compared to one managed by the primary surgeon failed to show differences in pain scores but did show some difference in the incidence of side effects (Stacey et al. 1997). There appears to be little question that any qualified medical professional can prescribe PCA. What makes PCA effective is the commitment to regular reassessment, intervention for ineffective pain relief, management of side effects, and prevention of adverse outcomes.

REFERENCES

Camu F, Van Aken H, Bovill JG: Postoperative analgesic effects of three demand-dose sizes of fentanyl administered by patient-controlled analgesia. *Anesth Analg* 1998;87:890–895.

Dresner M, Dean S, Lumb A, Bellamy M: High-dose ondansetron regimen vs droperidol for morphine patient-controlled analgesia. *Br J Anaesth* 1998;81:384–386.

Etches RC: Patient-controlled analgesia. *Surg Clin North Am* 1999; 79:297–312.

Keita H, Geachan N, Dahmani S, et al: Comparison between patient-controlled analgesia and subcutaneous morphine in elderly patients after total hip replacement. *Br J Anaesth* 2003;90:53–57.

Lavand'Homme P, De Kock M: Practical guidelines on the postoperative use of patient-controlled analgesia in the elderly. *Drugs Aging* 1998;13:9–16.

Lehmann KA: Modifiers of patient-controlled analgesia efficacy in acute and chronic pain. *Curr Rev Pain* 1999;3:447–452.

Pang WW, Mok MS, Lin CH, et al: Comparison of patient-controlled analgesia (PCA) with tramadol or morphine. *Can J Anaesth* 1999; 46:1030–1035.

Plummer JL, Owen H, Ilsley AH, Inglis S: Morphine patient-controlled analgesia is superior to meperidine patient-controlled analgesia for postoperative pain. *Anesth Analg* 1997;84:794–799.

Rapp SE, Egan KJ, Ross BK, et al: A multidimensional comparison of morphine and hydromorphone patient-controlled analgesia. *Anesth Analg* 1996;82:1043–1048.

Sidebotham D, Dijkhuizen MR, Schug SA: The safety and utilization of patient-controlled analgesia. *J Pain Symptom Manage* 1997; 14:202–209.

Smythe MA, MB Zak, O'Donnell MP, et al: Patient-controlled analgesia versus patient-controlled analgesia plus continuous infusion after hip replacement surgery. *Ann Pharmacother* 1996;30:224–227.

Stacey BR, Rudy TE, Nelhaus D: Management of patient-controlled analgesia: a comparison of primary surgeons and a dedicated pain service. *Anesth Analg* 1997;85:130–134.

Tramer MR, Walder B: Efficacy and adverse effects of prophylactic antiemetics during patient-controlled analgesia therapy: a quantitative systematic review. *Anesth Analg* 1999;88:1354–1361.

Trentadue NO, Kachoyeanos MK, Lea GJ: A comparison of two regimens of patient-controlled analgesia for children with sickle cell disease. *Pediatr Nurs* 1998;13:15–19.

Tsui SL, Tong WN, Irwin M, et al: The efficacy, applicability and side-effects of postoperative intravenous patient-controlled morphine analgesia: an audit of 1233 Chinese patients. *Anaesth Intensive Care* 1996;24:658–664.

Upton RN, Semple TJ, Macintyre PE: Pharmacokinetic optimisation of opioid treatment in acute pain therapy. *Clin Pharmacokinet* 1997;33:225–244.

Acute Herpes Zoster

ROBERT SPRAGUE

Acute herpes zoster (HZ) is an infectious disease involving reactivation of the varicella virus, which affects the dorsal root ganglia primarily. Immunocompromised individuals, whether due to age, malignancy, or other systemic illnesses, are most often affected. Children make up only 5% to 8% of cases, whereas patients older than 50 years of age account for 40% of cases. Presentation of symptoms, typically erythema, vesicular rash, and paresthesia and dysesthesia of distinct unilateral dermatomes occurs within 2 to 3 days of the start of viral replication. The distribution of dermatomes is primarily thoracic (55%) and cranial (25%), with sacral or generalized distributions occurring rarely. The goals of therapy are pain relief, decreasing viral replication, and prevention of postherpetic neuralgia (PHN).

A. A thorough history and physical examination are important for delineating the dermatomal distribution involved, as is the time since the onset of symptoms. Studies have shown dramatic alleviation of symptoms and prevention of PHN if oral antiviral agents are used within 72 hours of the onset. The physical examination may also uncover the underlying cause of the immunodeficiency, such as an occult malignancy.

B. Ocular HZ may lead to permanent blindness and should be treated by an ophthalmologist. Oral antiviral agents should be prescribed immediately if symptoms are less than 72 hours old. A stellate ganglion blockade may also be beneficial.

C. Oral antiviral agents have been shown in numerous studies to be effective in decreasing viral replication but only if administered within 72 hours of the onset of the rash. If acyclovir is used, adequate hydration must be ensured, as the kidney is the primary route of excretion. Some studies recommend antiviral agents only for patients less than 50 years of age. Most of the literature seems to support antiviral agents in any patient whose symptoms have been present less than 72 hours and who has moderate to severe pain.

D. Oral antiviral drug dosages are outlined in Table 1.

E. Analgesia is of the utmost concern to the patient as this syndrome is extremely painful. The course of the acute eruption is short, so oral narcotics may be administered in the short term, especially when combined with nonsteroidal antiinflammatory drugs (NSAIDs). If the pain is not as severe, NSAIDs or acetaminophen may be all that is needed.

F. Sympathetic blocks may provide pain relief and speed healing in patients with HZ and may prevent the onset of PHN by improving circulation to the affected nerve root. Epidural blockade, especially when combined with antiviral agents, has been shown to be extremely effective.

G. Intradermal injections of local anesthetics or saline with triamcinolone along the lines of distribution and in open lesions may provide temporary relief and speed healing of the vesicular eruptions.

H. Oral steroids have been used to treat HZ with mixed results. Pain and inflammation appear to be reduced, and some decrease in the incidence of PHN has been demonstrated. There is some concern of systemic HZ dissemination associated with the use of steroids in immunocompromised patients, such as those with acquired immunodeficiency syndrome.

I. Many anecdotal and retrospective adjuvant therapies for treating HZ have been discussed in the literature. Lidocaine gel 10%, ketorolac gel, chloroform with aspirin, ice/ethyl chloride spray, and various drying lotions have been used topically, with some relief of pain. Care must be taken, however, when using topical agents on open lesions because of systemic absorption. Topical antibiotics may be considered if any signs of local infection develop. Transcutaneous electrical nerve stimulation has also been used and has met with limited success.

REFERENCES

Beutner KR: Clinical management of herpes zoster in the elderly patient. *Comp Ther* 1996;22:183.

Hwang C: The effects of epidural blockade on the acute pain in herpes zoster. *Arch Dermatol* 199;135:1359.

Raj PP: Management of herpes zoster pain and post herpetic neuralgia. *Pain Dig* 1992;2:201.

Schmidt SI, Moorthy SS, Dierdorf SF, West R: Current therapy for herpes zoster and post herpetic neuralgia. *Anesthesiol Rev* 1991;18:35.

Stankus SJ: Management of herpes zoster and post herpetic neuralgia. *Am Fam Physician* 2000;61:2437.

TABLE 1
Oral Antiviral Dosage Regimens

Drug	Dosage regimen
Acyclovir	800 mg 5 times q day × 7 days
Valacyclovir	1000 mg 3 times q day × 7 days
Famciclovir	750 mg 3 times q day × 7 days

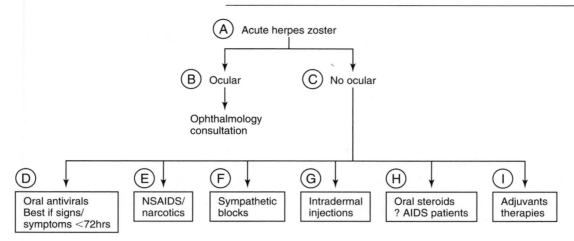

Acute Upper Extremity Pain

DOUGLAS M. ANDERSON AND JERRY A. BEYER

The upper extremities are common sites for acute pain or chronic pain with acute exacerbations. The most common etiologies of upper extremity pain include trauma, tumor, infection, and neuropathic pain (including radicular pain). Successful treatment of acute upper extremity pain usually involves a multifaceted approach utilizing medications, physical therapy (PT), and regional anesthesia.

A. Treatment of acute upper extremity pain is usually aided by the use of analgesic medications such as nonsteroidal antiinflammatory drugs (NSAIDs), acetaminophen, and opioids. Antispasmodic (muscle relaxants) medications may be considered if severe muscle spasms are a significant component of the pain. Optimal pharmacologic therapy often includes a combination of several medications.

B. Physical therapy is extremely important for the successful treatment of acute pain and the prevention of chronic pain and permanent disability. PT is often facilitated by medications and regional anesthetic techniques.

C. There are many effective regional anesthetic techniques available for relief and control of acute upper extremity pain. Prior to choosing a technique, the patient's specific needs must be determined by answering the following questions. Is the patient a suitable candidate? Which nerves are involved in the production of pain? Will a tourniquet be used? Is anesthesia or analgesia required? What are the potential complications associated with each technique? Would the patient benefit from a long-term regional technique such as a peripheral nerve catheter? Finally, what is your experience and expertise?

It may be difficult to determine which nerves are involved with the production of pain in an injured or painful extremity. The cutaneous innervation of an extremity is highly variable, with much overlap of adjacent nerves (Figure 1). In addition, the innervation of the underlying muscles (myotomes) and bones (sclerotomes) are often not the same as for the overlying skin. Always consider the differential innervation of the involved structures to avoid developing an unsatisfactory regional anesthesia plan (Table 1).

D. A cervical epidural is an excellent neuraxial technique for managing pain in the neck, shoulders, and upper extremities; it is particularly useful when both upper extremities are involved. Cervical epidurals offer many unique advantages and disadvantages. It is difficult or impossible to provide unilateral anesthesia or analgesia with neuraxial anesthetic techniques. Respiratory depression, hemodynamic instability, sedation, local anesthetic toxicity, epidural hematoma/ abscess, cord injury, accidental dural puncture, and pruritus are all potential complications or side effects. In addition, many anesthesiologists do not have experience with this technique.

E. It is useful to categorize nerve blocks of the upper extremity into two groups: blocks performed at the level of the brachial plexus and those performed at the level of the terminal nerve. Blocks at the level of the brachial plexus can be further subdivided by the specific approach utilized to perform the block (i.e., supraclavicular, infraclavicular, axillary).

F. There are many supraclavicular approaches to the brachial plexus including interscalene, subclavian perivascular, classic supraclavicular, and parascalene blocks. Blocks performed above the clavicle are highly successful owing to the condensed nature of the brachial plexus in this region. With these blocks, the local anesthetic can spread to adjacent structures. In the case of an interscalene block utilized for shoulder surgery, spread into the cervical plexus is desirable, whereas blockade of the phrenic nerve (i.e., with an interscalene, subclavian perivascular, or parascalene approach) is rarely desirable and, in fact, can be problematic in patients with underlying pulmonary disease. The incidence of recurrent laryngeal nerve block associated with interscalene blocks is 5% to 17%. Horner's syndrome is also a common side effect of supraclavicular approaches and would interfere in the neurologic evaluation of a patient with head trauma. The interscalene approach to the brachial plexus rarely blocks the lower roots of the brachial plexus (i.e., C8, T1) and is a poor choice for pain originating in the hand or medial aspect of the extremity. The intercostobrachial nerve (T2) and the medial cutaneous nerve of the arm (T1) innervate the medial aspect of the arm proximal to the elbow. These nerves are poorly anesthetized with many approaches to the brachial plexus, so a supplemental field block may be required to achieve analgesia or anesthesia (e.g., tourniquet pain). Supraclavicular approaches to the brachial plexus are highly effective for pain originating in the shoulder and arm. If the pain is originating in the shoulder and an interscalene approach is not used, it may be necessary to block the cervical plexus for skin analgesia. The most feared complication of the supraclavicular approaches to the brachial plexus is pneumothorax; the risk depends on the specific approach and the experience of the practitioner. Fortunately, with experienced practitioners the incidence of clinically significant pneumothorax is low.

G. Infraclavicular and axillary approaches to the brachial plexus are highly effective for relieving pain mediating from the hand, forearm, and arm. The literature describes many types of infraclavicular and axillary blocks. These approaches have enjoyed popularity owing to their favorable side effect and safety profiles. Infraclavicular approaches have become fashionable. Positioning the painful arm is not usually required,

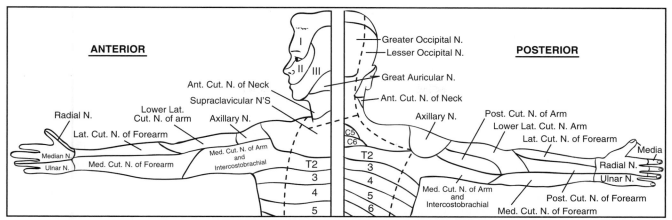

FIGURE 1 Cutaneous distribution of peripheral nerves. (Modified from Wright PE, Simons JCH: Peripheral nerve injuries. In: Edmonson AS, Crenshaw AH [eds] *Campbell's Operative Orthopaedics*, 6th ed. St. Louis, Mosby, 1980, p 1644, with permission.)

TABLE 1
Blocks for Nerves of Upper Extremities

Nerves of the Upper Extremities	Methods of Blocking (Cervical Epidural)
Cervical plexus	
Supraclavicular nerves (C3, C4)	Interscalene brachial plexus block (dependent on proximal spread to cervical plexus)
	Deep or superficial cervical plexus block
	Necessary to block for most shoulder procedures
Brachial plexus	
Musculocutaneous (C5—7)	Supra/infraclavicular approaches to brachial plexus block (most reliably blocked with supraclavicular approaches)
	Isolated musculocutaneous n. block in coracobrachialis muscle
Lateral cutaneous n. of forearm	Any type of musculocutaneous nerve block
	Proximal or midhumeral block
	Isolated lateral cutaneous n. of the forearm block in antecubital fossa
Axillary (C5, C6)	Supra/infraclavicular approaches to brachial plexus block
	Variable success with axillary approaches
Radial (C5—8)	Supra/infraclavicular approaches to brachial plexus block
	Axillary approach to brachial plexus
	Proximal or midhumeral block (not reliable for procedures above the elbow)
	Elbow/wrist block
Posterior cutaneous n. of arm	Supra/infraclavicular approaches to brachial plexus block
	Axillary approach to brachial plexus
Lower lateral cutaneous n. of arm	Supra/infraclavicular approaches to brachial plexus block
	Axillary approach to brachial plexus
	Proximal humerus block
Posterior cutaneous n. of forearm	Supra/infraclavicular approaches to brachial plexus block
	Axillary approach to brachial plexus
	Proximal or midhumeral block
Median (C6—8, T1)	Supra/infraclavicular approaches to brachial plexus block
	Axillary approach to brachial plexus
	Proximal or midhumeral block
	Elbow/wrist block
Ulnar (C8, T1)	Supra/infraclavicular approaches to brachial plexus block (not reliably blocked with interscalene block)
	Axillary approach to brachial plexus
	Proximal or midhumeral block
	Elbow/wrist block
Median cutaneous n. of forearm (C8, T1)	Supra/infraclavicular approaches to brachial plexus block (not reliably blocked with interscalene block)
	Axillary approach to brachial plexus
	Proximal or midhumeral block
	Elbow block
Median cutaneous n. of arm (T1)	Not reliably blocked by many approaches to the brachial plexus
	Field block of very proximal humerus in axilla
Intercostobrachial (T2)	
	Not blocked by any approach to brachial plexus
	Field block of very proximal humerus in axilla

and a catheter can be easily placed and fixed to the anterior chest wall. The intercostobrachial nerve (T2) and the medial cutaneous nerve of the arm (T1) often must be given supplements if analgesia is required for tourniquet or medial arm pain. With the axillary approach to the brachial plexus, it is possible to miss the musculocutaneous nerve, which leaves the fascial sheath prior to entering the axilla. If necessary, block the musculocutaneous nerve by injecting local anesthetic into the belly of the coracobrachialis muscle. The lateral cutaneous nerve of the forearm is a terminal branch of the musculocutaneous nerve.

H. Blocks performed at the elbow, wrist, and digits can be highly effective for relieving localized pain or "rescuing" an incomplete block. Many operations can be performed with a limited distal block, but prolonged tourniquet use (>20 minutes) may not be tolerated by the patient. Consider the combination of a proximal block with an intermediate-duration local anesthetic and a distal block with a long-duration local anesthetic; this protocol is extremely effective for managing postoperative pain with a limited distribution.

REFERENCES

Bonica JJ, Cailliet R, Loeser JD: General considerations of pain in the neck and upper limb. In: Loeser JD (ed) *Bonica's Management of Pain,* 3rd ed. Philadelphia, Lippincott Williams & Wilkins, 2001, pp 969–1002.

Brown DL: *Atlas of Regional Anesthesia,* 2nd ed. Philadelphia, WB Saunders, 1999.

Brown DL, Bridenbaugh LD: The upper extremity: somatic block. In: Cousins MJ, Bridenbaugh PO (eds) *Neural Blockade in Clinical Anesthesia and Management of Pain,* 3rd ed. Philadelphia, Lippincott-Raven, 1998, pp 345–371.

DeLaunay L, Chelly JE. Indications for upper extremity blocks. In: Chelly JE (ed) *Peripheral Nerve Blocks: A Color Atlas.* Philadelphia, Lippincott Williams & Wilkins, 1999, pp 17–27.

Vester-Andersen T, Christiansen C, Hansen A, et al: Interscalene brachial plexus block: area of analgesia, complications and blood concentrations of local anesthetics. *Acta Anaesthesiol Scand* 1981;25:81–84.

ACUTE UPPER EXTREMITY PAIN

Clinical evaluation
- History and physical examination
  - Detailed musculoskeletal history and exam
  - Consider possible occult systemic disease
  - Consider exacerbation of previous problem
- Pain history and characteristics
  - Speed of onset
  - Site of pain
  - Radiation
  - Intensity of pain
  - Character (quality) of pain
  - What provokes pain
- If etiology of pain is uncertain, consider studies

Laboratory evaluation
- Often not needed
- Useful in evaluating pain of unknown etiology
  - Cancer related bone pain
  - Rheumatologic disease
  - Joint aspirates: infection, gout, etc.

Radiographic evaluation
- Often not needed
- Useful in evaluating pain of unknown etiology
  - Cancer related bone pain
  - Rheumatologic disease

Treatment

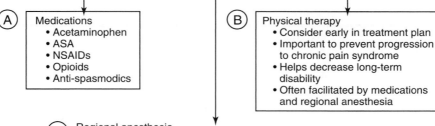

(A) Medications
- Acetaminophen
- ASA
- NSAIDs
- Opioids
- Anti-spasmodics

(B) Physical therapy
- Consider early in treatment plan
- Important to prevent progression to chronic pain syndrome
- Helps decrease long-term disability
- Often facilitated by medications and regional anesthesia

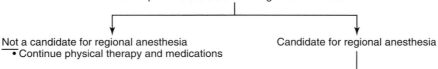

(C) Regional anesthesia
- Consider psychological and physiologic state of patient
  - Is the patient a candidate for regional anesthesia?

Not a candidate for regional anesthesia
- Continue physical therapy and medications

Candidate for regional anesthesia

Choosing a regional anesthesia technique
- Block needed for intra-op and post-op pain control
  - Place block before surgery for preemptive analgesia
  - Will a tourniquet be used for the operation?
  - Where and how long (>20 min.) will tourniquet be used?
- Consider contraindications to specific types of blocks
  - Coagulopathy, COPD, etc.
- Consider placing a catheter for long-term pain control

Local anesthetic choice
- See Chapter 87, p. 238 regarding local anesthetic choice

See table for guidance in choosing block(s)

Acute Lower Extremity Pain

DOUGLAS M. ANDERSON AND JERRY A. BEYER

The lower extremities are common sites for acute pain or chronic pain with acute exacerbations. The most common etiologies of lower extremity pain include trauma, tumor, infection, ischemia, and neuropathic pain (including radicular pain). Successful treatment of acute lower extremity pain usually involves a multifaceted approach utilizing medications, physical therapy (PT), and regional anesthesia (Table 1). In a nonsurgical patient, regional anesthesia might be useful for helping to break the pain cycle.

A. Treatment of acute lower extremity pain usually includes analgesic medications such as nonsteroidal antiinflammatory drugs, acetaminophen, and opioids. Antispasmodic (muscle relaxants) medications may be considered when severe muscle spasms are a significant component of the pain.

B. Physical therapy can play an important role in the successful treatment of acute pain and the prevention of chronic pain and permanent disability. PT may be the primary focus of the treatment plan, but it is often facilitated by the addition of medications and regional anesthesia techniques.

C. There are many effective regional anesthetic techniques available for relief and control of acute lower extremity pain. Prior to choosing a technique,

TABLE 1
Methods for Blocking Nerves of the Lower Extremities

Nerves of the Lower Extremities	Blocking Methods (Intrathecal or Epidural)
Lumbar plexus	
Lateral femoral cutaneous (L2, 3)	Isolated lateral femoral cutaneous nerve block
	3-in-1 Block
	Fascia iliaca block
	Psoas compartment block (posterior approach to lumbar plexus)
Femoral (L2–4)	Isolated femoral nerve block
	3-in-1 Block
	Fascia iliaca block
	Psoas compartment block (posterior approach to lumbar plexus)
Saphenous	Any type of femoral nerve block
	Isolated saphenous nerve block
	Subsartorial (trans-sartorial) block
	Femoral paracondylar block
	Below-knee field block
Obturator (L2–4)	Isolated obturator nerve block
	Mansour's parasacral sciatic block (nerve in same fascial plane)
	Psoas compartment block (posterior approach to lumbar plexus)
	3-in-1 Block (not reliable)
Sacral plexus	Mansour's parasacral sciatic block
Sciatic (L4–S3)	Multiple approaches to posterior sciatic nerve block
	Anterior approach to sciatic nerve block
	Lateral approach to sciatic nerve block
	Popliteal fossa block (performed knee joint line)
Common peroneal	Any type of sciatic nerve block
	Isolated common peroneal nerve block at fibular head
Lateral sural cutaneous	Sciatic or common peroneal nerve block
Superficial peroneal	Sciatic or common peroneal nerve block
	Part of classic ankle block
Deep peroneal	Sciatic or common peroneal nerve block
	Isolated deep peroneal nerve block at ankle
	Part of classic ankle block
Tibial	Sciatic nerve block
Plantar nerves of the foot	
Medial calcaneal branches	Sciatic nerve block
Sural (contribution from calcaneal peroneal)	Part of classic ankle block
Lateral calcaneal branches	
Posterior cutaneous n. of thigh (S1–3)	
	Isolated posterior cutaneous nerve of the thigh block
	Not a branch of the sciatic nerve
	More likely to block with higher approaches
	to sciatic nerve
	Most reliably blocked by Mansour's parasacral sciatic block

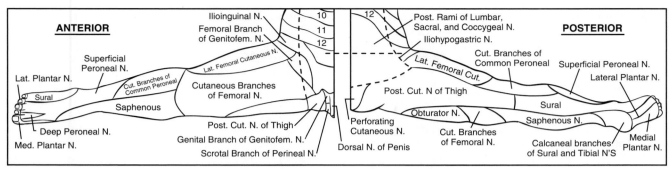

FIGURE 1 Cutaneous distribution of lower extremities peripheral nerves.

determine the patient's specific needs by answering the following questions: Is the patient a suitable candidate? Which nerves are involved in the production of pain? Will a tourniquet be used? Is anesthesia or analgesia required? What are the potential complications associated with each regional technique? Would the patient benefit from a long-term technique such as a continuous epidural or peripheral nerve catheter? What is your experience and expertise?

It may be difficult to determine which nerves are involved in the production of pain in an injured or painful extremity. The cutaneous innervation of an extremity is highly variable, with much overlap of adjacent nerves (Figure 1). In addition, the innervation of the underlying muscles (myotomes) and bones (sclerotomes) is often not the same as that of the overlying skin. Always consider the differential innervation of the involved structures to avoid developing an unsatisfactory regional anesthetic plan.

D. A subarachnoid block and lumbar epidural with local anesthetics or narcotics (or both) are effective methods for treating acute lower extremity pain, especially when both lower extremities are involved. A lumbar epidural can provide prolonged analgesia for hospitalized patients. Most practitioners and hospital staff are familiar with these techniques. The techniques do have some disadvantages, however. For example, it is difficult or impossible to provide unilateral anesthesia or analgesia with neuraxial anesthetic techniques. Respiratory depression, hemodynamic instability, urinary retention, sedation, postdural puncture headache, local anesthetic toxicity, epidural hematoma/abscess, and pruritus are potential complications or side effects associated with neuraxial anesthesia.

E. Pain involving the entire lower extremity can be effectively managed with a combined lumbar plexus and sciatic nerve block. This method provides better postoperative pain relief than general anesthesia and offers more hemodynamic stability than spinal or epidural anesthesia. There are several reliable, easy approaches to the lumbar plexus and the sciatic nerve block. The posterior approach to the lumbar plexus (psoas compartment block) offers many advantages, as it reliably blocks all three nerves of the lumbar plexus (femoral, lateral femoral cutaneous, obturator). This approach is preferred in patients who have had a prior operation near the femoral nerve or artery. The parasacral approach to the sciatic nerve has several advantages over other approaches and is technically easy to perform. This approach reliably blocks both the obturator nerve and the posterior cutaneous nerve of the thigh. Blockade of the obturator nerve can be helpful when treating hip or knee pain. Both the parasacral approach to the sciatic nerve and the posterior approach to the lumbar plexus allow placement of a catheter for continuous infusions of local anesthetic solutions.

F. Choose a more finely targeted block or combination of blocks for pain localized to a specific region of an extremity. A saphenous nerve block is highly effective for treating pain localized in the medial aspect of the leg. Several approaches for blocking the saphenous nerve have been described, but the subsartorial approach immediately above the knee is the easiest and most efficacious. A common peroneal nerve block is extremely effective for managing pain localized in the lateral aspect of the leg. A lateral femoral cutaneous nerve block is effective for treating pain localized in the lateral thigh. An isolated femoral nerve block effectively controls pain originating in the knee, femur, or hip. Preoperative placement of a femoral nerve block in patients with a fractured femur or hip can facilitate movement and positioning of a patient in the operating room. The addition of a lateral femoral cutaneous nerve block is helpful when managing the pain associated with the skin incision used for hip and femoral fractures.

REFERENCES

Bridenbaugh PO, Wedel DJ: The lower extremity: somatic blockade. In: Cousins MJ, Bridenbaugh PO (eds) *Neural Blockade in Clinical Anesthesia and Management of Pain*, 3rd ed. Philadelphia, Lippincott-Raven, 1998, pp 373–394.

Brown DL: *Atlas of Regional Anesthesia*, 2nd ed. Philadelphia, WB Saunders, 1999.

Chelly JE: General considerations for lower extremity blocks. In: Chelly JE (ed) *Peripheral Nerve Blocks: A Color Atlas*. Philadelphia, Lippincott Williams & Wilkins, 1999, pp 63–69.

ACUTE LOWER EXTREMITY PAIN

Clinical evaluation
- History and physical examination
  - Detailed musculoskeletal history and exam
  - Consider possible occult systemic disease
  - Consider exacerbation or previous problem
- Pain history and characteristics
  - Speed of onset
  - Site of pain
  - Radiation
  - Intensity of pain
  - Character (quality) of pain
  - What provokes pain
- If etiology of pain is uncertain, consider studies

Laboratory evaluation
- Often not needed
- Useful in evaluating pain of unknown etiology
  - Cancer related bone pain
  - Rheumatologic disease
  - Joint aspirates: infection, gout, etc.

Radiographic evaluation
- Often not needed
- Useful in evaluating pain of unknown etiology
  - Cancer related bone pain
  - Rheumatologic disease

Treatment

(A) Medications
- Acetaminophen
- ASA
- NSAIDs
- Opioids
- Anti-spasmodics

(B) Physical therapy
- Consider early in treatment plan
- Important to prevent progression to chronic pain syndrome
- Helps decrease long-term disability
- Often facilitated by medications and regional anesthesia

(C) Regional anesthesia
- Consider psychological and physiologic state of patient
  - Is the patient a candidate for regional anesthesia?

Not a candidate for regional anesthesia
- Continue physical therapy and medications

Candidate for regional anesthesia

Choose a regional anesthetic technique
- Block needed for intra-op and post-op pain control
  - Place block before surgery for preemptive analgesia
  - Will a tourniquet be used for the operation?
  - Where and how long (>20 min.) will be tourniquet be used?
- Consider contraindications to specific types of blocks
  - Coagulopathy, COPD, etc.
- Consider placing a catheter for long-term pain control

Local anesthetic choice
- Intermediate or long acting local anesthetic agents

See table for guidance in choosing block(s)

Acute Thoracic Pain

DOUGLAS M. ANDERSON AND JERRY A. BEYER

The etiology of acute thoracic pain usually is easily ascertained. However, referred pain from vital organs such as the heart and other thoracic structures can present as acute-onset musculoskeletal pain. When evaluating a patient with thoracic pain of unclear etiology, always consider nonmusculoskeletal causes. The management of acute thoracic pain can be challenging and is important for preventing chronic thoracic pain. Acute-onset thoracic pain may be the first clinical manifestation of a serious underlying chronic problem. A few of the causes of thoracic pain are myocardial ischemia, thoracotomy, mastectomy, trauma, herpes zoster, pneumonia, neoplasms (metastatic or primary lesions), costochondritis, costovertebral joint dysfunction, and degenerative disease of the spine. This chapter focuses on the treatment of acute thoracic pain secondary to trauma (i.e., postsurgical or accidental).

A. Several regional anesthetic techniques and medications [opioids, nonsteroidal antiinflammatory drugs (NSAIDs)] are used to treat acute thoracic pain, with varying degrees of success. Regional anesthetic options include intrapleural, epidural, paravertebral, and intercostal nerve blocks and cryoanalgesia. Each technique offers specific advantages and disadvantages in a given patient. The addition of regional anesthesia to the pain management plan generally increases patient satisfaction, improves pulmonary function, and results in lower pain scores. Aggressive control of acute thoracic pain may decrease the incidence of chronic thoracic pain. Approximately 50% of patients who have undergone a thoracotomy report chronic pain by 2 years after surgery. Although opioids (intravenous, subarachnoid, epidural) can partially relieve postthoracotomy pain, they do not improve postoperative respiratory function. The ideal therapeutic regimen probably includes a combination of opioids, NSAIDs, and regional anesthesia.

B. Management of thoracic pain with intrapleural local anesthetics can be effective. However, this technique has many drawbacks and is probably the least favorable regional technique. Risks include lung injury and pneumothorax. This risk is decreased if the patient already has a chest tube in place, but a patient with a chest tube requires frequent dosing of local anesthetic owing to loss through the chest tube and dilution of the local anesthetic by fluid present in the pleural space. The surface of the lung contains an extremely large vascular bed; and local anesthetic toxicity is a real concern with frequent dosing. Inflammatory processes of the pleura may contribute to local anesthetic toxicity by speeding absorption. It is suggested that application of local anesthetics to the diaphragm contributes to impaired respiratory function. The patient must be positioned such that the nerve roots innervating the painful region of the chest are exposed to the local anesthetic solution if analgesia is to be obtained.

C. Epidural anesthesia is the most widely used regional anesthetic technique for the management of acute thoracic pain. An epidural is most effective when the medication is administered in the middle of the involved dermatomes. The epidural approach is not without problems, however. The technique is complicated in the presence of coagulopathy, scoliosis, or a spinal fracture. In addition, thoracic epidurals can have major hemodynamic consequences that may necessitate intensive care monitoring.

D. Thoracic paravertebral blockade is an old technique that is once again gaining popularity. Several studies have shown this technique to be the most effective way to treat thoracotomy and mastectomy pain while preserving lung function. It is easy to perform and has fewer side effects than other regional techniques. This blockade can be achieved using various methods. Each spinal level can be blocked individually or with a large-volume single injection (multisegmental spread). A catheter can be placed in the paravertebral space for long-term pain relief. Depending on the local anesthetic chosen, a single injection can provide up to 24 to 36 hours of pain relief. Thoracic paravertebral blockade is rarely associated with a hemodynamically significant sympathectomy, even when performed bilaterally. The major potential complication is pleural puncture with subsequent injury to the lung, but it occurs only rarely and is reported to be clinically insignificant in most cases. Therefore some believe the paravertebral approach to be the best regional technique for managing acute thoracic pain.

E. Intercostal nerve blocks are relatively simple and effective for providing short-term thoracic pain relief. Blocks performed with long-acting local anesthetics rarely last more than 12 hours. "Intercostal" catheters can be placed for continuous infusions, but in most cases they act as paravertebral catheters, with spread of the local anesthetic within the paravertebral space. Serum levels of local anesthetic after intercostal nerve blocks are higher than after other regional techniques. This point is important when multiple injections are planned to manage postsurgical thoracic pain. The most feared complication of intercostal nerve blockade is pneumothorax, reported to occur in fewer than 1% of patients.

F. Cryoanalgesia is the result of destroying specific peripheral nerves by exposing them to extreme cold (60°C). The degree and duration of pain relief is highly variable, ranging from weeks to months. The equipment necessary is expensive and not readily available to the average practitioner. Complications include skin damage (full-thickness burns reported on a superficial lesion) and possible pneumothorax when intercostal nerves are blocked. Each nerve must

ACUTE THORACIC PAIN

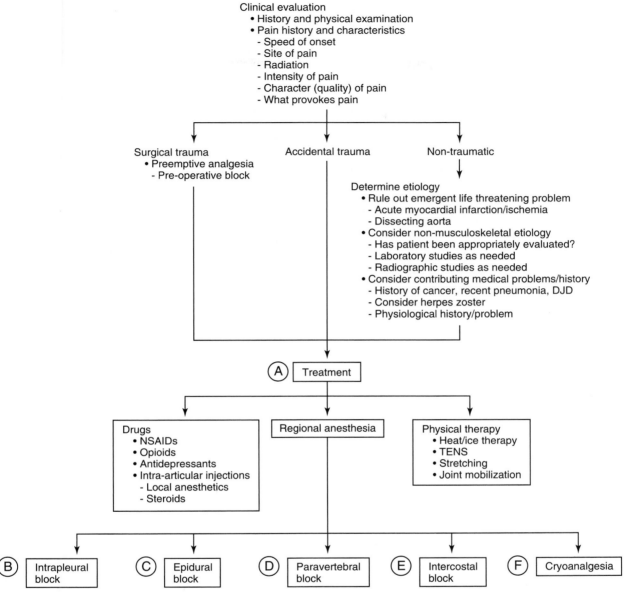

Clinical evaluation
- • History and physical examination
- • Pain history and characteristics
  - - Speed of onset
  - - Site of pain
  - - Radiation
  - - Intensity of pain
  - - Character (quality) of pain
  - - What provokes pain

Surgical trauma
- • Preemptive analgesia
  - - Pre-operative block

Accidental trauma

Non-traumatic

Determine etiology
- • Rule out emergent life threatening problem
  - - Acute myocardial infarction/ischemia
  - - Dissecting aorta
- • Consider non-musculoskeletal etiology
  - - Has patient been appropriately evaluated?
  - - Laboratory studies as needed
  - - Radiographic studies as needed
- • Consider contributing medical problems/history
  - - History of cancer, recent pneumonia, DJD
  - - Consider herpes zoster
  - - Physiological history/problem

(A) Treatment

Drugs
- • NSAIDs
- • Opioids
- • Antidepressants
- • Intra-articular injections
  - - Local anesthetics
  - - Steroids

Regional anesthesia

Physical therapy
- • Heat/ice therapy
- • TENS
- • Stretching
- • Joint mobilization

(B) Intrapleural block

(C) Epidural block

(D) Paravertebral block

(E) Intercostal block

(F) Cryoanalgesia

DJD, degenerative joint disease; NSAIDs, nonsteroidal antiinflammatory drugs; TENS, transcutaneous nerve stimulation.

be individually treated with a minimum of three freeze-thaw cycles, so the technique is time-consuming. Technologic improvements have resulted in smaller probes with built-in nerve stimulators. Such advancements may expand the use of cryoanalgesia in the future.

G. Rarely, despite the use of narcotics, NSAIDS, and regional blockade, patients continue to have excruciating postoperative pain. It is thought that the pain reaches the central nervous system via an unusual route. Sometimes one can palpate an extremely tender spot on the back, usually in the scapular area. In these cases, trigger point injection or scapular nerve block can result in immediate, dramatic relief. Phrenic nerve blockade has also been reported to provide pain relief in some patients. There are also reports of patients with resistant chronic postthoracotomy pain who obtain immediate, sustained pain relief from direct costovertebral joint manipulation.

REFERENCES

Alaya M, Auffray JP, Alouini T, et al: Comparison of extrapleural and intrapleural analgesia with bupivacaine after thoracotomy. *Ann Fr Anesth Reanim* 1995;14:249–255.

Hamada H, Moriwaki K, Shiroyama K, et al: Myofascial pain in patients with postthoracotomy pain syndrome. *Reg Anesth Pain Med* 2000;25:302–305.

Katz J, Jackson M, Kavanagh BP, Sandler AN: Acute pain after thoracic surgery predicts long-term post-thoracotomy pain. *Clin J Pain* 1996;12:50–55.

Richardson J, Sabanathan S, Shah R: Post-thoracotomy spirometric lung function: the effect of analgesia: a review. *J Cardiovasc Surg (Torino)* 1999;40:445–456.

Scawn ND, Pennefather SH, Soorae A, et al: Ipsilateral shoulder pain after thoracotomy with epidural analgesia: the influence of phrenic nerve infiltration with lidocaine. *Anesth Analg* 2001;93:260–264.

Acute Vertebral Pain

SOMAYAJI RAMAMURTHY

Severe acute pain overlying the spine can result from numerous causes. A thorough history; physical examination, especially neurologic examination; and appropriate laboratory tests and imaging studies are necessary to rule out referred pain from the viscera and intraabdominal or intrathoracic structures such as the esophagus, heart, aorta, pancreas, and so forth.

A. Trauma. Patients with acute vertebral pain following trauma should have neurologic examination and imaging studies. Patients with neurologic compromise; vertebral fractures, especially involving the neural arch; or instability should be evaluated by a spine surgical consultant for possible decompression and stabilization. Patients with stable nondisplaced fractures without neurologic compromise can be treated conservatively with bracing, heat, and analgesics. If the pain continues, thoracic medial branch blocks with local anesthetics may be beneficial. If the patient obtains only temporary relief of the pain, radiofrequency lesion of the medial branches may provide prolonged pain relief.

B. Osteoporosis. Elderly individuals, especially women with osteoporosis or patients who have been treated with steroids for asthma and rheumatoid arthritis or other conditions, can develop significant acute pain secondary to a vertebral compression fracture. These patients should receive conservative therapy with bracing, heat, and nonopioid and opioid analgesics. Patients with severe pain of less than 3 months' duration should be considered for vertebroplasty and/or kyphoplasty.

C. Infection and hematoma. Patients with a septic focus such as endocarditis or patients who have had surgical procedures or epidural injections can develop epidural or intravertebral abscess. Diagnosis is established by appropriate imaging such as computed tomography (CT) scans or magnetic resonance imaging (MRI). These patients need to be evaluated by spine surgery consultants for decompressive surgery along with antimicrobial treatment.

Patients with bleeding and clotting disorders and patients who are on anticoagulants can develop epidural hematoma following an epidural needle placement, with severe back pain. After diagnosis with neurologic evaluation and imaging studies, neurosurgical consultants should evaluate the patient for early (<24 hours) decompression to prevent long-term neurologic deficits.

D. Discogenic and mechanical pain. After the workup and diagnosis, patients with acute pain secondary to radicular involvement, facet joint pain, and discogenic and myofascial pain should be treated as outlined in Chapter 40, p. 110.

REFERENCES

Loeser JD: *Bonica's Management of Pain*, 3rd ed. Philadelphia, Lippincott Williams & Wilkins, 2001.

Diamond TH: Management of acute osteoporotic vertebral fractures: a randomized trial comparing percutaneous vertebroplasty with conservative therapy. *Am J Med* 2003; 114:257–265.

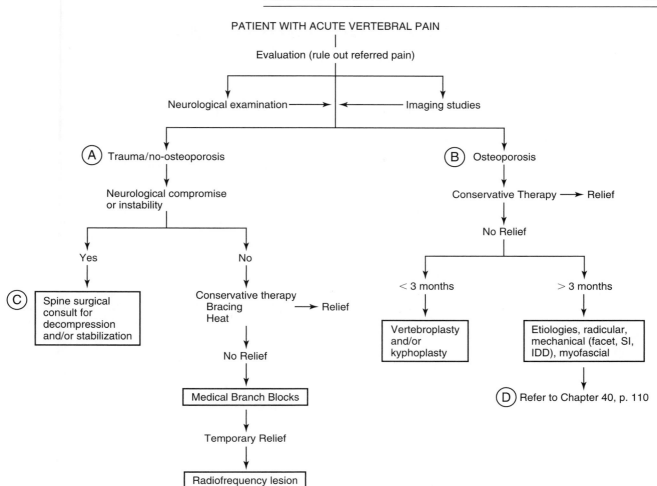

PATIENT WITH ACUTE VERTEBRAL PAIN

Evaluation (rule out referred pain)

Neurological examination ⟶ ⟵ Imaging studies

(A) Trauma/no-osteoporosis

(B) Osteoporosis

Neurological compromise or instability

Conservative Therapy ⟶ Relief

No Relief

Yes | No

< 3 months | > 3 months

(C) | Spine surgical consult for decompression and/or stabilization

Conservative therapy
Bracing
Heat ⟶ Relief

Vertebroplasty and/or kyphoplasty

Etiologies, radicular, mechanical (facet, SI, IDD), myofascial

No Relief

(D) Refer to Chapter 40, p. 110

Medical Branch Blocks

Temporary Relief

Radiofrequency lesion

Acute Abdominal Pain

KELLY GORDON KNAPE

Discomfort in the abdomen is common. It usually arises from the viscera or the parietal peritoneum, although referred pain from intrathoracic disease is also common, making the differential diagnosis difficult. Referred pain may be experienced in the skin and body wall, as with inguinal and testicular pain from ureteral stones. True visceral pain is early, dull and aching, vague, diffuse, and difficult to pinpoint, although it is usually described as being in the midline and deep despite the location of the involved organ. Visceral pain is due to spasm of the smooth muscles of hollow organs; contraction against an obstruction; sudden or extensive stretch of the organ or its capsule; inflammation or ischemia; chemical or mechanical irritation of inflamed membranes; stretch, traction, or twisting of the mesentery, ligaments, or vessels; and necrosis.

Parietal pain is sharp and sometimes stabbing, and it may be localized or referred. Both sources are accompanied by reflex guarding, tenderness, hyperalgesia, and (when severe) nausea and vomiting. Sympathetic stimulation including sweating or vagal stimulation with bradycardia is also possible.

A. The history should be complete to rule out systemic as well as extra-abdominal disease, such as diabetes, uremia, porphyria, sickle cell crisis, black widow spider bite, lead poisoning, lower rib fracture or dislocation of costochondral cartilage, acute myocardial infarction, pulmonary embolism, pneumothorax, tabes, spinal cord compression, herpetic problems, and psychological disorders. The duration of the pain is important: Severe pain lasting longer than 6 hours in a previously healthy patient is an "acute abdomen" and requires immediate diagnosis and possible surgical intervention. Onset should be classified as sudden (rupture, perforation, embolism), rapid (acute inflammation, colic, torsion, obstruction, toxic or metabolic disease), or gradual (chronic inflammation, ectopic pregnancy, tumor, infarct). The quality is described as sharp (cutaneous or somatic, including nerve root compression), burning (neuralgia, upper gastrointestinal inflammation of mucous membranes), tearing (dissecting aortic aneurysm, anal fissure), or vague (visceral disease). Temporal features (continuous: peritonitis, colicky stones, hernia; constant: cancer, migratory, emotional), factors that aggravate or relieve, the relation to other body functions (menstruation, defecation), and associated signs and symptoms (nausea, diarrhea, segmental distribution, spasm of rectus, abdominal distension) are also noted and must be specific. A menstrual history is obtained from all women. Any previous use of analgesics and other medications for associated symptoms is also documented. Earlier therapies may mask the intensity of the pain and other symptoms such as fever. Consult appropriate specialties (internal medicine, obstetrics/gynecology, general surgery) to confirm or assist with the diagnosis, treatment, and follow-up.

B. A complete physical examination is essential. Vital signs may suggest sepsis (fever, tachycardia, hypotension). Any distension or hernia, stillness (peritonitis) or restlessness (ureteral stones), and concomitant sweating or pallor (or both) should be noted. Gently palpate the abdomen, noting guarding (voluntary or involuntary) and the presence of rebound pain. Percussion detects organomegaly, ascites (fluid wave), or masses. Careful auscultation notes silence or hyperperistalsis. Perform a rectal or pelvic examination (or both) unless a specialist is available.

C. Clinical testing requires blood and urine sampling as well as radiography. Serum electrolyte as well as urine ketone and specific gravity tests suggest the degree of dehydration. Elevated white blood cell counts, especially with fever, suggest infection; and a low hematocrit suggests nonacute blood loss. Sample stool is collected for occult blood. Radiographs should include not only the chest but also abdominal views. An electrocardiogram is also helpful. Additional tests include peritoneal lavage (trauma) and a computed tomography scan.

D. If the pain is not useful for evaluation, initiate analgesia immediately. This may facilitate additional evaluation, especially that requiring patient cooperation. Nausea may be caused by pain, and adequate relief may be sufficient to treat it. Analgesics, especially opioids, do not mask pertinent findings, and a "constipating" effect may relieve pain secondary to peristalsis. Immobilization may offer temporary relief. Hydration must also be initiated early and the vital signs monitored. Respiratory therapy should be started early and is used to estimate the effectiveness of analgesia.

E. Infiltration of a local anesthetic by the surgeon or anesthetist at the end of the procedure is an effective alternative to analgesia, especially in outpatients (e.g., wound infiltration for inguinal herniorrhaphy). A long-acting agent such as bupivacaine can reduce the need for analgesics and promote mobilization.

F. Regional anesthesia can provide postoperative analgesia and other potential benefits. Continuous epidural infusions can be maintained for several days with an opioid, local anesthetic, or both. A local anesthetic provides sympathectomy to optimize perfusion, although orthostasis can occur and high concentrations may affect ambulation. Intraspinal opioids by epidural or intrathecal routes are effective, especially for visceral pain. Adding an opioid to a local anesthetic can improve the quality of analgesia, especially for mobilization and cough, and it reduces the dosage of each required. Recommended dosages include 0.03125% to 0.0625% bupivacaine with fentanyl 2 to 5 µg/kg/hr. A patient-controlled analgesia (PCA) device can be connected to an epidural catheter. Epidural or intrathecal administration of preservative-free morphine provides approximately 24 hours of superior

PATIENT WITH ACUTE ABDOMINAL PAIN

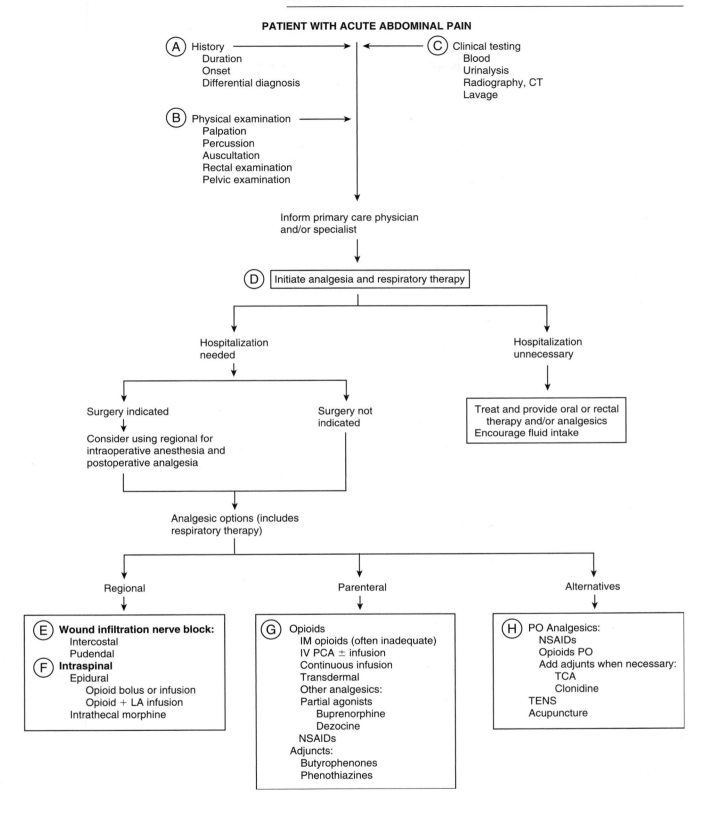

(A) History
   Duration
   Onset
   Differential diagnosis

(C) Clinical testing
   Blood
   Urinalysis
   Radiography, CT
   Lavage

(B) Physical examination
   Palpation
   Percussion
   Auscultation
   Rectal examination
   Pelvic examination

Inform primary care physician
and/or specialist

(D) Initiate analgesia and respiratory therapy

Hospitalization
needed

Hospitalization
unnecessary

Surgery indicated

Surgery not
indicated

Treat and provide oral or rectal
therapy and/or analgesics
Encourage fluid intake

Consider using regional for
intraoperative anesthesia and
postoperative analgesia

Analgesic options (includes
respiratory therapy)

Regional

Parenteral

Alternatives

(E) **Wound infiltration nerve block:**
   Intercostal
   Pudendal
(F) **Intraspinal**
   Epidural
      Opioid bolus or infusion
      Opioid + LA infusion
   Intrathecal morphine

(G) Opioids
   IM opioids (often inadequate)
   IV PCA ± infusion
   Continuous infusion
   Transdermal
   Other analgesics:
   Partial agonists
      Buprenorphine
      Dezocine
   NSAIDs
   Adjuncts:
      Butyrophenones
      Phenothiazines

(H) PO Analgesics:
   NSAIDs
   Opioids PO
   Add adjuncts when necessary:
      TCA
      Clonidine
   TENS
   Acupuncture

relief; the common side effects of pruritus and urinary retention are easily managed. Doses are 0.05 mg/kg and 0.002 to 0.005 mg/kg, respectively. Addition of fentanyl (100 µg) or sufentanil (10 to 30 µg) can speed up the slow onset of analgesia from epidural morphine. Postoperative epidural analgesia can reduce perioperative pulmonary complications in high-risk patients.

G. Administration of parenteral opioids is most efficacious when a PCA device is used. PCA pumps provide the patient with some control and independence. A "background" infusion can be added. Transdermal fentanyl is another sustained opioid alternative. "Balanced analgesia" can be provided by adding nonsteroidal anti-inflammatory drugs to reduce opioid requirements. The partial opioid agonists can be used with an efficacy similar to that of morphine, with a ceiling for side effects. Adjunctive agents such as promethazine can potentiate analgesia and reduce nausea, but sedation may result.

H. Oral adjuncts can be added (tricyclic antidepressants or clonidine), which when given at bedtime can improve sleep and provide analgesia. Transcutaneous electrical nerve stimulation and acupuncture have also been used.

REFERENCES

Bonica JJ: General considerations of acute pain. In: Bonica JJ, Loeser JD, Chapman CR, et al (eds) *The Management of Pain*, 2nd ed. Philadelphia, Lea & Febiger, 1990, pp 1146.

Dahl JB, Kehlet H: Non-steroidal anti-inflammatory drugs: rationale for use in severe postoperative pain. *Br J Anaesth* 1991;66:703.

Dahl JB, Rosenberg J, Hanssen BL, et al: Differential analgesic effects of low dose epidural morphine and morphine-bupivacaine at rest and during mobilization after major abdominal surgery. *Anesth Analg* 1992;74:362.

Gwirtz KH: Intraspinal narcotics in the management of postoperative pain. *Anesthesiol Rev* 1990;17:17.

Sinatra RS, Sevarine FB, Chung JH, et al: Comparisons of epidurally administered sufentanil, morphine, and sufentanil-morphine combination for postoperative analgesia. *Anesth Analg* 1991; 72:522.

Yamaguchi H, Watanabe S, Motokawa K, et al: Intrathecal morphine dose response data for pain relief after cholecystectomy. *Anesth Analg* 1990;70:168.

Acute Pancreatic Pain

LINDA TINGLE

Acute pancreatitis (AP) is an inflammatory reaction characterized by abdominal pain and extensive local and systemic effects. In 80% to 90% of cases in the United States, the cause is related to alcohol abuse or biliary tract disease. Drugs, infection, trauma, ischemia, and genetics can also cause AP. These various causative agents result in a similar inflammatory reaction, producing extensive local and systemic effects. Although the precise cellular mechanisms are not entirely characterized, there is activation and retention of enzymes, which injure acinar cells, releasing inflammatory mediators and activating the complement system. Hypotension, tachycardia, hypoxia, and capillary leak syndrome then occur. There is a varied clinical presentation ranging from mild symptomatic illness to a rapidly fatal condition.

A. Serum amylase levels are sensitive but nonspecific indicators. Computed tomography reveals diffuse enlargement of the pancreas as well as extrapancreatic fluid collection, pseudocysts, and abscesses. Ultrasonography is less sensitive for detecting pancreatic abnormalities but more sensitive for detecting biliary calculi. Endoscopic retrograde cholangio-pancreatography (ERCP) may identify treatable causes of AP.

B. Medical management of AP includes aggressive patient support to prevent death during the early phases of severe AP. Maintaining tissue perfusion with volume resuscitation, respiratory support, transfusion, prophylaxis against gastric stress ulcers, and early intravenous nutritional support are effective. Pain management is most often accomplished with narcotic analgesia. Meperidine is the preferred agent as it has less contractile action on the sphincter of Oddi than morphine. Nalbuphine or buprenorphine may be alternatives in patients who should not take meperidine.

C. Surgical intervention during the acute phase is discouraged as there is lack of benefit but a risk of infecting sterile phlegmon. An exception to this rule is when serious concomitant intraabdominal pathology is suspected. ERCP is also avoided during the early stages unless the patient has an obstructed common bile duct stone.

D. Epidural opioids provide excellent analgesia without biliary spasm. Epidural infusion of dilute local anesthetic provides pain relief, improves ventilation, and decreases reflex muscle spasm and any neuroendocrine response. Intrapleural injection of local anesthetics provides pain relief. Immunosuppression occurs with AP and alcoholism, so catheter insertion should be considered carefully (Heller et al. 2000). Celiac plexus block with local anesthetic and a steroid appears to hasten resolution of symptoms if used early in the course of therapy for AP (Kennedy 1983).

REFERENCES

Graham DD, Bonica JJ: Painful diseases of the liver, biliary system, and pancreas. In: Loeser JD (ed) *Bonica's Management of Pain*, 3rd ed. Philadelphia, Lippincott Williams & Wilkins, 2001.
Heller AR, Ragaller M, Koch T: Epidural abscess after epidural catheter for pain release during pancreatitis. *Acta Anaesthesiol Scand* 2000;44:102–108.
Isenhower HL, Mueller BA: Selection of narcotic analgesics for pain associated with pancreatitis. *Am J Health Syst Pharm* 1998; 55:480–486.
Kennedy SF: Celiac plexus steroids for acute pancreatitis. *Reg Anesth* 1983;8:39–40.
Vlodov J, Tenner SM: Acute and chronic pancreatitis. *Prim Care* 2001;28:607–628.

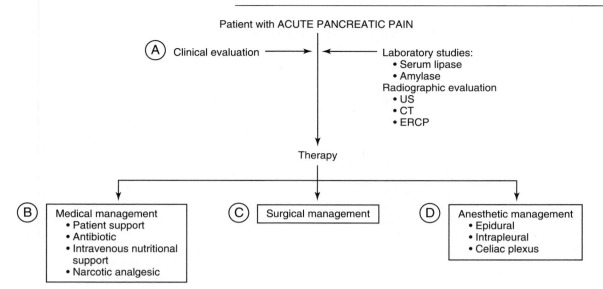

Obstetric Pain

SUSAN NOORILY

Labor is usually a painful experience, although it varies considerably from patient to patient. A recent survey of 1091 parturients reported that 80% described labor pain as "very severe" or "intolerable," and 50% noted that their pain management was inadequate. An ideal anesthetic would provide rapid pain relief lasting throughout the labor and delivery period and have no adverse effect on the mother, fetus, or progress of labor.

A. Labor pain has two components. During the first stage of labor, pain results from cervical dilatation and distension of the lower uterine segment with contractions. Pain is transmitted by small unmyelinated visceral afferent C fibers (passing through the paracervical plexus and lumbar plexus) and accompanying sympathetic fibers, terminating in the dorsal horn of the spinal cord from T10 to L1. Pain is referred to dermatomes T10 through L1. During the late first and second stages of labor, pain results from vaginal and perineal distension during fetal descent. This pain is transmitted by thin, myelinated, A-δ somatic sensory nerve fibers traveling in the pudendal nerve (S2, S3, S4) and entering the dorsal horn of the spinal cord. Ascending spinal cord tracts transmit afferent nociceptive impulses to the cortex. Several techniques have been used to target the pain pathways at all points, from the most distal (e.g., paracervical and pudendal nerve blocks) to the most proximal (e.g., systemic medications, psychotherapy).

B. A thorough preanesthetic evaluation is performed on any patient requesting analgesia for labor and delivery. In addition to a history and physical examination, the obstetric diagnosis, fetal status, and progress of labor are assessed; and pertinent laboratory information (e.g., coagulation studies in preeclamptic patients) is obtained.

C. Labor pain causes adverse physiological changes (e.g., hyperventilation, increased oxygen consumption, catecholamine release) that can be attenuated with analgesia. The analgesic options are discussed with the patient, counseling her regarding the risks and benefits of each. Education decreases anxiety and allows the parturient to give informed consent. Selection of the appropriate technique must be individualized. Some women prefer nonpharmacologic methods, whereas others request systemic medications. Some patients have medical contraindications to neuraxial analgesia techniques; for example, patients with abnormal hemostasis may be at risk for epidural hematoma formation after neuraxial instrumentation.

D. Nonpharmacologic methods of pain control during labor have several mechanisms of action, including competitive sensory stimulation, alteration of the biologic response to pain, and amelioration of negative psychological issues. The nonpharmacologic methods include natural childbirth, psychoprophylaxis (e.g., Lamaze), hypnosis, biofeedback, acupuncture, transcutaneous electrical nerve stimulation (TENS), hydrotherapy (e.g., warm water baths), and psychosocial support. These methods provide a safe alternative for all laboring patients.

E. Systemic medications, including opioids, sedatives (e.g., barbiturates), and amnestic drugs (e.g., ketamine), are available for use during labor. Of these agents, opioids are the most commonly used but have limited analgesic efficacy for labor pain and provide poor patient satisfaction. However, opioids may be the best option for women who cannot have neuraxial analgesia (NA) or who are in hospitals where NA is not available. Opioids interact with mu, delta, and kappa opioid receptors in the dorsal horn of the spinal cord, periaqueductal gray matter, and thalamus. High doses result in unwanted side effects in both the mother [i.e., nausea and vomiting (N/V), sedation, respiratory depression, disorientation, delayed gastric emptying] and baby (i.e., respiratory depression, low neurobehavioral scores). Newborn respiratory depression depends on the total dose and the interval of time between the dose and delivery. It is recommended that narcotics be avoided during the last 2 to 4 hours of labor, but this time frame may be difficult to judge. Meperidine is the narcotic most widely used during labor and is often given in conjunction with an antiemetic to prevent N/V. Morphine use fell into disfavor many years ago because of a concern regarding neonatal respiratory depression. Fentanyl is a more potent, highly lipid-soluble, rapid-acting narcotic that is useful for labor analgesia. Patient-controlled analgesia is available in some institutions.

F. Paracervical block provides excellent analgesia for a period of up to 2 hours during the first stage of labor. This block has the potential for severe complications (i.e., fetal bradycardia, distress, and death) and is not commonly used. Lumbar sympathetic block can provide analgesia for the first stage of labor. Pudendal nerve block is useful during the second stage of labor and to augment an epidural that does not provide good sacral analgesia.

G. Inhalation analgesia with a variety of agents (e.g., nitrous oxide, halothane, isoflurane, sevoflurane) and oxygen can be effective. Advantages include rapid action and minimal neonatal depression. However, this technique is associated with several risks (i.e., loss of consciousness, vomiting, aspiration, laryngospasm, hypoventilation, hypoxia, cardiac arrhythmias) and therefore is not commonly employed in the United States.

H. Neuraxial analgesia is the most effective method for providing analgesia during labor. In addition to excellent pain relief, regional analgesia (RA) helps decrease circulating catecholamine concentrations,

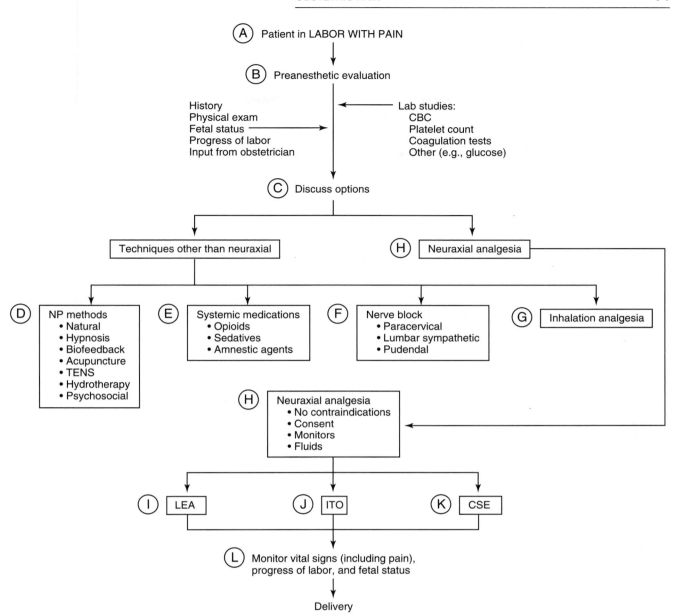

(A) Patient in LABOR WITH PAIN

(B) Preanesthetic evaluation

History
Physical exam
Fetal status
Progress of labor
Input from obstetrician

Lab studies:
 CBC
 Platelet count
 Coagulation tests
 Other (e.g., glucose)

(C) Discuss options

Techniques other than neuraxial

(H) Neuraxial analgesia

(D) NP methods
 • Natural
 • Hypnosis
 • Biofeedback
 • Acupuncture
 • TENS
 • Hydrotherapy
 • Psychosocial

(E) Systemic medications
 • Opioids
 • Sedatives
 • Amnestic agents

(F) Nerve block
 • Paracervical
 • Lumbar sympathetic
 • Pudendal

(G) Inhalation analgesia

(H) Neuraxial analgesia
 • No contraindications
 • Consent
 • Monitors
 • Fluids

(I) LEA

(J) ITO

(K) CSE

(L) Monitor vital signs (including pain),
progress of labor, and fetal status

Delivery

maintains adequate maternal and fetal oxygenation with a decrease in maternal hyperventilation, and decreases the incidence of maternal and fetal acidosis. Many high-risk obstetric patients benefit from RA techniques. RA is contraindicated in patients with frank coagulopathy, uncorrected hypovolemia, sepsis, infection at the needle entry site, increased intracranial pressure, and allergy to a local anesthetic (LA). If RA is chosen, obtain informed consent and prepare the patient. Place the appropriate monitors on the patient and administer intravenous fluids for preload.

I. Lumbar epidural analgesia (LEA) provides excellent pain relief throughout the course of labor and can be extended to provide anesthesia for an instrument delivery and cesarean section. LEA is instituted when labor is well established (e.g., 4 to 5 cm cervical dilatation). A continuous infusion of dilute LA (with the possible addition of lipid-soluble opioid to reduce the LA requirement) produces reliable analgesia with minimal motor blockade as well as a minimal effect on uterine activity and fetal well-being. Side effects are minimal. Potential complications include inadvertent dural puncture causing postdural puncture headache (PDPH), postpartum low back pain, nerve injury, infection, hematoma, hypotension, N/V, urinary retention, respiratory depression, pruritus, inadequate pain relief, and possibly an increased risk of prolonged labor and instrument or operative delivery (controversial). The risks of inadvertent subarachnoid or intravascular injection due to catheter malpositioning are prevented by careful test dosing.

J. Intrathecal opioids (ITOs) provide effective, rapid analgesia during early labor without motor or sympathetic blockade. Maternal hypotension, when it occurs, is likely due to analgesia and decreased circulating catecholamines. Several early case reports described sudden fetal bradycardia after administration of an ITO, but the changes were usually transient and resolved spontaneously. Other complications include pruritus, N/V, urinary retention, respiratory depression, risk of PDPH (1% to 2% with a pencil-point spinal needle), nerve injury, and infection. ITOs have a limited duration of action. A combination of an ITO with a small dose of an LA increases the duration of analgesia and provides perineal anesthesia. Other agents that have been investigated for intrathecal use include clonidine and neostigmine.

K. Combined spinal-epidural (CSE) analgesia for labor offers the advantages of both an ITO (i.e., rapid onset) and LEA (i.e., placement of a catheter). With this technique, the ITO injection takes place prior to threading an epidural catheter. A test dose must be administered before the LEA catheter is activated. The catheter can be used immediately or at a later time.

L. Patients who have been given labor analgesia must be carefully monitored. In all patients the progress of labor and the fetal status must be followed. Anesthetic requirements may change throughout labor, and some patients require assistance with pain management after delivery.

REFERENCES

Holdcroft A, Thomas TA: *Principles and Practice of Obstetric Anaesthesia and Analgesia.* Oxford, Blackwell Science, 2000.

Ranta P, Spalding M, Kangas-Saarela T, et al: Maternal expectations and experiences of labor pain: options of 1091 Finnish parturients. Acta Anaesthesiol Scand 1995;39:60–66.

Richardson MG: Regional anesthesia for obstetrics. Anesthesiol Clin North Am 2000;18:383–406.

Ward ME: Acute pain and the obstetric patient: recent developments in analgesia for labor and delivery. Int Anesthesiol Clin 1997; 35:83–103.

CHRONIC PAIN SYNDROMES

Myofascial Pain

Postherpetic Neuralgia

Complex Regional Pain Syndrome

Diabetic Neuropathy

Chronic Pancreatitis Pain

Neuropathic Pain

Central Pain Syndrome

Phantom Pain

Spinal Cord-Injured Patient

The Fibromyalgia Syndrome

Rheumatoid Arthritis

Osteoarthritis

Discogenic Back Pain

Nonsomatic Pain

Hiv-Aids

Sickle Cell Disease

Groin Pain

Pelvic Pain

Myofascial Pain

JOHN C. KING

The term myofascial pain has been used generically to refer to any muscular or fascial pain such as tendinitis. The term myofascial pain used here refers to a more specific condition in which an exquisitely tender, palpable, muscular taut band or nodule is palpated, with or without associated pain; when it is present, the pain is typically referred elsewhere as well. This specific condition is called the myofascial pain syndrome. Most often this disorder presents acutely in a focal area with typical referral patterns according to the site of the muscular nodule. When diffuse, involving all four quadrants (above and below the waist, left and right), the diagnostic criteria for fibromyalgia are often met. In patients with an extremely focal myofascial pain syndrome, though, there are many associated co-morbidities with fibromyalgia that typically are not present, at least on initial presentation. A palpable, tense area of highly tender muscle is required for the diagnosis; the presence of simple point tenderness, without palpatory findings, is not adequate. All muscles are susceptible, but certain muscles are more typically involved. Often this disorder can be traced to increased muscle tension or guarding secondary to another disorder, such as nearby degenerative joint arthritis or bursitis/tendonitis, but it can also result from strain due to poor posture or muscle tension associated with anxiety.

The myofascial pain syndrome frequently resolves upon effective treatment of an associated underlying disorder. The symptoms attributable to the tender muscular nodule and its referred pains can also be directly ameliorated by treatments directed at this secondary myofascial trigger point (TrP), similar to the treatment used for a suspected primary TrP (in which no other associated condition is found). Effective interventions include muscle energy techniques, stretching, modalities such as icing and ultrasound application with or without electrical stimulation, deep massage, and finally trigger point injections (TPIs).

A short-acting anesthetic agent can decrease the initial discomfort, but dry needling and saline are just as effective long term; steroids do not provide any additional benefit. Oral medications add only minimal benefit unless treating an underlying condition. Many of the typical muscle locations for TrPs are also classic acupuncture sites; and the burning sensation, or "Chi," described as an indication of good pain effect during acupuncture, is also typical of the immediate discomfort felt upon initial injection or dry needling of TrPs. The "local twitch response" or transient needle grabbing, which is prognostic of a good effect on TPIs, is also described in the acupuncture literature as a good sign.

A. There are many causes of pain localized to the musculoskeletal system, which includes referred visceral and neurologic pain. The palpatory findings are most helpful for distinguishing the myofascial pain syndrome from other sources of nociception.

B. If widespread, one should test for fibromyalgia diagnostic criteria and inquire about typical co-morbidities: a nonrestorative sleep pattern (awake feeling tired or "beat up"), transient morning stiffness, incapacitating fatigue, irritable bowel disorder, thyroid disorders, and interstitial cystitis, among others.

C. If there are no palpable findings, consider other etiologies. TrPs are often extremely tender (eliciting the "chandelier" sign), although "latent" TrPs may have the same palpatory consistency as an "active" TrP but are not tender and cause no pain.

D. Typical pain referral patterns often can guide the examiner to the correct muscle to palpate. The referral pain usually worsens significantly upon palpation of the eliciting TrP. Tender muscle bands without referral patterns may be true "spasms." A focal electromyography study may be both diagnostic (spasms are highly electrically active, whereas TrPs are relatively silent despite tense muscle) and therapeutic (dry needling). Muscle spasms usually occur acutely around a traumatically injured joint or limb.

E. Trigger points that return after the usual 2 to 3 weeks of relief after a TPI should be reassessed for possible perpetuating factors (i.e., an underlying disorder). If not resolved after two or three TPIs, the disorder should be treated similarly to fibromyalgia, with attention to the associated sleep disturbance, a home stretching program, and progressive aerobic conditioning despite the expected initial exacerbations of pain. Unfortunately, the benefit often is not seen until 6 to 9 weeks into the conditioning. If the patient is not compliant with this regimen and the condition is disabling, consider inpatient behavioral modification and reconditioning programs. In patients who have short-term relief after local anesthetic injections or in those who are unable to stretch muscles to normal length (prosthetic hip, contracture), long-term relief may be achieved by injecting botulinum toxin.

REFERENCES

Acupuncture. NIH Consensus Statement. 1997;15:1–34.

Fischer AA: Documentation of myofascial trigger points. *Arch Phys Med Rehabil* 1988;69:286–291.

Fricton JR, Esam AA: *Advances in Pain Research and Therapy: Myofascial Pain and Fibroneuralgia.* New York, Raven Press, 1990.

King JC, Goddard MJ: Pain rehabilitation. 2. Chronic benign pain and myofascial pain. *Arch Phys Med Rehabil* 1994;75:S9.

Mense S, Simons DG, Russel IJ (eds): *Muscle Pain: Understanding Its Nature, Diagnosis, and Treatment.* Philadelphia, Lippincott Williams & Wilkins, 2001.

Travell JG, Simons DG: *Myofascial Pain and Dysfunction. The Trigger Point Manual.* Baltimore, Williams & Wilkins, 1983.

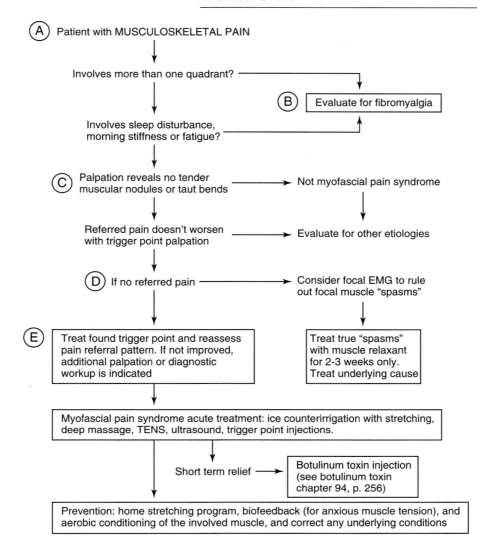

(A) Patient with MUSCULOSKELETAL PAIN

Involves more than one quadrant? ─────────────┐

(B) | Evaluate for fibromyalgia |

Involves sleep disturbance, morning stiffness or fatigue? ──────────┘

(C) Palpation reveals no tender muscular nodules or taut bends ──────→ Not myofascial pain syndrome

Referred pain doesn't worsen with trigger point palpation ──────→ Evaluate for other etiologies

(D) If no referred pain ──────→ Consider focal EMG to rule out focal muscle "spasms"

(E) | Treat found trigger point and reassess pain referral pattern. If not improved, additional palpation or diagnostic workup is indicated |

| Treat true "spasms" with muscle relaxant for 2-3 weeks only. Treat underlying cause |

| Myofascial pain syndrome acute treatment: ice counterirrigation with stretching, deep massage, TENS, ultrasound, trigger point injections. |

Short term relief ──────→ | Botulinum toxin injection (see botulinum toxin chapter 94, p. 256) |

| Prevention: home stretching program, biofeedback (for anxious muscle tension), and aerobic conditioning of the involved muscle, and correct any underlying conditions |

Postherpetic Neuralgia

EULECHE ALANMANOU

The true prevalence of postherpetic neuralgia (PHN) is not known. It is a complication of acute herpes zoster that is characterized by debilitating neuropathic pain following healing of the vesicular lesions or more than 6 weeks after the onset of the rash. The pain is typically present in dermatomal distribution with allodynia and other abnormal sensations.

The duration of PHN is less than 1 year in 78% of patients. Histopathologic studies have shown varying degrees of degenerative changes affecting nerve ganglia, nerve roots, and the central nervous system. However, the correlation with PHN pain is not always established.

It has been suggested that patients may be classified into three categories. A subset of patients with mechanical allodynia with minimal sensory loss have "irritable nociceptors" (sensitized cutaneous nociceptors). In these patients, topical capsaicin worsens pain, whereas topical local anesthetics provide pain relief. A second subset of patients have spontaneous pain, mechanical allodynia, and thermal sensory deficits secondary to synaptic plasticity or aberrant connections of preserved large-diameter Aβ fibers in the dorsal horn of the spinal cord, resulting from small-fiber (C fibers) deafferentation. The third subset of patients have severe spontaneous pain without allodynia or hyperalgesia. There is a loss of large and small afferent fibers. The pain with marked deafferentation is explained by the spontaneous activity in deafferented central neurons as a result of either release of inhibition or hyperactivity of central pain transmission neurons. An influence of sympathetic activity and catecholamines on sensitized and damaged primary afferents has also been suggested.

The difference in the relation between ongoing pain and allodynia induced by dynamic mechanical stimuli in patients with a duration of PHN of less than 1 year versus more than 1 year suggests that the mechanism of pain is mainly peripheral early in the disease and mainly central later, and that anatomic reorganization in the dorsal horn explains the allodynia.

A. The pathophysiology of PHN, then, involves central and peripheral mechanisms that evolve with time. Once PHN is established, it is difficult to treat. Prevention includes vaccination against varicella-zoster virus during childhood as well as early, aggressive treatment of acute herpes zoster.

   1. When treating PHN, begin with the safest and simplest approaches. The common first choice is a tricyclic antidepressant that provides analgesia via a norepinephrine and serotonin reuptake inhibiting effect. Using this approach, 50% of patients have pain relief without intolerable adverse effects. A trial of selective serotonin reuptake inhibitors is appropriate in case of contraindication or side effects to tricyclics.

   2. The anticonvulsants produce a membrane-stabilizing effect by blocking sodium and calcium channels. Gabapentin may have an effect on α2δ-type calcium channels. Studies suggest that gabapentin is useful for monotherapy and has a safer profile than phenytoin or carbamazepine. Its side effects include somnolence, dizziness, ataxia, and peripheral edema.

   3. Nonopioid analgesics are rarely efficacious in patients with PHN. Opioids may be useful, however, in some patients who do not respond to antidepressants or anticonvulsants. A combination of medications that have effects on several mechanisms might be required to address the patient's pain.

B. Topical local anesthetics, such as EMLA cream, have proven to relieve PHN pain, but the occlusive dressings used with topical agents are impractical for most patients. Subcutaneous lidocaine infiltration was reported to relieve PHN; but peripheral nerve, epidural, or sympathetic anesthetic blocks do not appear to be useful. Other modalities that have been used include intrathecal methylprednisolone, implanted spinal catheters and pumps, and a dorsal root entry zone lesion.

C. Behavioral therapy should always be considered in view of the complex nature of PHN.

REFERENCES

Fields HL, Rowbotham M, Baron R: Postherpetic neuralgia: irritable nociceptors and deafferentation. *Neurobiol Dis* 1998; 5:209–227.

Nurmikko TJ: Postherpetic neuralgia: a model for neuropathic pain? In: *Neuropathic Pain: Pathophysiology and Treatment. Progress in Pain Research and Management*, vol 21. Seattle, IASP Press, 2001.

Pappagallo M, Oaklander AL, Quatrano-Piancentini AL, et al: Heterogeneous patterns of sensory dysfunction in postherpetic neuralgia suggest multiple pathophysiologic mechanisms. *Anesthesiology* 2000;92:691–698.

Rowbotham MC, Fields HL: Postherpetic neuralgia: the relation of pain complaint, sensory disturbance, and skin temperature. *Pain* 1989;39:129–144.

POSTHERPETIC NEURALGIA

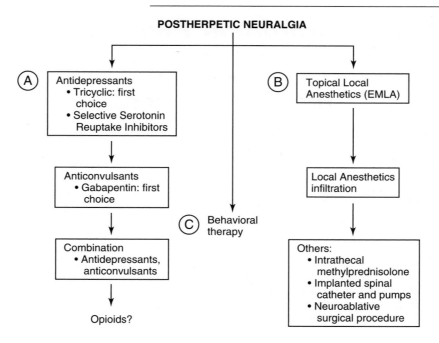

Complex Regional Pain Syndrome

MARK E. ROMANOFF

The clinical entity, complex regional pain syndrome (CRPS) has gone through multiple descriptive "namings" since it was first described by Mitchell during the Civil War in 1872. Prior to CRPS it was known as reflex sympathetic dystrophy (RSD) or causalgia. The clinical complex of symptoms are described in Table 1. Many theories have been formulated to explain the pathophysiology of CRPS and are divided into central nervous system and peripheral causes. Unfortunately, none has successfully accounted for all the symptoms seen in this syndrome.

The latest name change, in 1994, omitted "sympathetic" owing to the varying nature of the sympathetic component seen in patients. Most patients describe a burning pain in an extremity following trauma along with allodynia, hypersensitivity, edema, and vasomotor changes. CRPS I is not associated with known nerve damage, whereas CRPS II does have a discrete nerve injury.

A. The history and physical examination (H&P) comprise the primary means for identifying CRPS. The precipitating trauma can be as mild as prolonged walking or as severe as a gunshot wound. Approximately 60% of CRPS is caused by trauma, and 20% occurs after operative procedures. It is rare that *no* inciting event is elicited in the history. If the "trauma" was a myocardial infarction or a cerebrovascular event, usually the upper extremity is involved and the syndrome is described as "shoulder-hand syndrome."

1. The H&P should elicit the signs and symptoms described in Table 1. The symptoms are often varied; and although they are grouped by stages, patients may exhibit signs from more than one stage. Stages may last days or months, and the physician may not encounter the patient until the latter stages, making the diagnosis more difficult. Patients rarely present with "classic" symptoms. Axial or bilateral extremity CRPS is rare and is often quite challenging to diagnose and treat.

2. The differential diagnosis includes other neuropathic processes (diabetic neuropathy, nerve entrapment), Raynaud's disease, and acrocyanosis.

B. Diagnostic studies should confirm the suspicion of CRPS, but they rarely rule out the diagnosis. Another way to say this is that CRPS is a clinical diagnosis. Radiographs may show loss of density (Sudek's atrophy) or loss of trabecular densities. Magnetic resonance imaging (MRI) scans can reveal edema of muscles or soft tissue, muscle atrophy, or soft tissue enhancement. Some studies suggest that MRI has a positive predictive value of 100% but a negative predictive value of only 45%. Triple-phase bone scans evaluating blood and tissue flow have 60% sensitivity. Measurements of blood flow, such as Doppler studies or indirect measures utilizing temperature measurements (e.g., temperature probes, thermography), are also helpful. Some investigators have come up with a diagnostic criteria grading system that combines symptoms, signs, and diagnostic studies in an attempt to objectify the diagnosis of CRPS. Another diagnostic test is the patient's response to a sympathetic block. Improvement following a selective sympathetic block is pathognomonic of CRPS. Unfortunately, the lack of response to a sympathetic block cannot rule it out.

C. Physical therapy (PT) is a mainstay of treatment, providing desensitization and increased range of motion and function. PT alone has been shown to provide significant improvement in more than 50% of patients. Unfortunately, most patients cannot cooperate with PT because of pain, so pain relief must be provided to allow adequate participation. Iontophoresis can be used to deliver analgesic or antiinflammatory agents deep into the affected tissues. Transcutaneous electrical nerve stimulation may provide pain relief. Interventional therapy such as brachial plexus blocks or epidural injections can allow at least passive motion by a therapist, as these measures provide a sensory block. CRPS of the lower extremity is often easier to treat because most patients can do some weight-bearing and walking. Upper extremity involvement may lead to absolute immobility by the patient, which explains the "frozen" shoulder phenomenon.

D. Conservative treatment including medications, counseling, and biofeedback should be used as an adjunct to interventional therapy or in patients in whom injections are contraindicated (coagulation issues, anatomic abnormalities, patient preference). Biofeedback and imaging may help improve regional blood flow, reverse dystrophic changes, and provide pain relief. Counseling is necessary to address the personality issues and provide coping techniques.

TABLE 1
CRPS Symptoms by Stage

Stage 1: Acute Phase	Stage 2: Dystrophic Phase	Stage 3: Atrophic Phase
Burning pain	Constant pain	Pain moves proximally
Hypersensitivity	Indurated edema	Flexion contractures
Allodynia	Decreased temperature	Thickened fascia
Edema	Trophic changes (hair, nail, skin)	Continued loss of range of motion
Dependent rubor	Osteoporosis	Skin ulceration/ ischemia/infection
Increased temperature	Personality changes	—
Decreased range of motion	—	—

1. The use of antiinflammatory agents should be attempted, as many studies have shown that CRPS may be propagated by prostaglandins. High-dose corticosteroids have decreased symptoms but with attendant side effects. Antidepressants can be used for the mood disturbance as well as their nociceptive effects. Tricyclic antidepressants (TCAs) are perhaps the most studied medications. They are effective in up to 70% of patients.

2. Selective serotonin reuptake inhibitors have been shown to alleviate symptoms as well. Antiepileptic drugs such as gabapentin and lamotrigine are popular. They have been shown to be effective, but at this time their efficacy appears to be equivalent to that of TCAs.

3. Vasodilators, including nifedipine and phenoxybenzamine, can improve the outcome in patients with "cold" CRPS by improving blood flow. β-Blockers and clonidine, a central-acting α_2-agonist, reduce peripheral sympathetic tone and have shown promise. Many patients believe that wearing the clonidine patch over the affected area is effective.

4. Pentoxifylline, a phosphodiesterase inhibitor that makes red blood cell membranes more flexible, can improve blood flow. Substance P plays a role in CRPS, and topical capsaicin may reduce pain by reducing existing pools of substance P in the neurons.

5. Topical local anesthetics (EMLA, lidocaine) can also be used but may be limited by the appearance of methemoglobinemia and tachyphylaxis. N-Methyl-D-aspartate (NMDA) receptors can be blocked by topical ketamine or dextromethorphan. We have combined topical ketamine with ketoprofen (NSAIDs), amitriptyline (a TCA), and lidocaine with limited success.

6. Although CRPS and other neuropathic processes are often considered "resistant" to narcotics, these agents should be tried in resistant cases. We have found that higher doses are often necessary, but pain relief can be achieved. Narcotics alone or in combination with other medications are usually not sufficient to allow full participation in PT.

E. Sympathetic nerve blocks are often used for the purpose of diagnosis, and they are the mainstay of treatment. Upper extremity symptoms can be initially treated with a stellate ganglion block. As this is a "pure" sympathetic block, it is often used to confirm the diagnosis. Unfortunately, as many as 30% of patients do not experience an effective sympathetic block of the upper extremity. This is due to the cephalad location of the needle for a stellate ganglion block and the possible inability to anesthetize the lower sympathetic nerves to the arm (T1–T3). Measuring the temperature of the extremity after the block helps to confirm a successful injection.

1. If a temperature elevation of at least 1.5°C is not seen, a brachial plexus block is necessary to give a more complete sympathectomy. Upper arm symptoms should be treated with an interscalene approach and lower arm symptoms with an axillary approach. Obviously, a sensory and motor block accompanies the sympathetic block and makes using these blocks less specific as diagnostic tools. They often, however, provide more pain relief, especially for PT participation.

2. For lower extremity symptoms, I often begin treatment with an epidural injection performed with dilute local anesthetic at L2-3, where most of the sympathetic outflow to the legs originates. This block is easier to perform and is less painful than a lumbar paravertebral sympathetic block, but again it is not specific for the sympathetic chain. If the epidural injection is not successful, proceed to a paravertebral injection at L2. In some patients a block at L3 or even L4 is also necessary for a complete sympathectomy to the lower leg or foot. PT should be scheduled immediately after an injection. A series of blocks should continue weekly so long as improvement is demonstrated in PT (improved range of motion, less sensitivity, less pain).

F. Intravenous regional blockade can also be used to provide a sympathectomy. Many agents have been used, but the most experience has been with lidocaine, bretylium, guanethidine, and ketorolac. Ketamine and corticosteroids can be added to these mixtures. These blocks require additional equipment (double tourniquet), are labor-intensive, and are associated with an increased risk of seizures compared with traditional sympathetic blocks. They are currently being used less often than in previous years.

G. Limited success with single-shot sympathetic, epidural, or intravenous regional blocks should be followed by continuous techniques. An intensive PT program should be undertaken concurrently with these blocks. Brachial plexus, lumbar sympathetic, epidural, or intrathecal catheters can be placed and are usually dosed continuously with a small, portable, volumetric pump. Local anesthetics can be combined with narcotics or clonidine to provide pain relief along with a sympathectomy. Narcotics have been found to provide additional pain relief at peripheral sites and can be added to the brachial plexus catheters. This practice allows a lower dose of local anesthetic, in turn allowing more active participation in PT because of less motor block. Many providers send patients home after a 24-hour observation period in the hospital. These percutaneous catheters can be left in place up to 2 weeks with a low risk of infection. Long-term surgically tunneled catheters have been used for up to 3 years. In one study pain reduction of 60% to 100% was seen in 95% of patients.

H. Neurolytic sympathetic blocks should be considered if sympathetic blocks provide significant pain relief, but only for the duration of the local anesthesia. Stellate ganglion neurolytic blocks are rarely performed because of the potential damage to nearby structures and because a permanent Horner's syndrome would occur. Neurolytic lumbar sympathetic blocks can be performed easily under fluoroscopy. The neurolytic agent should be mixed with contrast agent so the spread of the agent can be limited to the sympathetic chain. This minimizes the risk of sensory or motor deficits due to lumbar plexus involvement. Increased pain from partial sympathetic denervation has been described, more commonly with absolute alcohol than with phenol.

I. Surgical sympathectomy is indicated if neurolytic techniques have failed or are contraindicated. Success rates are quite high if the diagnosis has been confirmed by sympathetic blocks before surgery. Eighty percent success rates have been documented long term. Postsympathectomy neuralgia has been seen in up to 40% of patients, although it is usually temporary. Thoracoscopy is used for upper extremity symptoms and allows a less invasive approach than traditional thoracotomy without the risk of Horner's syndrome. An open procedure is necessary for a lumbar sympathectomy and is associated with a longer recovery phase.

J. Spinal cord stimulators have been shown to be effective and appear to produce pain relief based on the gate control theory of Wall and Melzack. Providing large fiber afferents "closes the gate" and effects pain relief. Approximately 50% of patients reportedly experience an 80% reduction of pain.

1. Implanted intrathecal medication pumps have been used to provide pain relief when oral narcotics have been given, but their use is limited because of side effects. The addition of bupivicaine or clonidine is often helpful. Good to excellent pain relief is usually achieved in 75% of patients. Intrathecal baclofen has also been found to be effective in reducing dystonia symptoms in some patients.

2. Deep brain stimulation has been shown to provide pain relief in recalcitrant cases. However, the reported success rates have been no higher than 30%.

REFERENCES

Bogduk N: Complex regional pain syndrome. *Curr Opin Anaesthesiol* 2001;14:541–546.

Kemler MA, Barendse GAM, van Kleef M, et al: Spinal cord stimulation in patients with chronic reflex sympathetic dystrophy. *N Engl J Med* 2000;343:618–624.

Koltzenburg M, Scadding J: Neuropathic pain. *Curr Opin Neurol* 2001;14:641–647.

Mellegers MA, Furlan AD, Mailis A: Gabapentin for neuropathic pain; systematic review of controlled and uncontrolled literature. *Clin J Pain* 2001;17:284–295.

Melzack R, Wall PD: Pain mechanisms: a new theory. *Science* 1965;150:971–979.

Merskey H, Bogduk N (eds): *Classification of Chronic Pain*, 2nd ed. Seattle, IASP Press, 1994.

CRPS SUSPECTED

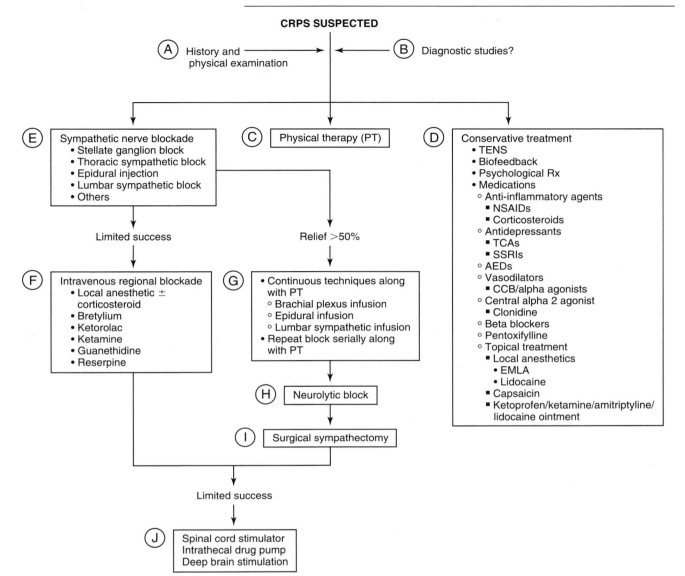

Diabetic Neuropathy

RICHARD BAROHN

Various types of peripheral neuropathies (PNs) occur in patients with diabetes mellitus (DM) and a number of painful diabetic PNs are usually treated symptomatically. No specific metabolic therapy provides any significant clinical benefit. However, tight glucose control is the most effective means to prevent the occurrence and progression of diabetic neuropathy. PNs associated with DM can broadly be classified into generalized/symmetric and focal/asymmetric types.

A. Compressive mononeuropathies occur frequently in DM and are clinically indistinguishable from those of cutting in nondiabetics. Carpal tunnel syndrome is the most common type. Initially, it is managed conservatively with nonsteroidal antiinflammatory drugs (NSAIDs) and wrist splints. If this fails, surgical decompression may be necessary.

B. Other mononeuropathies such as those involving cranial nerves (CNs) III, VI, and VII (Bell's palsy) are thought to be due to nerve ischemia and infarction. They tend to recover spontaneously over weeks or months. With CN III palsy, an aneurysm is unlikely if the pupil examination and the brain computed tomography (CT) scan are normal.

C. Diabetic lumbosacral radiculopathy (DLSRP), or diabetic amyotrophy, consists of leg weakness (often more prominent proximity) and severe back pain. DLSRP begins unilaterally but often the other leg becomes weak. It is presumably due to ischemia of the roots of the lumbosacral (LS) plexus. Weight loss frequently occurs. Therapy consists of reducing the pain with drugs and transcutaneous electrical nerve stimulation (TENS) as stated in G, H, and I, as well as aggressive physical therapy. Oral opioids are often required for temporary relief of severe pain. Reflex sympathetic dystrophy or chronic regional pain syndrome may occur and should be treated appropriately. The symptoms persist or progress for several months and then may slowly resolve spontaneously. The DLSRP that is most frequently missed is compressive radiculopathy, in which imaging studies of the LS spine are normal. Nevertheless, patients who may have DLSRP frequently undergo unnecessary LS spine surgery.

D. A limited form of diabetic radiculopathy can involve isolated thoracic routes. The differential diagnosis consists of herpes zoster but the rash never develops if diabetes mellitus is the cause. Treatment is outlined in E, F, and G. Cervical root involvement is rare, but can occur.

E. For symptoms of autonomic neuropathy, the primary treatment is midodrine (Pro Amatine). Hypotension can also be treated with elastic garments on the lower extremities and oral fludrocortisone (Florinef).

F. Generalized distal symmetric painful neuropathy (DSPN) predominantly alters sensory and/or autonomic function. Significant weakness in DSPN is rare, although some motor involvement is usually found on electromyography (EMG). DSPN usually consists of numbness and tingling in the toes and fingers. If pain is not present, the medications listed in G should not be used.

G. The DSPN may be associated with severe burning pain in the feet and occasionally in the hands. Drug therapy for the pain consists of the following options: (1) a tricyclic antidepressant (TCA) such as amitriptyline, 25 to 75 mg at bedtime; (2) gabapentin (Neurontin), 300 to 1200 mg three times a day; (3) duloxetine (Cymbalta), 30 to 60 mg daily (duloxetine was recently approved by the FDA for the treatment of painful diabetic neuropathy); (4) topiramate, 25 to 100 mg twice a day; (5) zonisamide (Zonegran), 100 to 400 mg at bedtime; (6) tiagabine hydrochloride (Gabitril), 4 to 12 mg twice a day; (7) lamotrigine (Lamictal), 25 to 100 mg twice daily (may be very effective in some patients but has been associated with rash and Steven Johnson syndrome); (8) carbamazepine, 200 mg three times a day or oxcarbazepine (Trileptal), 150 to 300 mg twice a day; (9) tramadol (Ultram), 50 to 100 mg twice a day; or (10) pregabalin (Lyrica), which has also recently been approved by the FDA for diabetic neuropathy, but has not been released on the market at this time.

H. Capsaicin cream (0.025% or 0.075%) applied three times per day may be helpful in painful DSPN. Lidocaine patches (Lidoderm) applied to the soles can occasionally be helpful.

I. TENS can be useful nonpharmacologic therapy for pain in some patients.

J. An unusual, purely sensory generalized PN can occur acutely. The burning pain may extend over all the limbs and trunk and the skin is extremely sensitive to touch. The neuropathy is associated with weight loss, hence the term *diabetic neuropathic cachexia*. Treatment consists of optimizing diabetic control and the measures outlined in G, H, and I. This PN is self limited and improves over many months.

REFERENCES

Backonja M, Beydoun A, Edwards KR, et al: Gabapentin for the symptomatic treatment of painful neuropathy in patient with diabetes mellitus. *JAMA* 1998;280:1831.

Barohn RJ, Sahenk Z, Warmolts JR, Mendell JR: The Bruns-Garland syndrome (diabetic amyotrophy). *Arch Neurol* 1991;48:1130.

Capsaicin Study Group: Treatment of painful diabetic neuropathy with topical capsaicin: a multicenter, double-blind vehicle-controlled study. *Arch Intern Med* 1991;151:2225–2229.

Eisenberg E, Lurie Y, Braker C, et al: Lamotrigine reduces painful diabetic neuropathy: a randomized, controlled study. *Neurology* 2001;57:505–509.

Harati Y, Gooch C, Swensen M, et al: Double-blind randomized trial of tramadol for the treatment of the pain of diabetic neuropathy. *Neurology* 1998;50:1842–1846.

Jackson CE, Barohn RJ: Diabetic neuropathic cachexia: reports of a recurrent case. *J Neurol Neurosurg Psychiatry* 1998;64:785.

Lesser H, Sharma Y, Lamoreaux L, Poole RM: Pregabalin relieves symptoms of painful diabetic neuropathy: a randomized controlled trial. *Neurology* 2004;63:2104.

Wolfe GI, Barohn RJ: Painful peripheral neuropathy. *Curr Treat Options Neurol* 2002;14:177.

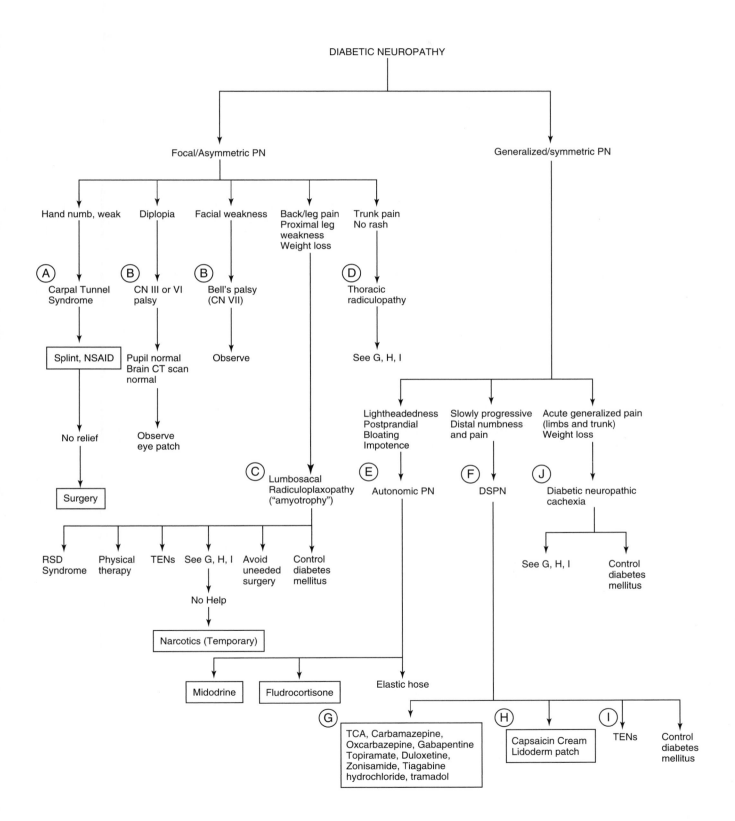

Chronic Pancreatitis Pain

LINDA TINGLE

Chronic pancreatitis (CP), an inflammatory disease of the pancreas, is hallmarked by chronic abdominal pain with exocrine and endocrine pancreatic insufficiency. Alcoholism is the most common cause of CP in the United States; malnutrition is a major cause worldwide. Cystic fibrosis and α_1-antitrypsin deficiency are other causes. Chronic abdominal pain is present as constant, gnawing epigastric pain that radiates to the back and is associated with alcohol ingestion. Non-alcohol-related pancreatitis results in episodes of severe pain with pain-free intervals.

A. Evaluation includes the patient's history, physical examination, psychological evaluation, and a review of laboratory and radiographic studies. Psychological evaluation with a focus on alcohol and narcotic use should precede interventions. Serum enzyme levels are nonspecific. Radiologic studies should include plain abdominal films (which may reveal calcific pancreas), computed tomography (CT), ultrasonography, and endoscopic retrograde pancreatography to help rule out malignancy. Endoscopic retrograde cholangiopancreatography (ERCP) is most invasive but most accurate.

B. Medical management of CP includes dietary restriction (low fat diet), abstinence from alcohol, pancreatic enzyme supplement, acid suppression, and nonnarcotic analgesics. Patients with severe pain respond to high-dose tramadol titration with fewer side effects than are seen with morphine (Wilder-Smith et al. 1999). Narcotic analgesics are often a mainstay of pain management and entail a long-term commitment that leads to physical dependence. The ability to evaluate the severity of pain is complicated in patients with chronic alcoholic pancreatitis who have an addictive personality.

C. Surgical approaches are effective in relieving pain but do not improve exocrine or endocrine function. Longitudinal pancreaticojejunostomy decompresses the pancreatic duct in patients with dilated ducts. About 60% to 80% of patients have significant pain relief with this procedure. Pancreatic resection is performed in patients with normal- or small-caliber ducts.

D. Differential neuraxial blockade using a thoracic epidural can differentiate patients with visceral versus nonvisceral pain. The patients with nonvisceral pain tend to respond to therapy, both surgical and non-surgical (Conwell et al. 2001). Thoracic epidural or left-sided interpleural (IP) catheter dosing is useful for acute exacerbations of CP. Daily injections of 0.5% bupivacaine (20–30 cc) through a left-sided IP catheter until the patient is pain-free or reaches a steady pain level may provide prolonged benefit (Reiestad et al. 1989). Immunocompromise occurs in patients with alcohol abuse. Therefore catheter insertion should be carefully considered (Heller et al. 2000). Celiac plexus block with steroids has been shown to have mixed results (Blanchard et al. 1988). It is difficult to justify neurolytic celiac plexus blocks for CP (Leung et al. 1983). The beneficial results of the neurolytic procedure are not permanent and may last only 2 to 4 months, necessitating numerous repeat procedures with the associated risks. Multiple injections of alcohol may result in fibrosis that obliterates the retroperitoneal fat plane, making future needle placement/injection impossible despite CT guidance (Pateman et al. 1990). There are concerns about producing a "silent abdomen": The alcoholic patient may return to imbibing, but the pain signifying an intraabdominal emergency may be absent.

REFERENCES

Blanchard J, Ramamurthy S, Hoffman J: Celiac plexus block with steroids for chronic pancreatitis. Reg Anesth 1988;13:34.

Conwell DL, Vargo JI, Zuccaro G, et al: Role of differential neuroaxial blockade in the evaluation and management of pain in chronic pancreatitis. Am J Gastroenterol 2001;96:431.

Heller AR, Ragaller M, Koch T: Case report: epidural abscess after epidural catheter for pain release during pancreatitis. Acta Anaesthesiol Scand 2000;44:1024.

Leung JWC, Bowen-Wright M, Aveling W, et al: Celiac plexus block for pain in pancreatic cancer and chronic pancreatitis. Br J Surg 1983;70:730.

Pateman J, Williams MP, Filshie J: Retroperitoneal fibrosis after multiple celiac plexus blocks. Anaesthesia 1990;45:309.

Reiestad F, McIlvaine WB, Kvalheim L, et al: Successful treatment of chronic pancreatitis pain with interpleural analgesia. Can J Anaesth 1989;36:713.

Wilder-Smith CH, Hill L, Osler W, O'Keefe S: Effect of tramadol and morphine on pain and gastrointestinal motor function in patients with chronic pancreatitis. Dig Dis Sci 1999;44:1107.

Patient with CHRONIC PANCREATITIS PAIN

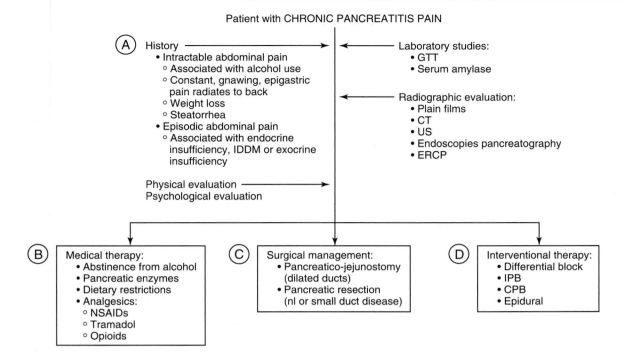

(A) History
- Intractable abdominal pain
  - Associated with alcohol use
  - Constant, gnawing, epigastric pain radiates to back
  - Weight loss
  - Steatorrhea
- Episodic abdominal pain
  - Associated with endocrine insufficiency, IDDM or exocrine insufficiency

Physical evaluation
Psychological evaluation

Laboratory studies:
- GTT
- Serum amylase

Radiographic evaluation:
- Plain films
- CT
- US
- Endoscopies pancreatography
- ERCP

(B) Medical therapy:
- Abstinence from alcohol
- Pancreatic enzymes
- Dietary restrictions
- Analgesics:
  - NSAIDs
  - Tramadol
  - Opioids

(C) Surgical management:
- Pancreatico-jejunostomy (dilated ducts)
- Pancreatic resection (nl or small duct disease)

(D) Interventional therapy:
- Differential block
- IPB
- CPB
- Epidural

Neuropathic Pain

MARK E. ROMANOFF

Neuropathic pain is described by the International Association for the Study of Pain as "pain following a primary lesion or dysfunction of the central or peripheral nervous system." This leads to grouping many varied, disparate pain processes, most with quite different etiologies, into the same category. The most common peripheral entities seen are diabetic neuropathy, peripheral neuropathy, postherpetic neuropathy, and human immunodeficiency virus-related neuropathy. Central causes are usually related to incomplete spinal cord injury, trigeminal neuralgia, and the poststroke condition. Central and peripheral syndromes are presented in Table 1. It appears that nerve injury inducing wallerian degeneration plays a role in pain generation. Recent research has suggested that the N-methyl-D-aspartate (NMDA) receptor, calcitonin gene-related peptide, and the capsaicin receptor VR_1 may be instrumental in nociceptive initiation and propagation. "Central sensitization" often occurs at the level of the spinal cord in wide-dynamic-range neurons producing prolonged, exaggerated symptoms and recruitment of noninvolved dermatomes.

A. The history and physical examination comprise an important first step in identifying neuropathic pain. All precipitating factors should be elicited (e.g., trauma, tumor, surgery, infection). The evaluation concentrates on the signs and symptoms of nerve injury. Burning pain is one of the cardinal descriptions of neuropathic pain. Other symptoms include hypersensitivity, numbness, lancinating pain, and sympathetic dysfunction. Dermatomal patterns of sensory/motor/sympathetic changes should be sought. Hyperpathia, allodynia, or hypesthesia should be present. The differential diagnosis includes all processes that can cause neuropathy and peripheral vascular disease, including complex regional pain syndrome and Raynaud's syndrome.

B. Laboratory studies should be performed to search for the most common causes of peripheral neuropathy. Thyroid function tests and assays for vitamin B_{12}, folate, and homocysteine should be performed if appropriate. Magnetic resonance imaging/computed tomography (MRI/CT) scans can locate cerebral and spinal cord lesions or plexus damage caused by tumor infiltration or compression. Vascular studies (Doppler sonography, angiography) may be necessary to evaluate blood flow to rule out peripheral vascular disease. Electromyography/nerve conduction velocity (EMG/NCV) tests can help confirm large-fiber damage.

C. Nerve blocks provide significant pain relief in many patients. The site of injection obviously depends on the location of the lesion. Central lesions may produce unilateral pain in the upper and lower extremities. Sympathetic blocks can be helpful in these cases. If bilateral lower extremity pain is noted, epidural injections or infusions can provide bilateral coverage. One study has shown that long-term (7–21 days) epidural infusions with bupivacaine and methylprednisolone significantly decreased the pain of postherpetic neuralgia. Weekly epidural injections (four injections) may provide the same level of pain relief. Compromise of the celiac plexus (pancreatic cancer) or the superior hypogastric plexus (pelvic tumors) can be treated by nerve block of the respective plexus. Neurolytic plexus injections are especially appropriate in these patients (see section F, below).

Injury confined to specific dermatomes are best treated by specific peripheral nerve blocks. Iliohypogastric, ilioinguinal, or genitofemoral nerve blocks markedly reduce pain in patients suffering neuropathic pain following herniorrhaphy. If peripheral nerve blocks are ineffective, sympathetic blocks should be considered, as described earlier. Somatic plexus blocks (brachial/lumbar) may be effective following trauma or after other damage to these areas.

D. Physical therapy can provide desensitization and increased range of motion and function. Iontophoresis can be used to provide analgesic or anti-inflammatory agents deeper into the affected tissues. A transcutaneous electrical nerve stimulation (TENS) unit may provide pain relief. In many cases however, providing large-fiber afferent stimulation by TENS may worsen the pain if wide-dynamic-range spinal cord neurons are already sensitized.

E. Oral medications can be combined to provide effective pain relief in conjunction with nerve blocks and physical therapy. The use of anti-inflammatory agents

---

TABLE 1
Causes of Neuropathic Pain

Peripheral conditions
  Diabetic neuropathy
  Peripheral neuropathy
  HIV-related neuropathy
  Alcoholic neuropathy
  Postherpetic neuralgia
  Tumor compression/plexopathy
  Cancer treatment (surgery/chemotherapy)
  Complex regional pain syndrome
  Phantom pain
  Trauma
  Trigeminal neuralgia
Central conditions
  Brain lesions (tumor/AVM)
  Stroke/cerebral vascular accident
  Multiple sclerosis
  Spinal cord injury/lesions
  Incomplete myelopathy
  Radiculopathy
  Failed back syndrome

HIV = human immunodeficiency virus; AVM = arteriovenous malformation.

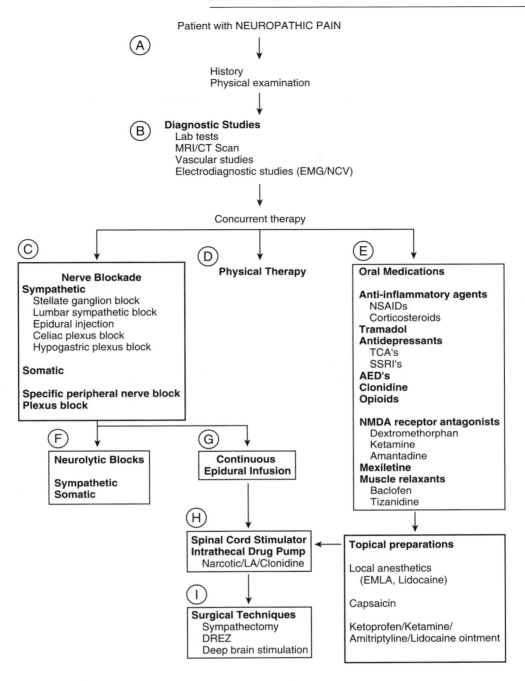

MRI-Magnetic resonance imaging; CT-Computed tomography; EMG-Electromyography; NCV-Nerve conduction velocity; TENS-Transcutaneous electrical nerve stimulation; NSAIDs-Nonsteroidal anti-inflammatory drugs; TCA-Tricyclic antidepressant; SSRI-Selective serotonin reuptake inhibitor; AED's-Anti-epileptic drugs; EMLA-Eutectic mixture local anesthetic; LA-Local anesthetic; DREZ-Dorsal root entry zone lesion.

should be attempted, as nociceptive activation occurs from prostaglandins. Tramadol may be used in patients with mild to moderate pain and has been shown to reduce allodynia significantly.

Tricyclic antidepressants (TCAs) are the "gold standard" of neuropathic pain treatment. Meta-analysis has shown significant pain relief. Unfortunately, their side effect profile [central nervous system (CNS) changes, dry mouth, cardiovascular symptoms] limit their use. Amytriptyline is the standard bearer in most studies. Selective serotonin reuptake inhibitors have been shown to alleviate symptoms in a small number of patients.

Antiepileptic drugs have shown great promise. Their efficacy is equivalent to that of the TCAs but often with fewer side effects. Gabapentin is effective but in many cases is associated with CNS side effects and unwanted weight gain. Zonisamide and topiramate are equally as effective and often contribute to weight loss. Clonidine, a central-acting α_2-agonist reduces peripheral sympathetic tone and has shown promise. Many patients believe that wearing the clonidine patch over the affected area is effective.

Neuropathic pain is thought to be opioid-resistant. One article has shown statistically significant pain relief for neuropathic pain with narcotics but only in fairly large dosages. The study was done with levorphanol, and the average daily dose for pain relief was 9 mg, although some patients required up to 16 mg/day. Oral morphine equivalents for the doses of levorphanol used range from 135 up to 480 mg/day.

NMDA receptors can be blocked by ketamine, dextromethorphan, or amantadine. We have compounded topical ketamine with ketoprofen (a nonsteroidal anti-inflammatory drug), amitriptyline (TCA), and lidocaine with limited success. Intravenous infusions of ketamine have also been described, and studies of intraspinal ketamine are underway. Oral dextromethorphan has decreased symptoms, but its use is limited to large doses of cough suppressant preparations. Oral amantadine has also been shown to be effective.

Mexiletine, a sodium channel blocker, is an oral analogue of lidocaine. It has been used with good success. We believe it is important to obtain a baseline electrocardiogram prior to treatment, as mexiletine is proarrhythmogenic in some patients. Some practitioners perform an intravenous lidocaine trial (up to 5 mg/kg) prior to starting mexiletine. In some cases, long-term pain relief has been seen with the infusions alone.

Baclofen is a γ-aminobutyric acid receptor agonist. It has been used successfully for neuropathic pain. Tizanidine, another centrally acting muscle relaxant, has also shown promise as an adjuvant agent.

Substance P plays a role in neuropathic pain, and topical capsaicin may reduce pain by reducing existing pools of substance P in the neurons. Topical local anesthetics (EMLA, lidocaine patch) can also be used but may be limited by their toxicity, including methemoglobinemia and tachyphylaxis.

F. Neurolytic sympathetic blocks should be considered if sympathetic blocks provide significant short-term pain relief. Stellate ganglion neurolytic blocks are rarely performed because of the potential damage to nearby structures and because a permanent Horner's syndrome would occur. Neurolytic lumbar sympathetic blocks can be performed easily under fluoroscopy. Neurolytic celiac plexus or superior hypogastric blocks are especially effective for cancer-related pain, with success rates of 90% reported. The neurolytic medication should be mixed with a contrast agent to visualize its spread so it can be limited to the sympathetic chain. This minimizes the risk of sensory or motor deficits.

Trigeminal neuralgia is a classic case where neurolytic injections have an excellent outcome. Gasserian ganglion injections can be dangerous if there is any spread into the surrounding cerebrospinal fluid. In peripheral causes of neuropathic pain, a neurolytic injection may be attempted if the nerve involved is predominantly sensory. The intercostal, iliohypogastric, and sural nerves are examples of nerves that can be ablated without significant motor deficits. However, these injections, when performed with absolute alcohol or phenol, can cause significant trauma to tissues and even skin sloughing that requires treatment. Increased pain from partial denervation has been described, most commonly with absolute alcohol use. Neurolytic blocks may not reproduce the pain relief of the trial injection for a number of reasons, including the volume of medication used, so this risk must be explicitly stated to the patient. Radiofrequency ablation and cryoanalgesia are also effective. They may be associated with fewer sensory/motor changes but have a similar risk of denervation pain.

G. Indwelling long-term epidural catheter infusions have been effective for many types of neuropathic pain. One study has shown significant pain reduction in postherpetic neuropathy patients with a 3-week duration of local anesthetic and methylprednisolone epidural infusions. For complex regional pain syndromes, the use of local anesthetic with or without narcotic or clonidine has been highly effective. This therapy should be combined with physical therapy. In one study, pain reduction of 60% to 100% was measured in 95% of patients.

H. If the following measures are not effective, more invasive procedures should be contemplated. Spinal cord stimulation has been shown to provide excellent pain relief. One review article reported 80% patient satisfaction after 2.5 years and 63% after 4 years. Intrathecal opioids have been shown to help in patients with refractory neuropathic pain. Morphine, dilaudid, and sufentanil have been used. The addition of bupivacaine provides pain relief in some patients. Clonidine may improve outcome as well. Long-term high-dose morphine (>15 mg/day) may lead to inflammation at the tip of the catheter. The addition of clonidine has been shown in animal studies to reduce the incidence of this side effect. Intrathecal baclofen has also been found to be effective in reducing dystonia symptoms in some patients.

I. Surgical techniques are indicated if neurolytic techniques or interventional techniques have failed or are contraindicated. Success rates for surgical sympathectomy are usually reasonable if pain relief has been confirmed by sympathetic blocks before surgery. Success rates of up to 80% have been documented long term. Postsympathectomy neuralgia has been seen in up to 40% of patients, although it is usually temporary. Thoracoscopy is used for upper extremity symptoms and allows a less invasive approach than traditional thoracotomy without the risk of Horner's syndrome. An open procedure is necessary for a lumbar sympathectomy and has a longer recovery phase. Deep brain stimulation has been shown to provide pain relief in recalcitrant cases. However, success rates over 30% have not been seen.

REFERENCES

Denkers MR, Biagi HL, O'Brien AM, et al. Dorsal root entry zone lesioning used to treat central neuropathic pain in patients with traumatic spinal cord injury: a systematic review. *Spine* 2002;27:E177–E184.

Koltzenburg M, Scadding J: Neuropathic pain. *Curr Opin Neurol* 2001;14:641–647.

Mellegers MA, Furlan AD, Mailis A: Gabapentin for neuropathic pain; systematic review of controlled and uncontrolled literature. *Clin J Pain* 2001;17:284–295.

Merskey H, Bogduk N (eds): *Classification of Chronic Pain*, 2nd ed. Seattle, IASP Press, 1994.

Rowbotham MC, Twilling L, Davies PS, et al: Oral opioid therapy for chronic peripheral and central neuropathic pain. *N Engl J Med* 2003;348:1223–1232.

Yaksh TL, Horais KA, Tozier NA, et al: Chronically infused intrathecal morphine in dogs. *Anesthesiology* 2003;99:174–187.

Central Pain Syndrome

SOMAYAJI RAMAMURTHY

Neuropathic pain resulting from the lesions of the central nervous system (CNS), known as central pain, is one of the most difficult pain syndromes to manage. Pain originating from the spinal cord is usually secondary to trauma and is commonly seen in young patients. Pain resulting from lesions in the brain is usually secondary to cerebrovascular accident (CVA) and is seen more commonly in older patients. Severe pain can also be associated with demyelinating lesions of the CNS such as multiple sclerosis. The mechanism of pain is unclear, no animal model is available, and hence it is very difficult to arrive at a rational treatment program. The pain can be a continuous burning or intermittent shooting sensation and is occasionally associated with allodynia and hyperpathia. It can also mimic visceral pain. Musculoskeletal pain can be of neuropathic origin or it can be secondary to deconditioning and disuse (for example: capsulitis of the shoulder). These patients can also have pain originating from the musculoskeletal structures, such as spasticity, autonomic dysreflexia, and urologic problems.

A. Thorough neurologic evaluation and diagnostic studies are essential before starting the treatment. Patients should be enrolled in an appropriate rehabilitation program including physical therapy and occupational therapy, exercises, and orthotics. Ongoing management of urologic problems, skin care, and wound care of the pressure sores should be included.

B. Pharmacotherapy directed at the management of neuropathic pain is the mainstay of the treatment. Tricyclic antidepressants such as amitriptyline are commonly utilized, as well as carbamazepine, gabapentin, valproic acid, lamictal, topiramate, zonisamide, Keppra, and other anticonvulsants. We prefer to start with gabapentin because of its favorable side effect profile before trying other anticonvulsants. Central pain is resistant to opioids. Methadone and N-methyl-D-aspartate (NMDA)-receptor blockers such as dextromethorphan, amantadine, ketamine, and magnesium have been reported to be useful in some patients.

C. In patients with acute pain, intravenous local anesthetics such as lidocaine administered intravenously (1.5 mg/kg) and used intermittently as needed have been very effective in controlling the pain; mexiletine may be used if intravenous lidocaine provides only temporary pain relief.

D. Spinal cord lesions: Patients with complete or incomplete spinal cord injury can complain of mild to severe pain even in the area where there is total sensory loss. Delayed onset pain is likely to be secondary to the development of syrinx and the patient should be appropriately investigated. Surgical treatment of the syrinx is necessary to prevent further progress of the pathology but 24% of patients may also obtain significant long-term pain relief.

E. Patients who have pain with allodynia in a nerve root distribution may benefit from percutaneous radiofrequency rhizotomy.

F. Incomplete lesion of the spinal cord: If a trial of epidural spinal cord stimulation is successful implantation of a spinal cord stimulation unit is indicated. Other surgical procedures such as cordotomy, cordectomy, and dorsal root entry zone (DREZ) lesions have been reported to be effective in some patients with lower extremity neuropathic pain.

G. Deep brain stimulation may be effective in patients who have continuous burning pain.

REFERENCE

Tasker RR: Central pain states. In: Loeser JD (ed) *Bonica's Management of Pain,* 3rd ed. Philadelphia, Lippincott Williams & Wilkins, 2001, pp. 433–457.

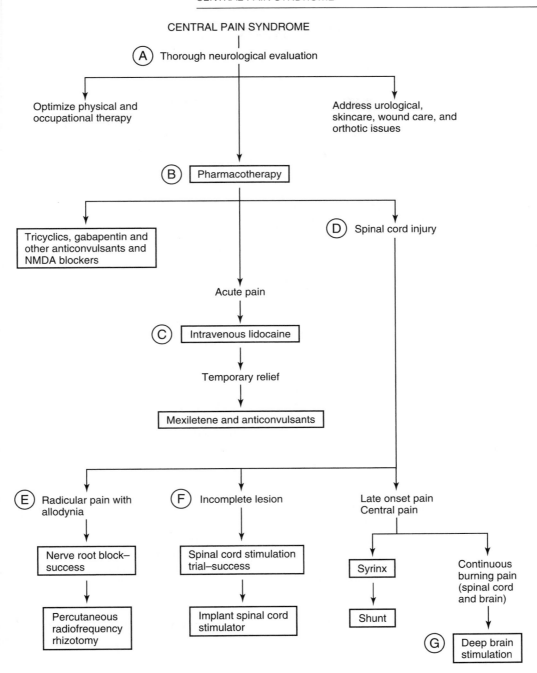

CENTRAL PAIN SYNDROME

Ⓐ Thorough neurological evaluation

Optimize physical and occupational therapy

Address urological, skincare, wound care, and orthotic issues

Ⓑ Pharmacotherapy

Tricyclics, gabapentin and other anticonvulsants and NMDA blockers

Ⓓ Spinal cord injury

Acute pain

Ⓒ Intravenous lidocaine

Temporary relief

Mexiletene and anticonvulsants

Ⓔ Radicular pain with allodynia

Ⓕ Incomplete lesion

Late onset pain Central pain

Nerve root block– success

Spinal cord stimulation trial–success

Syrinx

Continuous burning pain (spinal cord and brain)

Percutaneous radiofrequency rhizotomy

Implant spinal cord stimulator

Shunt

Ⓖ Deep brain stimulation

Phantom Pain

TED GINGRICH

A. Phantom pain can occur in any amputated body part including the limbs, breasts, nose, and genitalia, among others. It is important to distinguish between three entities: (1) stump pain, which is specifically located in, and does not extend beyond, the stump; (2) phantom pain, which is pain in the amputated body part; and (3) phantom sensation, which is by definition not painful. As with all pain evaluations, the provider must elicit specifics of the syndrome including the intensity of the pain, its pattern of radiation, its character, temporal factors, exacerbating and remitting factors, and the response to previous therapy. The role for preemptive neuraxial analgesia is debatable according to the literature. The first goal for all lower extremity amputees should be early prosthetic fitting and ambulation.

B. The incidence of stump pain may be as high as 71%. It may occur alone or along with phantom sensations or pain. Long-term stump pain may increase the incidence of phantom limb pain. The pain may be continuous or intermittent, focal or diffuse, and triggered by stimulation or emotions. The pain may be of a cramping, burning, aching, hot, or cold character and may be associated with myoclonic jerks and contractions.

   1. After careful examination of the stump for proper prosthetic fit, the patient is evaluated for potential surgical or medical pathology (skin lesions, bone spurs, osteomyelitis, deep abscess, circulatory insufficiency).
   2. Trigger point injections are effective for myofascial pain. The provider should examine the stump for neuromas, which if present can be injected with local anesthetic for diagnosis and treatment. Transcutaneous electrical nerve stimulation may provide relief through localized vasodilatation. Sympathetic blocks may be effective for burning, "causalgic" pain. Psychological strategies such as biofeedback and relaxation training should be made available to patients with a significant emotional trigger. Repeated neuroma resection and reamputation for pain should be only cautiously considered.

C. Phantom pain is a well recognized problem in a fraction of amputees, with a reported incidence of 2% to 97% (Table 1). Of those with phantom pain, 27% have pain for more than 20 days per month, more than 15 hours per day, or both. Most develop the pain within the first month, with only 10% of patients developing phantom pain more than a year after amputation. Typical descriptors of phantom pain are burning, aching, cramping, crushing, twisting, grinding, and stabbing. Up to 4% of patients have described abnormal positions: extreme flexion or a tightly

---

TABLE 1
Phantom Pain: Pathology, Nerve Injury, and Central Responses

Local pathology
Surgical trauma/postoperative pain
Ischemia
Inflammation/stitch abscess
Skin infection or trauma
Bone spurs
Local scarring
Ill-fitting prosthesis
Osteomyelitis
Myofacial pain/trigger points

Nerve injury and central responses
Neuromas
Major nerves

Small nerves in skin and deeper structures
Autonomic system abnormality
CRPS I- and II-type symptoms
Spinal cord/central structures

---

clenched fist with fingernails cutting into the palm. Ten percent of patients complain of spasms or jerking of the phantom limb, and 82% of the pain is in the distal aspect of the extremity (below the ankle or wrist).

   1. Several hypotheses have been proposed regarding the development of phantom pain, including peripheral, spinal, central, and psychological mechanisms. The literature is voluminous and often contradictory, and no single theory fully explains all the clinical characteristics of this condition.
   2. Experimental studies have shown that prior noxious conditioning may generate long-term changes in the central nervous system (CNS). It is argued that pain creates a nonerasable imprint in memory structures. Several clinical studies have suggested that phantom pain is more likely in patients who had pain prior to the amputation. This is an argument for preemptive analgesia prior to amputation. A history of phantom pain is a relative contraindication to regional anesthesia, as there are reports of pain recrudescence after spinal anesthesia.
   3. The usual course is for the pain to remain unchanged or to diminish with time. If it worsens, new etiologies should be considered, such as herniated discs and lower extremity radicular symptoms, angina with left upper extremity referral, recurrence of cancer, or herpes zoster, among others. The physical examination is usually unrevealing. Again, look for stump pain etiologies and trigger points.

PHANTOM PAIN

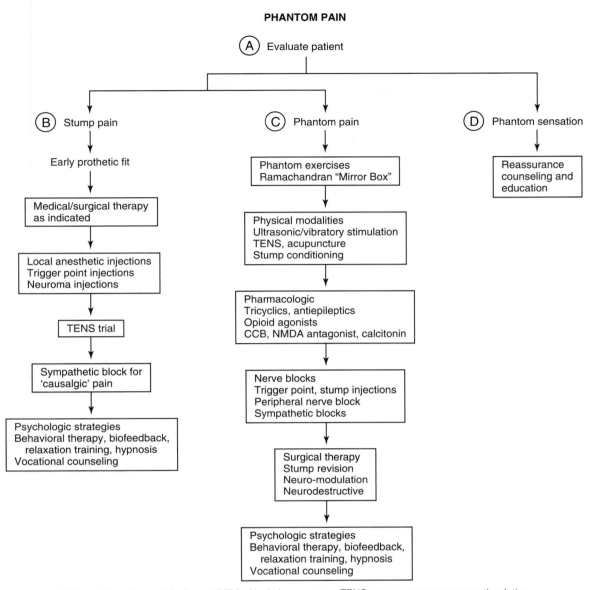

(A) Evaluate patient

(B) Stump pain

Early prothetic fit

Medical/surgical therapy
as indicated

Local anesthetic injections
Trigger point injections
Neuroma injections

TENS trial

Sympathetic block for
'causalgic' pain

Psychologic strategies
Behavioral therapy, biofeedback,
relaxation training, hypnosis
Vocational counseling

(C) Phantom pain

Phantom exercises
Ramachandran "Mirror Box"

Physical modalities
Ultrasonic/vibratory stimulation
TENS, acupuncture
Stump conditioning

Pharmacologic
Tricyclics, antiepileptics
Opioid agonists
CCB, NMDA antagonist, calcitonin

Nerve blocks
Trigger point, stump injections
Peripheral nerve block
Sympathetic blocks

Surgical therapy
Stump revision
Neuro-modulation
Neurodestructive

Psychologic strategies
Behavioral therapy, biofeedback,
relaxation training, hypnosis
Vocational counseling

(D) Phantom sensation

Reassurance
counseling and
education

CCB, calcium channel blockers; NMDA, N-ethyl-D-aspartate; TENS, transcutaneous nerve stimulation.

4. Phantom exercise has been long advocated. If the patient has voluntary control of the limb, isometric exercises can be extremely helpful. Some patients experience involuntary movements in their phantom limb, such as clenching spasms of the hand; voluntary unclenching can be difficult if not impossible. Ramachandran and Hirstein (1998) described construction of a mirror box, which conveys the visual illusion that the phantom limb has been "resurrected," enabling voluntary movements of the limb and relief of pain.

5. Physical therapy strategies include conditioning the stump and early prosthesis use. Ultrasonic and vibratory stimulation, stump percussion, heat, cold, and massage therapy, although rarely effective in and of themselves, should be considered as part of the treatment plan. Transcutaneous nerve stimulation provides good to excellent transient relief in approximately 25% of patients (contralateral stimulation is effective as well). Few reports in the Western literature address the role of acupuncture, but anecdotal evidence of its usefulness exists.

6. Pharmacologic therapies include tricyclic anti-depressants and antiepileptic drugs (AEDs), both of which have been thoroughly studied in models of neuropathic pain. Consider the AEDs for lancinating or shooting pain. β-Blockers, calcitonin, and N-methyl-D-aspartate (NMDA) antagonists (through their diminution of CNS hyperexcitability) have had anecdotal success with phantom pain. Although classically considered to be ineffective, opioid analgesics (specifically methadone) have been shown to be effective in some patients.

7. Trigger point injections, stump neuroma injections, peripheral nerve blockade, major conduction blocks, and sympathetic blocks have all been used to treat phantom limb pain. However, only 14% report a significant temporary change, and only 5% of patients demonstrate any permanent improvement or cure of pain. Consider sympathetic blocks in those with a causalgic description of the pain. Trigger points in the stump and on the contralateral side may be tried as well.

8. Surgical therapies include stump revision, neuromodulation (spinal cord stimulation), and neuroablation. Stump revision is indicated for infection or vascular insufficiency. For the 20% of patients with palpable neuromas that are resected, only 50% have improvement. Spinal cord stimulation may be considered in selected patients without drug addiction or psychological disturbances. There are various reports with 30% to 50% of patients having more than 50% reduction of their pain. Neuroablation (dorsal rhizotomy, dorsal column tractotomy, anterolateral cordotomy, thalamotomy, cortical resection) have produced mixed results in limited series.

9. Psychological strategies include explanation and reassurance, hypnosis, behavioral therapy, biofeedback, and relaxation training. Diseases such as depression and posttraumatic stress disorder must be treated aggressively. Vocational counseling and training may provide substantial benefit, as people who have something to do do not experience as much pain.

D. Phantom sensation is a nonpainful, vivid, highly articulated image of the lost part, described with definite volume and length. The sensation may be exteroceptive (surface sensations), kinesthetic (distortion of positional sensation), or kinetic (sensation of movement, willed or spontaneous). The phenomenon of "telescoping" involves gradual reduction of the phantom length and volume. The last part to disappear is the area with the highest cortical representation; for example, a patient with an upper arm amputation describes a phantom hand attached directly to the stump, with loss of all forearm sensation. The incidence increases with the patient's age: Only 20% of patients 2 years old and younger have a phantom sensation compared to nearly 100% of patients older than 8 years of age. Congenitally absent limbs are less likely to produce phantoms. Most sensations gradually resolve within the first 24 months unless they become associated with pain. Although by definition this sensation is not painful, it can be frightening to an unprepared patient. Therefore it is necessary to begin preamputation counseling and education, possibly arranging meetings with rehabilitated amputees. Assure patients that these sensations are normal, natural, and *not* a sign of mental illness.

REFERENCES

Jensen TS, Krebs B, Nielsen J: Immediate and long-term phantom limb pain in amputees: incidence, clinical characteristics and relationship to pre-amputation limb pain. *Pain* 1985;21:267–278.

Melzack R: From the gate to the neuromatrix. *Pain* 1999(Suppl)6:S121–S126.

Ramachandran VS, Hirstein W: The perception of phantom limbs: the D.O. Hebb lecture. *Brain* 1998;121(Pt 9):1603–1630.

Sherman RA: Stump and phantom limb pain. *Neurol Clin* 1989;7:249–264.

Spinal Cord-Injured Patient

MICHELE L. ARNOLD

In many patients with spinal cord injury (SCI), pain can be as much a handicap as the neurologic impairment and can be a limitation to functional recovery. According to the literature, the prevalence of pain with an SCI ranges from 34% to 90% (average 65%). Historical data that correlate with pain in the SCI patient include SCIs due to gunshot wounds, incomplete lesions, spasticity, more-caudal neurologic levels of injury, inactivity or bed rest, and depression and adjustment disorder after the injury.

Countless classification systems have failed to elucidate a concise approach to diagnosing or managing pain in the SCI patient. Hence a lack of consistent nomenclature has clouded research efforts to identify successful treatment strategies.

A. A detailed history and physical examination assists in classifying the pain as nociceptive, visceral, or neuropathic.

B. The neurologic level of the SCI is defined as the most caudal level with normal motor and sensory function. At-level pain is localized within two dermatomes above or below the neurologic level of the SCI.

C. Autonomic dysreflexia can be a life-threatening emergency characterized by reflexive hypertensive crisis in response to a noxious stimulus below the neurologic level of injury. Appropriate immediate management is first to have the patient sit upright and then search for and eliminate any noxious stimuli, such as tight clothing or bladder or bowel distension. Bite-and-swallow nifedipine or topical nitroglycerin paste is indicated to control hypertension while the investigation ensues.

D. Overuse syndromes are a frequent cause of upper extremity pain in paraplegics. In the SCI patient the shoulder joint bears the weight of the body while he or she is mobile, whether via wheelchair propulsion, transfers, or aide-assisted ambulation. This predisposes to muscle strain, bursitis, tendinitis, or rotator cuff tendinopathy. Excessive wear can result in glenohumeral degenerative joint disease. The wary practitioner should recall, however, that visceral pathology may also masquerade as shoulder pain.

E. Heterotopic ossification (HO) is a risk during the months immediately following the SCI. When present, it is located below the neurologic level of the SCI, most commonly involving the hip. Useful laboratory data include an elevated erythrocyte sedimentation rate and elevated C-reactive protein and alkaline phosphatase levels. A triple-phase bone scan detects HO even during its early stages. Etidronate or radiation therapy is indicated; alternatively, nonsteroidal antiinflammatory drugs may be given, or the HO may be resected surgically if it is refractory to other treatments.

F. Segmental transitional zone pain refers to a band of neuropathic pain localized to a 2 to 4 segment region at the border of the sensate/anesthetic skin. Central (deafferentation or dysesthetic) pain refers to neuropathic pain below the level of the injury, and it is notoriously difficult to treat.

G. Lesioning of the dorsal root entry zone (DREZ) is proposed to reduce neuropathic pain by interrupting the abnormal neuroelectrical activity. It is most effective for localized neuropathic segmental transitional zone pain, radicular at-level pain, or following failed shunt placement in the presence of syringomyelia.

H. The most common presenting symptom of syringomyelia is delayed onset of pain for more than 1 year following the SCI. Magnetic resonance imaging demonstrates a cystic cavity within the cord, typically at or above the neurologic level of the injury. Surgical approaches include detethering or lysis of arachnoid adhesions or placing a syringeal-subarachnoid or syringeal-peritoneal shunt. Neuropathic pain agents such as tricyclic antidepressants or antiepileptic drugs are helpful if pain persists following collapse of the syrinx, and DREZ may be of benefit.

I. Spinal cord stimulation (SCS) may play a role in the treatment of segmental transitional zone pain and postcordotomy pain in patients with an incomplete SCI. SCS might also play a role in the treatment of intractable complex regional pain syndrome (CPRS). Most studies report a decline in efficacy over time.

J. Deep brain stimulation has demonstrated some early relief in the treatment of below-level neuropathic central pain, but it has exhibited poor long-term efficacy.

K. The use of cordectomy and cordotomy remains controversial, although they may alleviate segmental transitional zone pain or unilateral below-level neuropathic central pain. They are typically reserved for end-stage cancer patients because of their potential serious complications.

REFERENCES

Bockenek WL, Stewart PJB: Pain in patients with spinal cord injury. In: Kirshblum S, Campagnolo JI, DeLisa JA (eds) *Spinal Cord Medicine.* Philadelphia, Lippincott Williams & Wilkins, 2002, pp 389–408.

Bryce TN, Ragnarsson KT: Pain management in persons with spinal cord disorders. In: Lin VW (ed) *Spinal Cord Medicine: Principles and Practice.* New York, Demos Medical, 2003, pp 441–460.

Burchiel KJ, Hsu FPK: Pain and spasticity after spinal cord injury. *Spine* 2001;26:S146–S160.

Siddall PJ, Loeser JD: Pain following spinal cord injury. *Spinal Cord* 2001;39:63–73.

Yarkony GM, Gittler MS, Weiss DJ: Pain syndromes following spinal cord injury. In: Monga TN, Grabois M (eds) *Pain Management in Rehabilitation.* New York, Demos Medical, 2002, pp 59–72.

PAIN IN THE PATIENT WITH SPINAL CORD INJURY

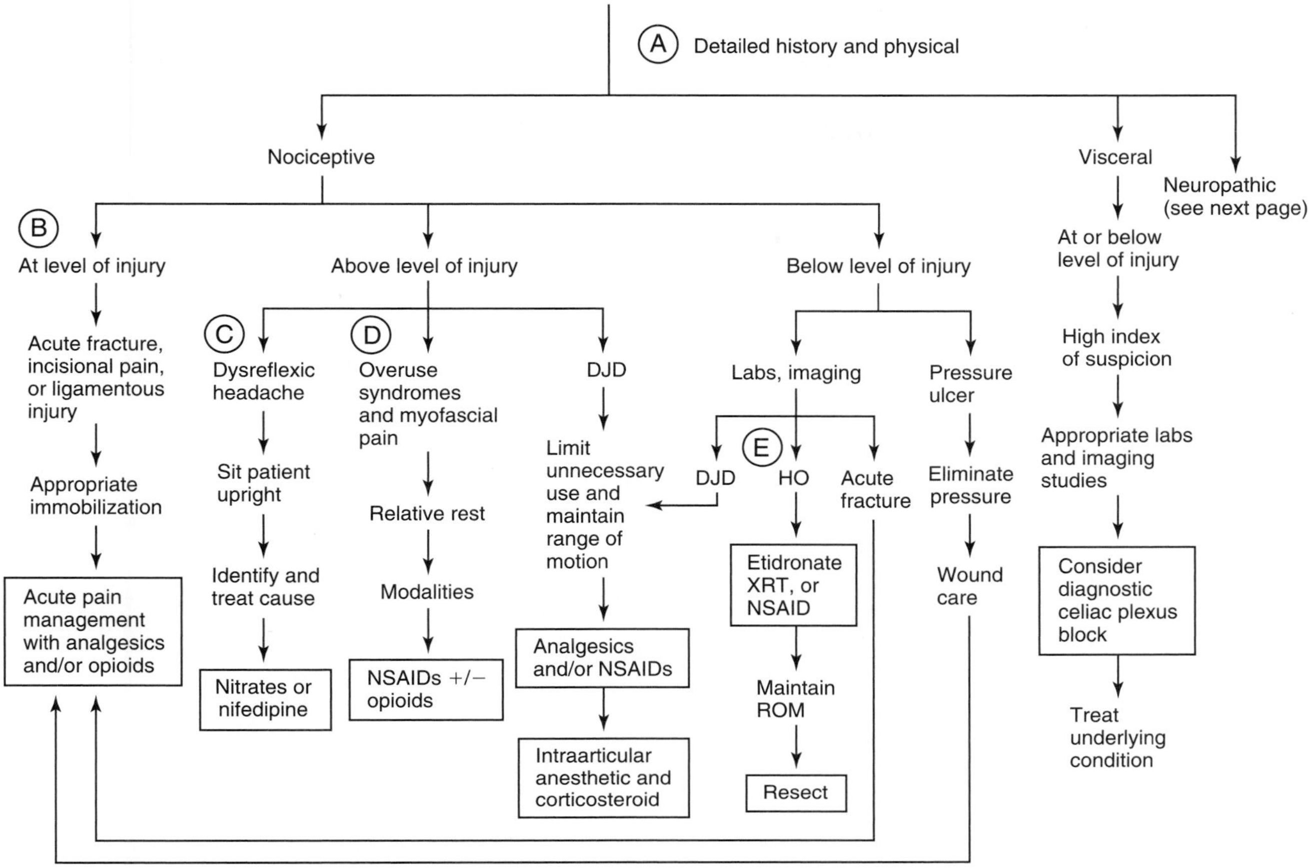

(A) Detailed history and physical

Nociceptive

(B) At level of injury

Acute fracture, incisional pain, or ligamentous injury

↓

Appropriate immobilization

↓

Acute pain management with analgesics and/or opioids

Above level of injury

(C) Dysreflexic headache

↓

Sit patient upright

↓

Identify and treat cause

↓

Nitrates or nifedipine

(D) Overuse syndromes and myofascial pain

↓

Relative rest

↓

Modalities

↓

NSAIDs +/− opioids

DJD

↓

Limit unnecessary use and maintain range of motion

↓

Analgesics and/or NSAIDs

↓

Intraarticular anesthetic and corticosteroid

Below level of injury

Labs, imaging

(E) DJD　　HO　　Acute fracture

Etidronate XRT, or NSAID

↓

Maintain ROM

↓

Resect

Pressure ulcer

↓

Eliminate pressure

↓

Wound care

Visceral

At or below level of injury

↓

High index of suspicion

↓

Appropriate labs and imaging studies

↓

Consider diagnostic celiac plexus block

↓

Treat underlying condition

Neuropathic (see next page)

(Continued)

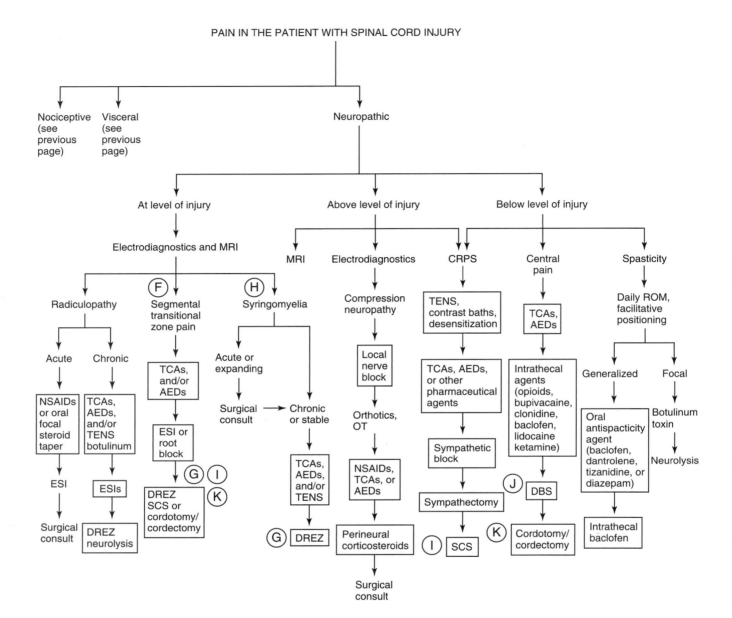

The Fibromyalgia Syndrome

I. JON RUSSELL

Fibromyalgia syndrome (FMS) is an idiopathic disorder characterized by a reproducible constellation of painful symptoms and unusual tenderness to deep somatic pressure. Its consistent epidemiologic pattern and a predictable prognosis distinguish it from a variety of other painful conditions. Associated signs and symptoms can include severe muscle contraction, headache, depression, anxiety, lightheadedness, cognitive dysfunction, insomnia, fatigue, exercise intolerance, neuroendocrine dysfunction, autonomic system dysfunction, irritable bowel-like symptoms, and irritable bladder.

Management of the pain associated with FMS has properly become a multimodal, multidisciplinary process that cannot be approached effectively without an integrated understanding of the condition and the affected individual. Given those resources, the approach should be guided by general principles but then be individualized to the patient. The therapeutic plan will undoubtedly be influenced by many variables, such as the physical plant of the practice, the availability of skilled health care professionals, the financial resources of the patient, and the willingness of the patient to actively participate in his or her treatment. The following discussion and algorithm outline an approach that should be feasible in most practice environments.

A. Attitude. If the physician's attitude is that "fibromyalgia does not exist," that it is a "diagnosis by exclusion," or that it is a "somatic manifestation of self-induced affective psychopathology" there probably is little value in that clinician's working with patients who have chronic pain. There are realistic limits to the range of diagnoses and kinds of care a physician can assume in modern medicine. Some physicians are uncomfortable with pain complaints, feel threatened by not knowing everything, or have a temperament characterized by a short irritability fuse. Fortunately for such individuals, medicine has a variety of branches that involve little or no direct patient contact, where skilled professionals can effectively use their talents and will probably enjoy life more. Despite that, there is no place for statements such as "the bane of my existence," "clean the refuse out of your practice," "another whining misfit," "a bunch of complaining crocks," or "its all in your head, lady" in the language of a health care professional. The physician who does not want to see patients with painful conditions or specifically FMS should be kind but frank in declining to assume care, without being accusatory or demeaning of the patient. On the other hand, for the physician who is willing to approach body pain with an inquisitive mind, one who is open to understanding the patient's perception of his or her symptoms, FMS can be very gratifying to diagnose and to manage. There is reason to expect that this objectively supportable disorder is exactly what the patients perceive it to be and that research will eventually define its pathogenesis sufficiently to focus therapy specifically on the cause.

There is a similar responsibility of attitude on the part of the patient, the patient's family, the employer, and the community. It is not yet possible to cure FMS. The goals of treatment must be hopeful but realistic. When the patient's expectations of health care professionals are unrealistic, there will be a failure of the relationship and potential benefits will remain frustratingly beyond reach. The patient must realize that treatment options are limited and carry with them the potential risk of adverse effects. The patient must accept a substantial portion of the responsibility for achieving the best possible outcome. The task is not easy but there is reason for exerting the necessary effort. Continued participation in all of life's activities, including gainful employment, should be among the objectives but often that is not possible, and a step down from many forms of usual activity seems to be necessary in some FMS patients.

B. History, examination, and tests. The classification of nonmalignant, painful musculoskeletal conditions includes more than 100 types of arthritic conditions and an even larger number of soft tissue pain syndromes. The arthritic conditions can be strategically divided into monoarticular, oligoarticular, and polyarticular diseases, indicating the involvement of one, several, or many joints, respectively. In a similar manner, the soft tissue pain syndromes can be classified either as localized, regional, or generalized pain conditions. Having the patient fill out a brief questionnaire indicating the location of the pain on a "body pain diagram" will identify which of these categories is relevant to a given patient. That knowledge will guide the direction of history-taking, the physical examination, and laboratory testing. Additional types of useful subjective information that the patient can provide on a simple one-page questionnaire could include the severity of the pain on a Visual Analog Scale, the severity of the insomnia, the duration of morning stiffness, and the level of physical dysfunction. In addition to the standard information to be obtained from a general physical examination, the FMS examination should determine the severity of the tenderness at each of the standard FMS tender points (TePs) (Wolfe et al. 1990), and document the status of muscles, nerves, and joints. A simple but valuable panel of laboratory screening tests should include the complete blood count, erythrocyte sedimentation rate, chemistry panel, thyroid function, vitamin B_{12}, red cell folate, antinuclear antibody, rheumatoid factor, and urinalysis. All of the usual health maintenance assessments indicated by age or gender would apply. Abnormal tests should be followed up in the

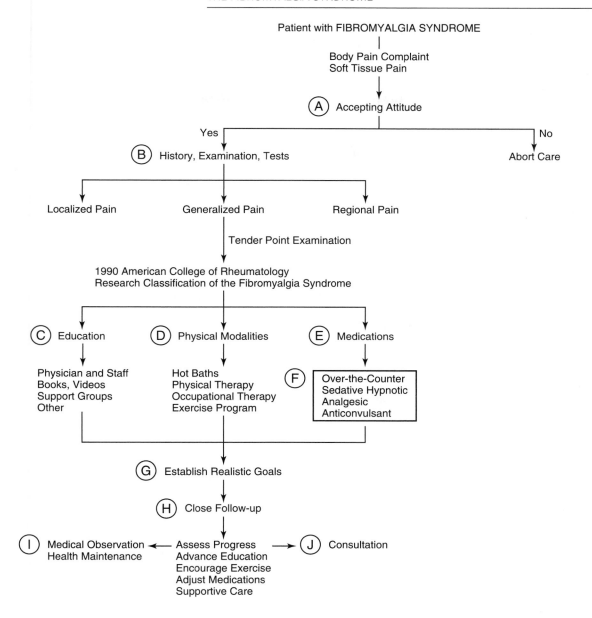

standard manner. The issue of compressive myelopathy has been raised in the public press. The question for the clinician is when magnetic resonance imaging should be performed in seeking evidence for Chiari malformation or compression of the cervical cord. The answer is: when a careful neurologic examination is abnormal.

Diagnosis. When a clinician evaluates an individual with a history of body pain, the interview and the examination should carefully assess the joints for evidence of arthritis and the soft tissue structures around the joints for sites of painful tenderness. In most patients with FMS, nearly all of the anatomically defined "tender point sites" will be symptomatic and painful to palpation at the first clinical presentation, meeting the published criteria for research classification as FMS (Wolfe et al. 1990). Occasionally, a patient will present with a single painful area ("chest pain" and "sciatica") but on examination will be

found to exhibit widespread tenderness at most of the other tender points, of which he or she may even have been unaware. At times, the generalized pain at presentation or follow-up can be so dramatic that it is referred to as a "flair" or as a "fibromyalgia storm."

The clinician's observational and diagnostic skills will be challenged to sort out a myriad of symptoms that represent or mimic other clinical disorders. Patients with FMS are subject to the same medical conditions prevalent among the general community, so the recognition of FMS does not exclude other current or future emergent or overlapping conditions. When FMS coexists with another condition, both disorders should be evaluated and managed as separate entities because the FMS in those situations is not clinically very different from "primary FMS" and there is still no clear evidence that the other conditions are the cause of the FMS, as implied by the term "secondary FMS." The diagnosis of both conditions should be made confidently, on the basis of established criteria, and treated accordingly. In the case of some inflammatory conditions, such as rheumatoid arthritis or systemic lupus erythematosus, many of the FMS symptoms have been observed to respond to treatment that was successfully directed specifically at the associated condition.

C. Education. Making a confident diagnosis of FMS usually has the effect of reducing that patient's utilization of medical resources such as emergency visits and expensive imaging tests. That benefit results principally from the patient's better understanding of his or her symptoms. Education may not reduce the severity of the pain experienced but can decrease the patient's concern that another condition such as cancer has been missed. Women who are being subjected to "wife battery" will benefit from proper referral. Accurate reading materials, video programs, and support group interaction resources are increasingly available to assist the health care provider in this area, but there is no substitute for quality physician time. The first couple of visits should be used to instill confidence in the diagnosis and to directly involve the patient in responsibility for the outcome of the FMS care program. It is important to inform the patient up front that a cure is not available but that teamwork between clinician and patient can usually result in substantial and sustained benefit. In some institutions, psychologists are available to offer biofeedback modalities (Ferraccioli et al. 1987) or cognitive behavioral therapy (Bradley 1989; Nielson et al. 1992; White and Nielson 1995).

D. Physical modalities. Research has established that physical exercise is important to the maintenance of physical functions in patients with FMS (McCain et al. 1988; Mengshoel et al. 1992; Clark et al. 2001; Jentoft et al. 2001). The problem is that unaccustomed physical exertion can induce severe body pain for a FMS patient, which will result in near incapacitation for several days thereafter. Gradual adaptation to a routine progressive exercise program such as alternate day bicycle ergometry, walking, or water exercise will usually be well tolerated. Most patients report benefit from heat in the form of a hot bath or from a professional modality such as hydrocollator packs or ultrasound. The hot bath or shower is a resource that patients will usually have access to at home and at any time of day. It is not uncommon for patients who benefit from this modality (as most do) to take three or more hot showers or baths per day. Gradual introduction of deep sedative massage is similarly appreciated by most patients after they adapt to it (massage is often painful at first) but the benefits last only a few days and there is limited research to objectively support its use. The roles of acupuncture and laser therapy are still uncertain.

For patients with very troublesome fatigue, especially toward the end of the day, an alternating work and rest program can be helpful. The actual details of the program should be determined by trial and error. The patient could begin by setting a timer in the morning for perhaps 1 hour of work. When the timer

rings, he or she would rest for a period of time, perhaps 10 minutes. The timer would then be reset for the next cycle. No matter what is happening at the end of the timed work period, the patient would stop and rest. At the end of the day, the results should be assessed and adjusted for the next day until a workable program has been found. Many women with FMS who do their work at home have found that 20 to 30 minutes of work followed by 10 minutes of rest is an effective schedule for them. Adapting this to a workplace setting is obviously more problematic but could be arranged in some settings if there is a will to do so.

E. Medication. Even though most patients with FMS regularly use one or more oral medications, none of those in common use can be said to be specific for FMS and none are dramatically effective. The development of specific therapy will necessitate a better understanding of the underlying biochemical abnormalities. In an earlier book chapter (Russell 2000), I predicted that in the future medications would be found to increase platelet serotonin, increase serum insulin-like growth factor-1 (IGF1), or decrease spinal fluid substance P concentration to effect more specific symptomatic benefit. There is now evidence to suggest that all three of these futuristic goals have evidence in fruition. Alprazolam seems to increase the average platelet serotonin level by blocking breakdown by platelet activation factor (Kornecki et al. 1984; Baer and Cagen 1987; Russell et al. 1991); parenteral administration of human growth factor increases serum IGF1 and reduces the severity of many FMS symptoms (Bennett 1995, 1998); and tizanidine therapy of FMS patients has now been shown to decrease the elevated levels of spinal fluid substance P in FMS patients (Russell 2001). Such successful prediction was more the result of insider information than a prophetic gift. The importance of these findings, however, can be accepted as evidence that there is now, and will increasingly be, biochemical logic for the medications that provide benefit in FMS.

F. Over-the-counter remedies. Many patients are influenced by advertisements for or even purposely seek out so-called "natural remedies" for their ailments. Several over-the-counter medications are available for which there is supportive research to indicate efficacy.

In FMS patients, two glycolytic pathway enzymes that depend on thiamine pyrophosphate (vitamin B_1) as a cofactor appear to require higher than normal levels of the vitamin for optimal activity (Basu et al. 1974; Eisinger and Ayavou 1990; Eisinger et al. 1996). It is not clear that administration of large doses of the vitamin will correct that problem but a trial (thiamine HCl 100 mg/day) might be reasonable considering its safety profile. Dosages higher than 300 mg/day pose a serious risk of inducing neuropathy.

A proprietary combination of malic acid and magnesium (Super Malic, 200 mg of malic acid and 50 mg of magnesium per tablet) was found to reduce fatigue from exertion when taken in fairly high doses (600 to 1200 mg bid) (Russell et al. 1995). The dosage limiting factor may be loose stools due to the magnesium. Caution is also advised when administering magnesium to any patient with renal insufficiency, because the levels of magnesium can rise and cause severe skeletal muscle (including diaphragmatic) weakness.

Topical capsaicin cream appeared to be beneficial in FMS (McCarty et al. 1994) and could be used on locally painful areas in addition to a regimen of oral agents. The limiting factor seems to be the cutaneous burning sensation, which tends to decrease with use and may respond to topical lidocaine or a eutectic mixture of local anesthetics (EMLA) cream. Patients should be advised to use rubber gloves when applying capsaicin cream to the skin and to avoid getting it in the eyes or delicate mucous membranes.

St. John's wort has been used by some patients (dosage recommended by the manufacturer) as a mood modifier and antidepressant. There is evidence to suggest that the mechanism may be a combination of reuptake inhibition and inactivation of monoamine oxidase. As such, it would be expected to increase the availability of serotonin and perhaps norepinephrine to synaptic effector receptors.

The most convincing research evidence for benefit in FMS from a nonprescription medication relates to 5-hydroxytryptophan (5-HTP) (Caruso et al. 1990). Concern about a contaminant in commercial preparations of 5-HTP causing eosinophilia myalgia syndrome (Klarskov et al. 1999) has apparently been averted by an alteration in the method of preparation. Administration of 100 mg three times daily resulted in improvement of many of the symptoms associated with FMS (Caruso et al. 1990). Our experience in San Antonio suggests that this therapy takes 2 to 3 months to show benefit and then remains effective while the dosage is being maintained, but the symptoms return when it is discontinued.

Sedative hypnotics and antidepressants. The most commonly advocated medications program in the past still bears considerable merit. Low-dose, tricyclic, sedative, hypnotic medications are inexpensive and often are dramatically effective in fostering restful sleep when they are first administered. There is evidence for benefit from amitriptyline and cyclobenzaprine (Goldenberg et al. 1986; Quimby et al. 1989; Bengtsson et al. 1990; Carette et al. 1994), which are really very similar chemical formulas even though one was marketed as an antidepressant and the other as a muscle relaxant. It has been hypothesized that these agents increase serotonin availability to downregulate nociception. A typical maintenance regimen might include amitriptyline (10 to 35 mg hs) or cyclobenzaprine (2.5 to 10 mg hs). There is no logical reason to use both in the therapy of a given individual patient.

Several potential adverse effects can limit the usefulness of tricyclic drug therapy. Most patients have some trouble with anticholinergic effects such as dry mouth, which can be managed with frequent sips of water or glycerin swabs, but tachycardia can be intolerable. A frequent error is initiating therapy at too high a dosage. The chronically tired FMS patient may sleep continuously for 2 or more days after a single first dose of 10 to 25 mg of amitriptyline or 5 to 10 mg

of cyclobenzaprine and then discontinue the drug without an adequate trial.

Tachyphylaxis with either amitriptyline or cyclobenzaprine is another problem that appears to occur in most patients after 90 to 120 days of continuous use. Taking a 2- to 4-week holiday from the drug may reestablish more normal nerve cell reuptake receptor density and seems clinically to restore effectiveness. When the tricyclic drugs are discontinued for a "holiday," it seems logical that all serotonin reuptake drugs (including fluoxetine, paroxetine, cyclobenzaprine, tramadol, etc.) should also be held to allow central nervous system readaptation. During the holiday from the tricyclic drugs, or when they are poorly tolerated, alprazolam (0.5 to 1.0 mg hs) has been a useful substitute since its mechanism of action is quite different. Clonazepam or Sinemet have been advocated especially when the insomnia is due to nocturnal myoclonus. The beneficial action of carisoprodol (SOMA, 350 mg hs) may also relate to sedation. Zolpidem (Ambien), in low dosage, has proven beneficial for the insomnia associated with FMS (Moldofsky et al. 1996; Rothschild 1997) but because of its tendency to induce rebound insomnia if used constantly for weeks, we recommend that it be taken only three nights per week. Its mere availability for the worst nights tends to increase a patient's confidence in his ability to cope with his insomnia.

Since one of the theoretical goals of treatment with the tricyclic drugs was to increase the availability of serotonin, it seemed likely that the new highly selective serotonin reuptake inhibitors (SSRI drugs) might also be useful. To date, only the first drug approved in this class (fluoxetine HCl, Prozac) has been formally tested (Wolfe et al. 1994; Goldenberg et al. 1996a; Arnold et al. 2002) but most have been tried clinically. In the first study conducted with this agent (Wolfe et al. 1994), fluoxetine reduced the overall severity of depression in the treatment group but did not significantly alter the painful symptoms. One hypothetical explanation might be that the muscarinic, histaminergic, or α_1-adrenergic receptors, which are more substantially influenced by the tricyclic drugs than by fluoxetine, may be important to the mechanism of benefit. In a more recent study (Arnold et al. 2002), both depression and subjective pain were improved but there was no effect on the tender point examination findings. When given to patients with FMS, fluoxetine should be given in the morning to avoid worsening the insomnia. There is evidence to suggest that a combination of fluoxetine (10 to 20 mg) in the morning followed by amitriptyline (10 to 35 mg) in the evening provides more relief from pain than either agent alone (Goldenberg et al. 1996b), while avoiding the nighttime insomnia or daytime grogginess that can characterize each separately.

A more than theoretic concern relates to the use of multiple medications with the potential to alter the metabolism of serotonin in synergistic ways (Gillman 1998; Gordon 1998; Carbone 2000; Dams et al. 2001). The effect of administered 5-HTP would be to increase the production and thus the release of serotonin at the synapse. The tricyclics, the SSRIs, and tramadol inhibit the reuptake of serotonin. The monoamine oxidase inhibitor drugs and St. John's wort inhibit the metabolic inactivation of serotonin in the synapse. A combination of each of these mechanisms could result in a flood of unopposed serotonin at the effector receptors and cause the (hyper)serotonin syndrome. This toxic syndrome, which resembles the malignant neuroleptic syndrome, is characterized by mental status changes, autonomic instability, fevers, gastrointestinal dysfunction, and myoclonus. Gradual introduction of medications make it less likely that the syndrome would become severe before discovery. Treatment would require discontinuation of one or more of the offending medications.

Analgesics. Patients with FMS traditionally have been given antiinflammatory level dosages of nonsteroidal antiinflammatory drugs (NSAIDs). Our experience has suggested that the propionic acid NSAIDs are more useful than other classes of NSAIDs, but that has not been proven by comparative study. While there appeared to be some synergy with NSAIDs and sedative hypnotic drugs, such as amitriptyline (Goldenberg et al. 1986) and alprazolam (Russell et al. 1991), these agents have not proven to be independently effective (Yunus et al. 1989). Some clinicians have followed the typical chronic pain therapy sequence, beginning with mild narcotics in combination with acetaminophen and progressing to daily morphine or methadone, but there are no convincing clinical trials to indicate benefit from narcotic therapy in FMS. There is also the potential to cause a dependency with growing tachyphylaxis that will require supervised withdrawal in a person with nonmalignant chronic pain. In my San Antonio practice, I have considered it wise to avoid using narcotic drugs for FMS patients.

In a recently completed study (Russell et al. 2000), tramadol was used in divided dosages ranging from 50 mg to 400 mg per day. It was tolerated poorly by about 20% of FMS patients who experienced nausea, somnolence, dizziness, pruritus, constipation, or headache. For those who tolerated at least 50 mg/day, relief from pain was quite uniform and persisted for at least 6 weeks with continued therapy. In the past year or two, this drug has been the most commonly prescribed analgesic medication for FMS patients. Tramadol may facilitate sleep by relieving the pain but it is not very sedating. The author usually adds amitriptyline 10 to 25 mg hs or occasional zolpidem 5 to 10 mg hs to the daily therapy with tramadol. Tramadol has been shown to be synergistic with acetaminophen; that combination therefore is also available. Many questions about the use of tramadol in FMS remain to be established. For example, will it be subject to tachyphylaxis and, thus, benefit from periodic "holidays" as seen with the tricyclic drugs?

Anticonvulsants and others. A wide range of other medications used in the treatment of painful neuropathic conditions could be considered but research to define their role in FMS is lacking. They include other tricyclic antidepressants not formally tested in FMS

(imipramine, doxepin, desipramine, nortriptyline, amoxapine, trazodone); anxiolytics (buspirone); anesthetics (lidocaine, mexiletine); α_2-agonists (clonidine); γ-aminobutyric acid agonists (baclofen); anticonvulsants (clonazepam, carbamazepine, gabapentin); neuroleptics (fluphenazine, chlorpromazine, pimozide); and calcitonin. As already mentioned, opioid analgesics including codeine admixtures with non-narcotic analgesics are currently not recommended in the treatment of FMS because of the perceived risk of habituation in patients with chronic pain. Human growth hormone is expensive and requires parenteral administration but there is convincing evidence from a single study that it is helpful for many of the symptoms associated with FMS.

G. Establish goals. A therapy program needs to have goals that are achievable and will mark progress in the right direction. Some goal of therapy with a readily measurable outcome should be identified and clearly understood by both the patient and the physician. A publication about clinical evidence (Anon. 2001) advocates the utilization of outcomes that matter to patients, meaning that those patients themselves are aware of, such as symptom severity, quality of life, level of physical dysfunction, or walking distance. That same source has, however, so far avoided the vexing question of what constitutes a clinically important change in a clinical outcome measure. For an FMS patient, the goal could be a defined improvement in the ability to sleep through the night, or to accomplish the tasks of the day without unbearable pain. Readily available measures of severity could be the Modified Health Assessment score, the Visual Analog Scale score for pain, or the duration of morning stiffness that can be easily recorded by the patient while waiting to see the doctor. Making the patient aware of any improvement in these subjective measures can be encouraging for both the patient and the physician.

H. Follow-up. It is difficult to extrapolate what may be optimal follow-up in a variety of physician–patient relationships and in other health care delivery settings. It is generally observed that FMS patients appreciate access to the physician at fairly frequent intervals (perhaps every 1 to 2 months for three visits) immediately after diagnosis and then do well with less frequent visits (perhaps every 3 to 4 months) thereafter. Visits can be used to document the severity of the tender point pain, to supportively monitor the patient's progress with the exercise program, the use of medications, the quality of sleep, and efforts toward self-education. The tone of the interaction should not be: patient—"I'm not better, what are you going to do about it?" but rather: physician—"You are still having quite a bit of trouble, lets see how we can work together more effectively to make the most of the limited numbers of proven treatment options available."

I. Health maintenance. Many physicians involved in the care of FMS patients have the persistent disquieting feeling that there might be something that has been missed. Could the patient have cancer, myelopathy, or vasculitis as the cause of such severe pain? That concern is probably born of both a true concern for the patient and a fear of being sued because something was not discovered in time. There is no clear evidence of an association between FMS and any form of malignancy. It seems prudent to maintain a standard health maintenance program but to focus on the management of the most troublesome symptoms.

J. Consultation. At present, between 5 and 25 million people in the United States have FMS. About 6% to 10% of the patients in the general medical or family physicians' waiting rooms are individuals with FMS. Considering these statistics, consultant physicians cannot provide care for all of them. The primary care physician should develop an understanding of the disorder and follow a systematic approach to providing care for these patients. Recognizing that a cure is not available, most physicians should be able to provide ongoing supportive care for the majority of FMS patients. However, some patients will exhibit symptoms out of proportion to the rest or unusual complications that require consultation. The referral should be directed to the physician with the most experience and success in dealing with such challenges in FMS patients or the subspecialist best fitting the reason for the referral if it involves an organ system.

REFERENCES

Anon.: *Clinical Evidence.* London, BMJ, 2001, p. xvi.

Arnold LM, Hess EV, Hudson JI, et al: A randomized, placebo-controlled, double-blind, flexible-dose study of fluoxetine in the treatment of women with fibromyalgia (see comments). *Am J Med* 2002;112:191–197.

Baer PG, Cagen LM: Platelet activating factor vasoconstriction of dog kidney. Inhibition by alprazolam. *Hypertension* 1987;9:253–260.

Basu T, Dickerson J, Raven R, Williams DC: The thiamin status of patients with cancer as determined by the red cell transketolase activity. *Int J Vitam Nutr Res* 1974;44:53–58.

Bengtsson A, Ernerudh J, Vrethem M, Skogh T: Absence of autoantibodies in primary fibromyalgia. *J Rheumatol* 1990;17:1682–1683.

Bennett RM, Clark SR, Burckhardt CS, Cook D: IGF-1 assays and other GH tests in 500 fibromyalgia patients. *J Musculoskelet Pain* 1995;3(Suppl 1):109 (Abstr).

Bennett RM, Clark SC, Walczyk J: A randomized, double-blind, placebo-controlled study of growth hormone in the treatment of fibromyalgia. *Am J Med* 1998;104:227–231.

Bradley LA: Cognitive-behavioral therapy for primary fibromyalgia (review). *J Rheumatol* 1989;19:131–136.

Carbone JR: The neuroleptic malignant and serotonin syndromes (review). *Emerg Med Clin North Am* 2000;18:317–325.

Carette S, Bell JJ, Reynolds WJ, et al: Comparison of amitriptyline, cyclobenzaprine, and placebo in the treatment of fibromyalgia: a randomized, double-blind clinical trial. *Arthritis Rheum* 1994; 37: 30–40.

Caruso I, Sarzi Puttini P, Cazzola M, Azzolini V: Double-blind study of 5-hydroxytryptophan versus placebo in the treatment of primary fibromyalgia syndrome. *J Int Med Res* 1990;18:201–209.

Clark SR, Jones KD, Burckhardt CS, Bennett R: Exercise for patients with fibromyalgia: risks versus benefits. *Curr Rheumatol Rep* 2001;3:135–140.

Dams R, Benijts TH, Lambert WE, et al: A fatal case of serotonin syndrome after combined moclobemide-citalopram intoxication. *J Anal Toxicol* 2001;25:147–151.

Eisinger J, Ayavou T: Transketolase stimulation in fibromyalgia. *J Am Coll Nutr* 1990;9:56–57.

Eisinger J, Ayavou T, Zakarian H, Plantamura A: Abnormalities of thiamin dependent enzymes in fibromyalgia. Unpublished manuscript, 1996.

Ferraccioli G, Ghirelli L, Scita F, et al: EMG-biofeedback training in fibromyalgia syndrome. *J Rheumatol* 1987;14:820–825.

Gillman PK: Serotonin syndrome: history and risk (review). *Fund Clin Pharmacol* 1998;12:482–491.

Goldenberg DL, Felson DT, Dinerman H: A randomized, controlled trial of amitriptyline and naproxen in the treatment of patients with fibromyalgia. *Arthritis Rheum* 1986;29:1371–1377.

Goldenberg D, Mayskiy M, Mossey C, et al: A randomized, double-blind crossover trial of fluoxetine and amitriptyline in the treatment of fibromyalgia. *Arthritis Rheum* 1996a;39: 1852–1859.

Goldenberg DL, Mayskly M, Mossey C, et al: The independent and combined efficacy of fluoxetine and amitriptyline in the treatment of fibromyalgia. *Arthritis Rheum* 1996b;39: 1852–1859.

Gordon JB: SSRIs and St.John's wort: possible toxicity? *Am Fam Physician* 1998;57:950.

Jentoft ES, Kvalvik AG, Mengshoel AM: Effects of pool-based and land-based aerobic exercise on women with fibromyalgia/chronic widespread muscle pain. *Arthritis Care Res* 2001;45:42–47(Abstr).

Klarskov K, Johnson KL, Benson LM, et al: Eosinophilia-myalgia syndrome case-associated contaminants in commercially available 5-hydroxytryptophan. *Adv Exp Med Biol* 1999;467:461–468.

Kornecki E, Ehrlich YH, Lenox RH: Platelet-activating factor-induced aggregation of human platelets specifically inhibited by triazolobenzodiazepines. *Science* 1984;226:1454–1456.

McCain GA, Bell DA, Mai FM, Halliday PD: A controlled study of the effects of a supervised cardiovascular fitness training program on the manifestations of primary fibromyalgia. *Arthritis Rheum* 1998; 31:1135–1141.

McCarty DJ, Csuka M, McCarthy G, Trotter D: Treatment of pain due to fibromyalgia with topical capsaicin: a pilot study. *Semin Arthritis Rheum* 1994;23:41–51.

Mengshoel AM, Komnaes HB, Forre O: The effects of 20 weeks of physical fitness training in female patients with fibromyalgia. *Clin Exp Rheum* 1992;10:345–349.

Moldofsky H, Lue FA, Mously C, et al: The effect of zolpidem in patients with fibromyalgia: a dose ranging, double blind, placebo controlled, modified crossover study (see comments). *J Rheumatol* 1996; 23:529–533.

Nielson WR, Walker C, McCain GA: Cognitive behavioral treatment of fibromyalgia syndrome: preliminary findings. *J Rheumatol* 1992; 19:98–103.

Quimby LG, Gratwick GM, Whitney CD, Block SR: A randomized trial of cyclobenzaprine for the treatment of fibromyalgia. *J Rheumatol* (Suppl) 1989;19:140–143.

Rothschild BM: Zolpidem efficacy in fibromyalgia (letter; comment). *J Rheumatol* 1997;24:1012–1013.

Russell IJ: Fibromyalgia. In: Loeser JD (ed) *Bonica's Management of Pain*, 3rd ed. Philadelphia, Lippincott Williams & Wilkins, 2001, pp. 543–559.

Russell IJ, Fletcher EM, Michalek JE, et al: Treatment of primary fibrositis/fibromyalgia syndrome with ibuprofen and alprazolam. A double-blind, placebo-controlled study. *Arthritis Rheum* 1991; 34:552–560.

Russell IJ, Michalek JE, MacKillip F, et al: Treatment of fibromyalgia syndrome with malic acid and magnesium: a randomized, double-blind, placebo-controlled, cross-over study. *J Rheumatol* 1995; 22:953–958.

Russell IJ, Kamin M, Bennett RM, et al: Efficacy of tramadol in treatment of pain in fibromyalgia. *J Clin Rheumatol* 2000;6:250–257.

Russell IJ, Michalek J, Xiao YM, et al: Effects of tizanidine HCl tablets on cerebrospinal fluid substance P in human subjects with fibromyalgia syndrome. *J Musculoskelet Pain* 2001;9(Suppl 5):96 (Abstr).

White KP, Nielson WR: Cognitive behavioral treatment of fibromyalgia syndrome: a followup assessment. *J Rheumatol* 1995;22:717–721.

Wolfe F, Smythe HA, Yunus MB, et al: The American College of Rheumatology 1990 Criteria for the Classification of Fibromyalgia. *Arthritis Rheum* 1990;33:160–172.

Wolfe F, Cathey MA, Hawley DJ: A double-blind placebo controlled trial of fluoxetine in fibromyalgia. *Scand J Rheumatol* 1994;23:255–259.

Yunus MB, Masi AT, Aldag JC: Short term effects of ibuprofen in primary fibromyalgia syndrome: a double blind, placebo controlled trial [published erratum appears in *J Rheumatol* 1989 Jun;16:855]. *J Rheumatol* 1989;16:527–532.

Rheumatoid Arthritis

BERT BLACKWELL

Rheumatoid arthritis (RA) is a systemic autoimmune disorder. The ensuing inflammatory changes are almost uniformly associated with pain. Erosion of articular surfaces is a prominent feature, and new bone formation and remodeling are noticeably absent (unlike osteoarthritis). Synovial proliferation is a common feature of RA. Pain may vary with the stage of the illness and may arise from complications of therapy (e.g., steroid-associated avascular necrosis). Physical examination findings are highly variable and do not show good correlation with the pain complaints.

A. Each joint should be carefully evaluated to assess joint effusion, synovial thickening, erythema, or warmth. Joint stability and deformity should also be noted.

B. Evaluation should include the erythrocyte sedimentation rate and rheumatoid factor (RF) and antinuclear antibody (ANA) assays. There is as much as a 5% false-positive rate associated with the RF and ANA testing, so the history and physical examination results must be carefully reviewed before basing the diagnosis on laboratory testing. Radiographs show typical inflammatory changes; but unlike osteoarthritis, new bone formation and remodeling features are conspicuously absent.

C. Pain in RA patients is highly correlated with psychological stress relating to fears of debility, loss of self-image, and change in lifestyle. Education and counseling has been shown to reduce pain by up to 19% in this population. Energy conservation and joint protection techniques can help reduce the severity and frequency of exacerbations while allowing relatively normal functioning.

D. Nonsteroidal antiinflammatory drugs (NSAIDs) have been the primary pharmacologic treatment for RA pain. Side effects such as platelet inactivation, gastrointestinal (GI) ulceration, and renal toxicity have been problematic and have led to the development of cyclooxygenase-2 (COX-2) selective agents. Although COX-2 agents produce significantly less platelet inactivation, and there is slightly less risk of GI ulceration, renal toxicity is still prevalent. Also, the risk of cardiovascular events is increased with the use of COX-2 inhibitors. NSAIDs alone are rarely effective for treating pain in RA patients. Treatment almost always involves the use of disease-modifying antirheumatic drugs. Systemic steroids are especially useful for treating inflammatory flare-ups but are not desirable for long-term treatment secondary to side effects. Tramadol or opioid analgesics may be needed when satisfactory relief is not obtained. Complex regimens and new drug developments often necessitate a rheumatology consult early in the course of disease.

E. Numerous modalities for treating RA pain have been attempted, including hydrotherapy, transcutaneous nerve stimulation, paraffin dips, diathermy, ultrasound application, fluidotherapy, hot packs, and ice. The success of these treatments was largely based on patient satisfaction. Recent studies have shown that application of heat may actually facilitate the inflammatory response. For this reason, it is recommended that heat application be avoided when possible. When unavoidable, the duration of heat application should be limited to 5 to 10 minutes.

F. Intraarticular steroid injections can provide excellent results and specifically target and modulate the pathologic inflammatory response. By giving local injections, the deleterious systemic side effects are largely avoided. However, such procedures are not without risk of infection and atrophy, especially in structures already compromised by an autoimmune disease process.

G. More than 90% of patients with severe, incapacitating RA have shown excellent pain relief following total hip or knee replacement. Surgery should be entertained as an option whenever the patient has intractable pain, severe deformity, or joint instability.

REFERENCES

Bellamy N, Bradley L: Conference summary: workshop on chronic pain, pain control, and patient outcomes in rheumatoid and osteoarthritis. *Arthritis Rheum* 1996;39:357.

Klippel JH (ed): *Primer on Rheumatic Diseases.* Atlanta, Arthritis Foundation, 1997.

Oosterveld FG, Rasker JJ: Treating arthritis with locally applied heat or cold. *Semin Arthritis Rheum* 1994;24:82.

Rice JR, Pietsky DS: Pain in the rheumatic diseases. *Rheum Dis Clin North Am* 1999;25:15.

RHEUMATOID ARTHRITIS

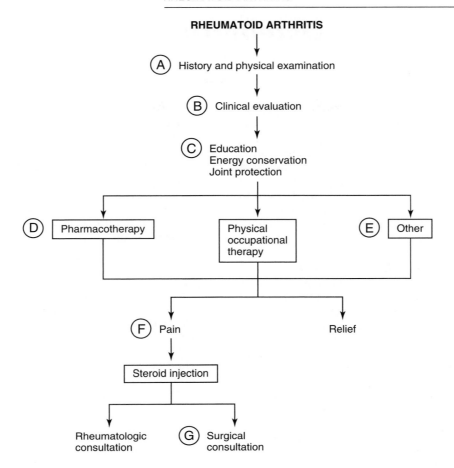

Osteoarthritis

BERT BLACKWELL

Osteoarthritis (OA) is the most common joint disease, affecting 80% of people over age 50. Until recently OA was thought to be noninflammatory in nature and was described as a degenerative joint disease. Recent studies have shown ongoing low-grade inflammation. The exact etiology remains unclear. The pathologic process results in destruction of cartilage and bony overgrowth adjacent to the joint. Joint deformity without swelling of the distal interphalangeal joints and first metacarpal joints is often seen.

A. Clinical evaluation includes plain radiographs, which almost always show joint space narrowing. Osteophytes, subchondral cysts, and osteosclerosis may also be seen. Laboratory tests are of little value except when used to exclude similar conditions. Crepitus and decreased range of motion are common findings. None of these diagnostic findings shows good correlation with pain.

B. Education is key to slowing progression of the disease and preventing exacerbations. Joint protection and energy conservation strategies can provide a great deal of symptomatic relief. Obesity has been shown to correlate with an increased incidence of hip and knee OA. Even modest weight reduction can have a significant positive impact on disease progression.

C. Joint instability can be extremely problematic in that it not only exacerbates pain but can be unsafe in weight-bearing joints, leading to debility. Bracing may allow increased safety with weight-bearing and prevent further deleterious joint changes. When bracing is ineffective or impossible (especially in weight-bearing joints), surgery should be considered.

D. Therapies are directed at maintaining functional range of motion, strengthening muscles crossing affected joints, and preventing debility.

E. Heat and cold have each been shown to be effective for symptomatic pain relief. Neither modality has been shown to be superior. The modality chosen should be based on patient response.

F. Nonsteroidal anti-inflammatory drugs (NSAIDs) and acetaminophen are the mainstays of OA pharmacotherapy. NSAIDs are associated with the risk of gastrointestinal (GI) toxicity, although it can be minimized by concurrent misoprostil administration. Cyclooxygenase-2 (COX-2) selective inhibitors produce somewhat less GI toxicity and have considerably less antiplatelet activity. When satisfactory pain relief cannot be attained by the aforementioned, consideration should be given to using tramadol or opioid analgesics. Tramadol is not associated with renal or GI toxicity like NSAIDs and is less constipating than opioids. Long-acting opioid preparations are preferred and should be administered on a scheduled rather than as-needed basis. Chronic opioid use necessitates a bowel program to prevent constipation. Oral naloxone administration can be used to reverse opioid-induced constipation without systemic effects as it is not absorbed from the GI tract.

G. Intra-articular steroid injection can be extremely effective for relieving pain, particularly if inflammation is present. Injections are not without risk, however, and should be used judiciously only when other avenues of treatment have been unsuccessful.

H. Surgery can provide dramatic pain relief. Removal of structures affected by disease lead to prompt cessation of pain generation. The excellent success rate of hip and knee replacement procedures and the relatively small risks merit consideration of surgery early in the disease progress.

REFERENCES

Braddom RL: *Physical Medicine and Rehabilitation*. Philadelphia, Saunders, 1996.

McCarberg BH, Herr KA: Osteoarthritis: how to manage pain and improve patient function. *Geriatrics* 2001;56:14.

Meissner W, Schmidt U, Hartmann M, et al: Oral naloxone reverses opioid-associated constipation. *Pain* 2000;84:105.

Rice JR, Pietsky DS: Pain in the rheumatic diseases. *Rheum Dis Clin North Am* 1999;25:15.

OSTEOARTHRITIS

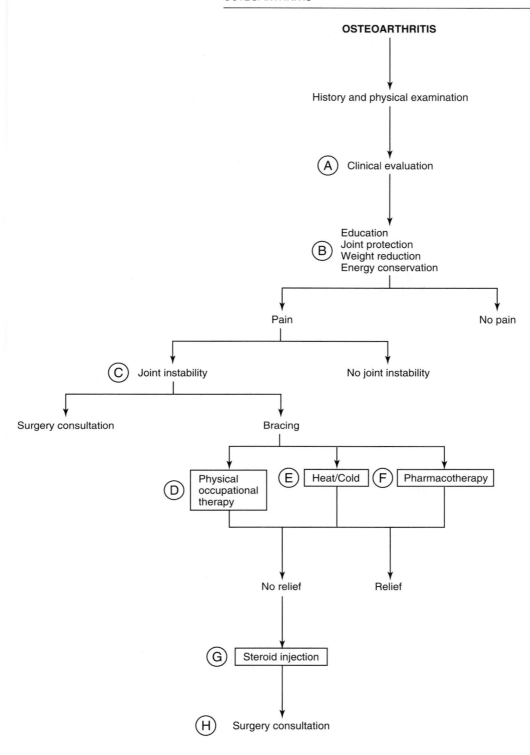

History and physical examination

(A) Clinical evaluation

(B) Education
Joint protection
Weight reduction
Energy conservation

Pain   No pain

(C) Joint instability   No joint instability

Surgery consultation   Bracing

(D) Physical occupational therapy   (E) Heat/Cold   (F) Pharmacotherapy

No relief   Relief

(G) Steroid injection

(H) Surgery consultation

Discogenic Back Pain

OCTAVIO CALVILLO AND IOANNIS SHARIBAS

One of the greatest challenges for physicians is accurately diagnosing the cause of low back pain. Discogenic pain can be categorized into three entities: internal disc disruption (IDD), degenerative disc disease, and segmental instability. This chapter deals predominantly with IDD as a source of axial lumbar pain. IDD is not to be confused with disc herniation or disc degeneration.

The etiology of IDD has not been definitively established, but it probably results from a compression injury causing an end-plate fracture; this in turn triggers inflammatory degradation of the nucleus pulposus and eventually of the annulus fibrosus in the form of annular fissures. The disc becomes painful as a result of chemical irritation of nerve endings in the outer annulus. The external perimeter of the disc remains intact and essentially normal. For this reason the condition is not evident on computed tomography (CT) or magnetic resonance imaging (MRI) scans, and it does not cause neurologic symptoms. The term internal disc disruption was coined by Crock (1970). The concept was based on a retrospective analysis of a large number of patients who continued to complain of disabling back and leg pain following operations for disc prolapse. With IDD the spinal nerve may not be mechanically compressed, but there is neurogenic inflammation due to leakage of nuclear material through annular fissures. The condition is characterized by alterations of the internal structure and metabolic functions of the intervertebral disc, usually following severe trauma to the spine. The clinical syndrome may include axial lumbar pain with variable radiation patterns and diffuse aching leg pain aggravated by physical activity, particularly activities that increase the compressive forces on the spine. In some patients, a profound loss of energy, reduction of body weight, and clinical depression may also ensue.

Patients may have limited flexion and extension secondary to pain. Nerve root tension signs are negative. The neurologic examination is usually normal. Motor, sensory, and reflex changes are uncommon.

Diagnostic evaluation by plain radiography or CT scans is usually noncontributory. MRI scans play an important but not exclusive role in the diagnosis of IDD.

Correlation studies of MRI and cryomicrotome specimens have improved our understanding of annular fissures. Three types of annular tear have been described: type I, concentric outer annular tears; type 2, radial annular tears; type 3, transverse annular tears. These fissures can be demonstrated on MRI scans with the use of gadolinium. A high-intensity zone on T2 echography has been demonstrated to correlate with annular fissures and pain during discography (April and Bogduk 1992). MRI scanning can be used as a screening tool prior to performing discography.

Discography, a diagnostic procedure designed to ascertain whether a disc is intrinsically painful, is the single most important test for diagnosing IDD. Since its introduction, discography has been a controversial subject, and it has undergone some modifications. The introduction of discography utilizing manometry, has added a significant degree of objectivity to the procedure. The specificity of discography has been demonstrated in various studies. Discography is an accepted diagnostic test for evaluating the intervertebral disc. The diagnosis of IDD requires a demonstration of pain during discography associated with a grade 3 or more annular tear seen on the CT scan after discography (Moneta et al. 1994).

A commonly recommended treatment for IDD is interbody fusion. This surgical approach may be satisfactory in well selected patients, but it is associated with a high failure rate. Nonsurgical percutaneous intradiscal treatments for IDD have been devised and are discussed in Chapter 114, p. 306.

REFERENCES

April C, Bogduk N: High intensity zone: a diagnostic sign of painful lumbar disc on magnetic resonance imaging. *Br J Radiol* 1992;65:361–369.

Crock HV: A reappraisal of intervertebral disc lesions. *Med J Aust* 1970;1:983–989.

Moneta GB, Videman T, Kaivantok, et al: Reported pain during lumbar discography as a function of annular ruptures and disc degeneration: a reanalysis of 833 discograms. *Spine* 1994;19:1968–1974.

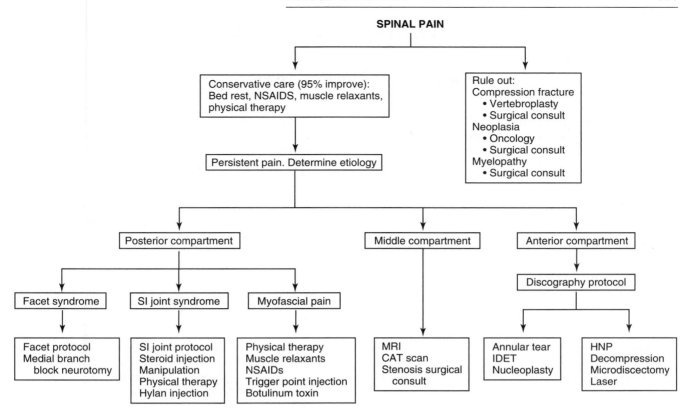

SPINAL PAIN

Conservative care (95% improve):
Bed rest, NSAIDS, muscle relaxants,
physical therapy

Rule out:
Compression fracture
• Vertebroplasty
• Surgical consult
Neoplasia
• Oncology
• Surgical consult
Myelopathy
• Surgical consult

Persistent pain. Determine etiology

Posterior compartment

Middle compartment

Anterior compartment

Facet syndrome

SI joint syndrome

Myofascial pain

Discography protocol

Facet protocol
Medial branch
  block neurotomy

SI joint protocol
Steroid injection
Manipulation
Physical therapy
Hylan injection

Physical therapy
Muscle relaxants
NSAIDs
Trigger point injection
Botulinum toxin

MRI
CAT scan
Stenosis surgical
  consult

Annular tear
IDET
Nucleoplasty

HNP
Decompression
Microdiscectomy
Laser

Nonsomatic Pain

LAWRENCE S. SCHOENFELD AND TRACY SLOAN

Treatment for chronic pain can be planned effectively only after distinguishing between patients whose pain has a primarily somatic etiology and those with nonsomatic pain. By further differentiating the nonsomatic pain patients into primary subgroups (malingering/factitious, somatoform, mood disorders, drug-seeking), target psychological-social-economic issues can be resolved. Although this protocol has limitations and is costly, it helps reduce unwarranted somatic interventions, iatrogenic injury, and abnormal illness behavior. Etiology is quickly established through a collaborative evaluation with an anesthesiologist and mental health professional (psychologist or psychiatrist).

A. Two diagnostic techniques (diagnostic epidural opioid method and the intravenous Pentothal test) are helpful for identifying the patient with chronic nonsomatic pain. The diagnostic epidural opioid technique may identify patients with chronic pain primarily under operant control. In the nonsomatic pain patient, the Pentothal pain test often dramatically demonstrates the absence of a pain response under Pentothal using maneuvers that had demonstrated significant pain behavior before the Pentothal induction.

B. A pain-psychological evaluation investigates motivation, cognition, and mood associated with the chronic pain condition. Under Amytal sedation, conflict areas can be further explored. Low-dose Amytal produces relaxation and improvement in patients with somatoform and mood disorders and worsening of pain complaints (with increased anxiety) in malingerers. With moderate-dose Amytal, the patient with a somatoform disorder demonstrates significant physical improvement, often with spontaneous abreaction, whereas the malingerer often complains about the test, demonstrates guarding behavior, and may become hostile.

   1. Typically, cognitive-behavioral therapy or the use of antidepressants (or both) effectively reduces chronic pain behaviors. Establishing a cooperative therapeutic relationship usually requires special physician attention to enhance treatment cooperation and compliance.

C. Malingering patients are informed that there is nothing significantly wrong with them physically or psychologically. They are encouraged to return to normal activities. Primary gains should not be supported by medical attention, treatment, or medical excuses. It is difficult to engage patients with malingering/factitious disorders in treatment because most discontinue the treatment when discovered or confronted.

D. A somatoform disorder (pain disorder) may develop in response to a variety of conflicts, including difficulties dealing with sexuality, marital dysfunction, and job-related stress. An interdisciplinary pain management program provides a setting in which pain patients usually are able to accept psychological intervention. Randomized trials support the efficacy of both individual and group cognitive-behavioral therapy for reducing distress and disability.

E. Depression often continues after an injury or peripheral illness has resolved, resulting in further disuse and associated chronic pain. Mobilizing the patient's coping strategies with antidepressant medication, activity programs, and psychotherapy (group and individual cognitive-behavioral therapy, interpersonal psychotherapy, psychodynamic psychotherapy) results in a successful treatment outcome.

F. Drug-seeking behavior should be confronted openly and detoxification programs offered. Successful treatment requires periodic drug screening and supportive psychological therapy.

REFERENCES

Cherry DA, Gourlay GK, McLachlan M, Cousins MJ: Diagnostic epidural opioid blockade and chronic pain. *Pain* 1985;21:143.

Ellis J, Ramamurthy S, Schoenfeld LS, et al: Diagnostic epidural opioid technique. *Clin Pain* 1989;5:21.

Russo MR, Brooks FR, Fontenot JP, et al: Sodium Pentothal hypnosis: a procedure for evaluating medical patients with suspected psychiatric comorbidity. *Milit Med* 1997;162:215.

Schoichet RP: Sodium amytal in the diagnosis of chronic pain. *Can Psychiatr Assoc J* 1978;23:219.

Simon GE: Management of somatoform and factitious disorders. In: Nathan PE, Gorman JM (eds) *A Guide to Treatments that Work.* New York, Oxford University Press, 1998, p 423.

Simon EP, Dahl LF: The sodium pentathol hypnosis interview with follow-up treatment for complex regional pain syndrome. *J Pain Symptom Manage* 1999;18:132.

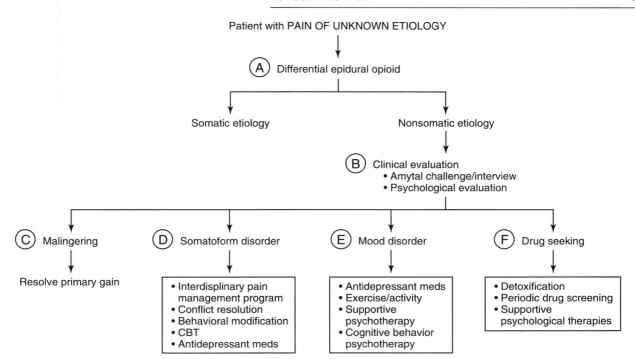

Patient with PAIN OF UNKNOWN ETIOLOGY

(A) Differential epidural opioid

Somatic etiology

Nonsomatic etiology

(B) Clinical evaluation
• Amytal challenge/interview
• Psychological evaluation

(C) Malingering

Resolve primary gain

(D) Somatoform disorder

• Interdisplinary pain
  management program
• Conflict resolution
• Behavioral modification
• CBT
• Antidepressant meds

(E) Mood disorder

• Antidepressant meds
• Exercise/activity
• Supportive
  psychotherapy
• Cognitive behavior
  psychotherapy

(F) Drug seeking

• Detoxification
• Periodic drug screening
• Supportive
  psychological therapies

HIV-AIDS

NIKESH BATRA

People with human immunodeficiency virus (HIV) infection suffer pain that is comparable to cancer pain. This pain, however, is often not recognized or is undertreated. This situation occurs mainly because physicians often neglect pain management and focus instead on other problems, such as life-threatening opportunistic infections. There is an inability to assess pain properly and limited knowledge of current pharmacotherapeutic approaches. Furthermore, there is an overzealous trepidation about the addiction potential and the adverse effects of the strong opioids required for adequate pain control. The patients also have limited expectation regarding pain relief and are reluctant to bring up pain as a focus of care.

The most common pain syndromes encountered in patients with acquired immunodeficiency syndrome (AIDS) include, but are not limited to, painful sensory peripheral neuropathy, headache, oral and pharyngeal pain, extensive Kaposi's sarcoma, abdominal pain, chest pain, arthralgias and myalgias, and painful skin conditions. These syndromes may be due to the direct effects of the HIV infection and immunosuppression to the medications used to treat AIDS. These patients also may have concomitant medical problems causing their pain.

Headache is one of the most common pains encountered in the HIV-infected patient. Mostly the headache is the stress/tension type, but it may be related to more portentous conditions, such as HIV encephalitis, toxoplasmosis, or lymphoma. Central nervous system infections should especially be kept in mind when CD4 counts fall below 200. Headache may also be related to azidothymidine (AZT) therapy.

About 30% of patients with HIV develop predominantly sensory neuropathy characterized by pain and numbness in the toes and feet; ankles, calves, and fingers are involved in more advanced cases. On physical examination these patients have reduced sharp pain and vibratory sensation, reduced or absent deep tendon reflexes especially ankle jerks, and sometimes allodynia in the affected area. Electromyography/nerve conduction velocity tests show a predominantly axonal neuropathy. Other neuropathies seen in HIV patients include toxic neuropathy, where the clinical features are the same as above but they occur after initiation of anti-HIV medications such as dideoxyinosine (ddi), dideoxycytidine (ddc), and stavudine (d4t). HIV-infected patients may also suffer from other peripheral neuropathies, such as tarsal tunnel syndrome, HIV-associated myopathy/AZT myopathy, polyradiculitis, vascular myelopathy, and inflammatory demyelinating polyneuropathies.

Abdominal pain in AIDS patients may be accompanied by changes in bowel habits (more often diarrhea) and may be due to infections such as cryptosporidiosis, which may lead to organomegaly and obstruction. A variety of rheumatologic conditions have been reported in AIDS patients, ranging from Reiter's syndrome to psoriatic arthritis, septic arthritis, vasculitis, Sjögren's syndrome, polymyositis, AZT myopathy, and dermatomyositis. Oropharyngeal ulcers may cause pain, and extensive Kaposi's sarcoma may cause local skin pain.

Pain in the pediatric HIV population may be caused by *Candida* dermatitis, oral and esophageal candidiasis, Herpes zoster infection, *Mycobacterium avium intracellulare* infection, cryptosporidiosis induced intestinal infections, dental caries, various abscesses and cellulitis, hepatosplenomegaly, and encephalopathic spasticity.

AIDS patients with pain have significantly more depression, more hopelessness, and greater overall psychological distress, including more suicidal ideation, than AIDS patients without pain.

The impact of a diagnosis of HIV seropositivity is devastating and argues that optimal pain management be multimodal and multidisciplinary in nature. Such an approach calls for access to pharmacologic, psychotherapeutic, cognitive-behavioral, anesthetic, neurosurgical, and rehabilitative interventions. A careful initial assessment would include determining the qualitative features of the pain, its time course, and the maneuvers that improve or worsen it. Pain intensity and pain descriptors play a role in the treatment of pain.

Although the World Health Organization approach to cancer pain has not yet been systematically validated for AIDS, the approach has been recommended for that purpose by the Agency for Health Care Policy and Research panel and other clinical authorities in the field of AIDS pain management. The pharmacologic management of pain in AIDS patients should include judicious use of nonsteroidal antiinflammatory drugs and weak and strong opioids administered around the clock and as needed. Adjuvant agents are added to enhance pain control. The important adjuvants include antidepressants, anticonvulsants, oral local anesthetics, corticosteroids, neuroleptics, anxiolytics, psychostimulants, laxatives, and antiemetics.

A variety of physical and psychological therapies may also prove useful in the management of HIV-related pain. Physical interventions range from cutaneous stimulation (heat cold and massage) to transcutaneous nerve stimulation to acupuncture. Patient information, as for all chronic pain syndromes, plays an important role in AIDS patients. Psychological interventions such as hypnosis, biofeedback, and reframing by a trained psychologist also play an important role.

Procedures such as nerve blocks, cordotomy, and intrathecal delivery of analgesics are options for patients whose pain cannot be managed by oral medications and other modalities.

Physicians treating HIV-infected patients should be extraordinarily careful when diagnosing the various pain syndromes and recognizing the potentially treatable ones. Pain should be treated aggressively in these patients to reduce the co-morbid psychological conditions and to enhance their quality of life.

REFERENCES

Breitbart W: Pain in human immunodeficiency virus disease. In: Loeser JD (ed) *Bonica's Management of Pain*, 3rd ed. Philadelphia, Lippincott Williams & Wilkins, 2001.

Breitbart W, McDonald MV: Pharmacological pain management in HIV/AIDS. *J Int Assoc Physicians AIDS Care* 1996;2:17–26.

Larue F, Fontaine A, Colleau SM: Underestimation and under-treatment of pain in HIV disease: multicentre study. *BMJ* 1997; 314:23–28.

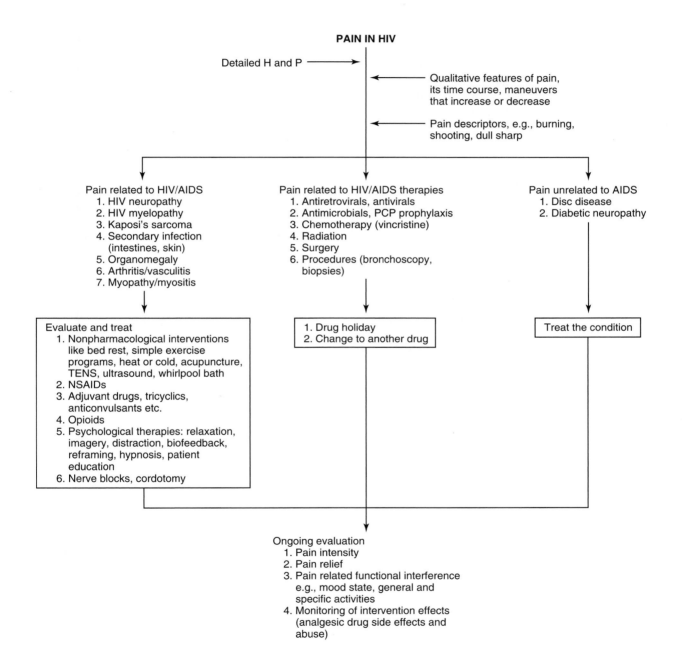

Sickle Cell Disease

SOMAYAJI RAMAMURTHY

Sickle cell disease results from an autosomal dominant related disorder of a single gene resulting in the abnormality of the hemoglobin B chain. This disease is more prevalent in the populations of African, Middle Eastern, and Mediterranean countries. This results in an abnormal sickle shape of the red blood cells (RBCs). The hemoglobin S in the presence of low oxygen saturation produces sickling of RBCs and occlusion of blood vessels, leading to ischemia of tissues and organs. This leads to chronic anemia, splenic infarctions, renal dysfunction, etc. Chronic pain with very severe episodes of acute pain is common in 60% to 80% of patients. Severe pain is the cause of 90% of hospital admissions. Pain is usually related to ischemia resulting in perivascular necrosis of the bone marrow, causing bone pain that may lead to osteomyelitis. Priapism requiring surgical intervention, abdominal pain secondary to splenic and mesentric infarcts, gallbladder disease, chest wall pain, strokes, renal failure, and skin ulceration contribute to severe pain and also to the significant morbidity and mortality.

Pain, which starts at an early age, significantly interferes with normal childhood, education, and employability. This creates a socioeconomic situation that makes it difficult to afford suitable medical care. Psychologic impairment associated with severe pain and the socioeconomic condition results in frustration, depression, and psychiatric impairment. The above conditions further impede the appropriate pain management with opioids.

Sickle cell disease is usually managed with nonsteroidal antiinflammatory drugs (NSAIDs), analgesics, hydroxyurea, and blood transfusions. Bone marrow transplantation has been very effective.

A. Thorough history, physical examination, and review of records are necessary before instituting therapy.
B. A multidisciplinary approach is needed, especially to evaluate the psychologic and social issues that are very commonly associated in patients with sickle cell disease.
C. NSAIDs and mild opioids may be sufficient to control the mild to moderate pain.

When the patient is admitted with severe pain, intravenous patient-controlled analgesia (PCA) with opioids is likely to be most effective. Continuous regional blocks may be appropriate when there is severe localized pain such as priapism or extremity pain. Meperidine should be avoided because of its propensity to produce seizure secondary to its metabolite normeperidine, which is likely to accumulate with chronic use, especially in the presence of renal impairment.

Patients treated in day hospitals appear to obtain significant pain control with decreased hospital admissions and associated cost savings. Patients with significant organ failure and severe pain are good candidates for palliative care to address psychologic, social, quality of life, and spiritual issues and adequately address functional restoration.

REFERENCES

Payne R: Pain management in sickle cell anemia. *Anesthesiol Clin North Am* 1997;15:305.

Brookoff D, Polomano R: Treating sickle cell pain like cancer pain. *Ann Intern Med* 1992;116: 364.

Benjamin LJ, Swinson GI, Nagel RL: Sickle cell anemia day hospital: an approach for the management of uncomplicated painful crisis. *Blood* 2000;95:1130–1136.

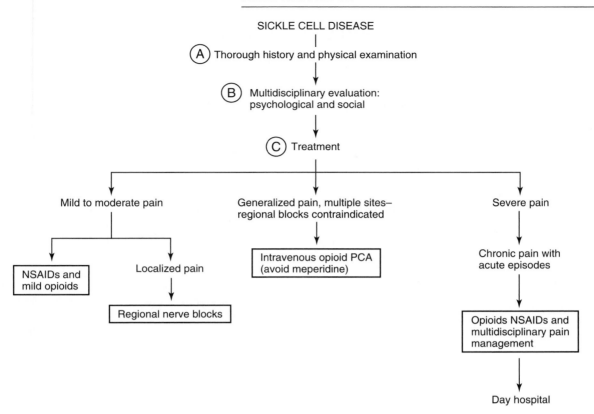

Groin Pain

SOMAYAJI RAMAMURTHY

A. Chronic pain in the groin can present a significant diagnostic challenge as it can be caused by numerous structures. Moreover, it may be referred pain from various intra- and extra-abdominal structures. A thorough review of the patient's history and medical records, previous surgical therapies, and psychosocial and sexual history is essential to be certain that gastrointestinal, urologic, gynecologic, and other intra-abdominal sources of referred pain had been adequately evaluated.

1. Gastrointestinal origin: A number of structures can produce groin pain. Inguinal hernia is one of the most common causes of groin pain; others are femoral hernia, Crohn's disease, and tumors of the colon.

2. Urogenital origin: Diseases of the kidney, ureter, bladder, testis, epidydemis, and vas deferens may cause groin pain.

3. Gynecologic origin: Diseases of the uterus, fallopian tubes, or ovaries or endometrial deposits in the pelvis or inguinal canal and round ligament may be the origin of groin pain.

4. Musculoskeletal origin: Patients with hip joint or sacroiliac joint disease sometimes complain of groin pain. Frequently, patients with knee joint or lumbar facet joint problems complain of pain in the groin. Other causes of groin pain are femoral trochanteric fractures, osteitis of the pubis and symphysis pubis, osteomyelitis of the pubis, Paget's disease, tendonitis of the iliopsoas or rectus femoris adductor longus, and bursitis over the iliopsoas, rectus femoris, and pectineus. Myofascial pain of longissimus, iliocostalis, and adductor muscles of the thigh may be referred to the groin.

5. Athletic injury: Inguinal and femoral hernia as well as tendonitis, bursitis, and osteitis (described above) are frequently diagnosed in young athletes. Injury to the external oblique aponeurosis with entrapment of the ilioinguinal nerve and the obturator nerve by the internal obturator muscles has also been reported.

6. Infection: Chronic infection in the lower extremity or the pelvic and perineal area can produce painful lymph nodes in the groin. Osteomyelitis of the pubis has been reported in athletes.

7. Malignancy: Malignant lesions of the urogenital, gastrointestinal, and gynecologic systems, the femur, and the hip joint can produce referred pain; or there may be pain due to involvement of the lymph nodes because of extension of the tumor.

8. Vascular origin: Aneurysms of iliac and femoral vessels, vascular injury, or hematoma secondary to catheterization may cause pain in the groin.

9. Neurologic origin: L1-2 radiculopathy may be a source of groin pain, as may neuralgias of the femoral, lateral femoral cutaneous, iliohypogastric, obturator, and genitofemoral nerves.

10. Postsurgical condition: About 15% to 28% of the patients who undergo herniorrhaphy continue to have pain at the 3- to 5-year follow-up. Suprapubic incisions for prostate or bladder surgery, cesarean section, and any other surgical procedures that require an incision in the groin can lead to chronic groin pain.

B. Diagnostic studies include the following.

1. Imaging: Herniography has been extremely useful for diagnosing occult hernias. Ultrasonography, magnetic resonance imaging, and computed tomography are often able to diagnose such conditions as hematoma and bursal enlargements, which may not be evident by plain radiography.

2. Injections: Pain relief following local anesthetic injection into the hip joint, sacroiliac joint, or facet joints, diagnostic nerve blocks of the ilioinguinal, iliohypogastric, and genitofemoral nerves, and infiltration of the spermatic chord, scar, or trigger areas in the muscles, tendons or bursae may be diagnostic.

C. Treatment. Once the diagnosis is established, appropriate treatment modalities, such as treatment of the infection, bursitis, arthritis, myofascial pain syndromes, tendonitis, or primary or secondary malignancy, may result in resolution or control of the symptoms or the disease process. Surgical correction such as tenotomy may be required in patients who have tendonitis and muscle spasms. If the neuropathic pain syndromes are not adequately controlled with conservative measures, neurolytic procedures may be considered. The use of alcohol and phenol in the management of nonmalignant pain syndromes may result in neuritis pain worse than that originally present. Cryoanalgesia or pulsed radiofrequency blocks may provide significant pain relief without impairing function or producing neuritis. Surgical resection of the ilioinguinal, iliohypogastric, and genitofemoral nerves proximal to the inguinal canal has been reported to provide pain relief.

REFERENCES

Cohen SP, Foster A: Pulsed radiofrequency as a treatment for groin pain and orchialgia. *Urology* 2003;61:645.

Courtney CA, Duffy K, Serpell MG, O'Dwyer PJ: Outcome of patients with severe chronic pain following repair of groin hernia. *Acta Radiol* 2002;43:603–608.

Kesek P, Ekberg O, Westlin N: Herniographic findings in athletes with unclear groin pain. *Br J Surg* 2003;90:367–368.

Lee CH, Dellon AL: Surgical management of groin pain of neural origin. *J Am Coll Surg* 200;191:137–142.

GROIN PAIN

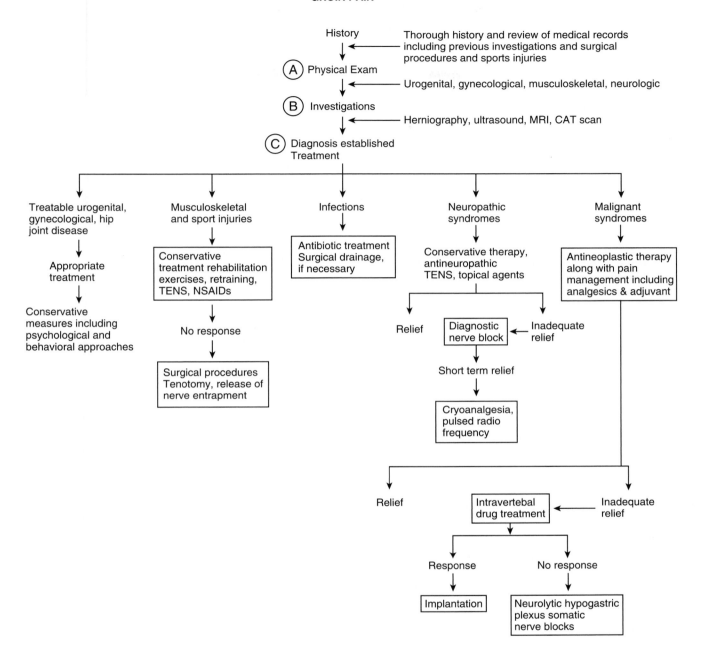

History — Thorough history and review of medical records including previous investigations and surgical procedures and sports injuries

(A) Physical Exam — Urogenital, gynecological, musculoskeletal, neurologic

(B) Investigations — Herniography, ultrasound, MRI, CAT scan

(C) Diagnosis established Treatment

Treatable urogenital, gynecological, hip joint disease

Appropriate treatment

Conservative measures including psychological and behavioral approaches

Musculoskeletal and sport injuries

Conservative treatment rehabilitation exercises, retraining, TENS, NSAIDs

No response

Surgical procedures Tenotomy, release of nerve entrapment

Infections

Antibiotic treatment Surgical drainage, if necessary

Neuropathic syndromes

Conservative therapy, antineuropathic TENS, topical agents

Relief

Diagnostic nerve block — Inadequate relief

Short term relief

Cryoanalgesia, pulsed radio frequency

Malignant syndromes

Antineoplastic therapy along with pain management including analgesics & adjuvant

Relief

Intravertebal drug treatment — Inadequate relief

Response

No response

Implantation

Neurolytic hypogastric plexus somatic nerve blocks

Pelvic Pain

SOMAYAJI RAMAMURTHY

Pelvic pain is a very common pain syndrome, especially in women. The pain is usually secondary to the involvement of the organ systems in the genitourinary or gastrointestinal system. Mechanical, musculoskeletal, and neurologic etiologies can cause pain even without a history of trauma. In a very high percentage of patients (10% to 50%), no causative factor can be established despite thorough investigations including imaging, laparoscopy, and surgical procedures such as hysterectomy. The lack of diagnosis leads to frustration and depression. In addition, because of the sociocultural taboos associated with pelvic and perineal pain, patients have a tendency not to bring it to the attention of family members. A significant number of patients complaining of the perineal and pelvic pain have a history of sexual abuse in childhood.

A. A study of history and medical records should be thoroughly reviewed to ascertain that correctable genitourinary and gastrointestinal pathology has been adequately investigated and treated. The sexual history may reveal dyspareunia, which is a very common and frustrating accompaniment. A thorough review of psychosocial history and testing is essential because of the high incidence of sexual abuse history, anxiety, depression, and frustration.

B. Physical, neurologic, and musculoskeletal examination should specifically look for the possibility of referred pain from the sacroiliac joint and the coccyx. Examination of the genitalia may reveal redness, blisters, and allodynia. Rectal or vaginal examination may reveal specific areas of tenderness, muscle spasm, and trigger points with the production of a patient's pain.

C. Diagnostic local anesthetic nerve blocks may be valuable in establishing nerve pathways conducting the pain and also the possibility of sympathetic pain syndrome. Transvaginal or transperineal pudendal nerve block may be helpful in diagnosing pudendal nerve entrapment syndrome. Sacroiliac joint injection, ganglion impar block, coccygeal nerve block, and superior hypogastric plexus block may be diagnostic.

D. Pelvic and perineal pain due to nonmalignant conditions is best managed with multimodal and multidisciplinary conservative approaches. Pharmacological approaches include nonsteroidal anti-inflammatory agents (NSAIDs), antidepressants, and anticonvulsant drugs to manage neuropathic pain. Physical therapy, pelvic floor exercises, and massage biofeedback are very helpful in improving pelvic support and using the muscle spasm. Psychological counseling and adequate management of depression other than psychological distress will be significantly beneficial to reduce the pain and discomfort.

E. Pain due to malignancy is managed with analgesics and adjuvants. Neurolytic hypogastric plexus and ganglion impar block may provide significant long-term pain relief. In patients who have lost bladder and bowel control, neurolytic subarchnoid block may provide excellent pain relief. Patients with neurologically intact bowel and bladder function may be good candidates for an intrathecal drug delivery system after a successful trial.

F. Local anesthetic nerve blocks of the pudendal nerve, sacral nerve roots, superior hypogastric plexus, ganglion impar, and trigger points may be very helpful in interrupting the pain cycle and facilitating physical therapy. Patients who have significant hypersensitivity may benefit from the application of a local anesthetic grain such as a eutectic mixture of local anesthetics (EMLA). Neurolytic block of the sacral nerve roots is not an option in patients who have intact bladder and bowel function. Stimulation of the sacral nerve roots either transsacrally or retrograde translumbar leads will provide significant pain relief in neuropathic pain and in selected patients with interstitial cystitis.

REFERENCES

Burnett AI, Wesselmann U: Neurobiology of the pelvis and perineum: principles for a practical approach. *J Pelvic Surg* 1999;5:224–232.

Kucharski A, Nagda N: Pelvic pain. In: Warfield CA, Bajwa ZH (eds) *Principles and Practices of Pain Medicine,* 2nd ed. New York, McGraw-Hill, 2004, pp. 359–368.

McDonald JS: Chronic pelvic pain. In: Copeland IJ, Jarell JF (eds) *Textbook of Gynecology.* Philadelphia, WB Saunders, 2000, pp. 741–758.

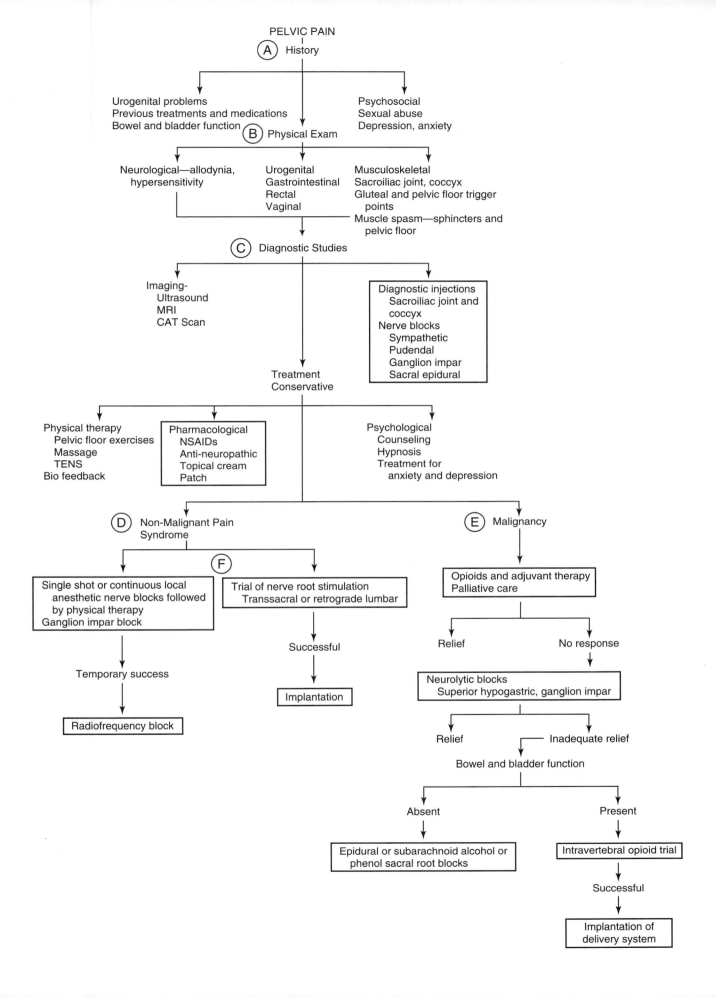

CANCER PAIN

PATIENT EDUCATION
MEDICAL MANAGEMENT OF CANCER PAIN
METASTATIC CANCER PAIN
NEUROLYTIC BLOCKS
HOSPICE CARE AND PALLIATIVE CARE

Patient Education

JAY ELLIS

Patient education on pain management is an often-neglected aspect of a pain management program. Much information exists on patient misconceptions about pain management, and published articles describe attempts to correct these misconceptions. However, patient education is not a "one size fits all" program. Educational programs for patients with cancer pain differ from those for patients with postoperative pain, which in turn differ from those for patients with chronic back pain, and so on. To complicate matters further, different populations of patients have different styles of learning. Some patients embrace computer-assisted learning, others prefer videotape instruction, some want a printed instruction sheet, and still others require one-on-one instruction (Barlow et al. 2002; Jonas and Worsley-Cox 2000). Age, educational background, and culture influence learning as well.

In addition to the difficulty of creating an effective patient education program, there is conflicting evidence as to the value of education programs in terms of improving patient pain scores, complications, or hospital length of stay (Chang et al. 2002; Griffin et al. 1998; Knoerl et al. 1999; Lam et al. 2001; McDonald et al. 2001; Pellino et al. 1998; Watt-Watson et al. 2000). Add to the mix the cost and time of creating an effective program, and one may wish to forget the program altogether. Despite the controversy, there is overwhelming evidence that patients have misconceptions about the risks, benefits, and side effects of pain management therapies; and they want more information (Carr 2002; Chumbley et al. 2002; Ferrel and Juarez 2002). In addition, many of the studies looking at the efficacy of educational programs did so as an isolated intervention. Patient education alone cannot solve poor pain management practice, but poor patient education can certainly hinder effective strategies for obtaining pain relief.

Despite the seemingly insurmountable problems of creating an effective educational program, there are several key features necessary for an effective program. First, patients must be taught an effective pain assessment tool to describe their pain and its intensity. The Verbal Rating Score, Visual Analog Scale, and Pediatric FACES assessment tool are just a few examples of pain assessment methods. No matter which tool is chosen, patients must be instructed on its effective use. For example, patients asked to rate pain on a scale of 1 to 10 sometimes respond, "It's an 11." Although descriptive in the sense that it is clear the patient is experiencing severe pain, it demonstrates a lack of understanding that there is no pain greater than 10. Education is best done before patients develop severe pain or at a time when pain has been brought under control.

Second, patients must understand that controlling pain is not just a comfort measure but an important part of their recovery from illness. They should have an expectation of effective pain control. Knowing the physiological and psychological consequences of untreated pain can make patients more willing to request pain relief.

Third, the educational program should debunk the myth that the use of opioids for pain treatment leads to addiction or can cause other serious harm. Patients have an exaggerated sense of the risks of opioid therapy, and they often refuse medication even when it is offered because of their fear of addiction or injury (Carr 2002).

Fourth, patients should learn to request pain medication at the time of the onset of pain to avoid situations where the pain is out of control. Patients must understand that there is a delay from the time when the medication is administered until the onset of analgesia.

Lastly, patients should have an understanding of the common side effects and complications of their analgesic regimen. They should also learn how to avoid them if possible and manage them when they are unavoidable.

How to deliver this information differs with the clinical setting and the population involved. The easiest method is a printed sheet given to a patient at the time of entry into the health system. However, a patient's ability to comprehend the printed material varies widely from one individual to another. Furthermore, giving the patient the material in no way ensures that the material is ever read and understood. A more effective approach is to have a staff member review the printed material with the patient at the time it is distributed. This ensures that the patient has the material, reviewed it at least once, and had an opportunity to ask questions. The printed material is then available for future reference. Videos and computer-assisted instructions are also an option; but whether they work the same, better, or worse than a printed sheet is not known nor is the efficacy of one-on-one instruction. It is unlikely that any one approach would work for all individuals all of the time.

Knowing that there are problems with the delivery of information indicates the need for a feedback mechanism for an educational program. There must be some measure of the effectiveness of that program. The most common assessment method is a test to see if patients retained important information. Tests have a negative connotation for most patients, though, and they are not always well received. Other methods of feedback are having patients demonstrate the appropriate use of an analgesic device, such as a patient-controlled analgesia pump, or to recite back to the instructor the important information received. Another form of feedback is a survey of the patient and staff after treatment to assess the patient's level of participation and effective use of analgesic therapy. This has the advantage of measuring the actual desired outcome: patient participation and degree of pain relief. It has the disadvantage, however, of being labor-intensive and time-consuming; moreover, it does not indicate whether poor pain relief is due to lack of education, poor staff performance, or other factors. No matter what feedback method is chosen, it must be used to guide the educational program continuously toward better patient outcomes.

REFERENCES

Barlow JH, Cullen LA, Rowe IF: Educational preferences, psychological well-being and self-efficacy among people with rheumatoid arthritis. *Patient Educ Couns* 2002;46:11–19.

Carr EC: Refusing analgesics: using continuous improvement to improve pain management on a surgical ward. *J Clin Nurs* 2002;11:743–752.

Chang MC, Chang YC, Chiou JF, et al: Overcoming patient-related barriers to cancer pain management for home care patients: a pilot study. *Cancer Nurs* 2002;25:470–476.

Chumbley GM, Hall GM, Salmon P: Patient-controlled analgesia: what information does the patient want? *J Adv Nurs* 2002;39:459–471.

Ferrell BR, Juarez G: Cancer pain ducation for patients and the public. *J Pain Symptom Manage* 2002;23:329–336.

Griffin MJ, Brennan L, McShane AJ: Preoperative education and outcome of patient controlled analgesia. *Can J Anaesth* 1998;45:943–948.

Jonas D, Worsley-Cox K: Information giving can be painless. *J Child Health Care* 2000;4:55–58.

Knoerl DV, Faut-Callahan M, Paice J, Shott S: Preoperative PCA teaching program to manage postoperative pain. *Medsurg Nurs* 1999;8:25–33.

Lam KK, Chan MT, Chen PP, Kee WD: Structured preoperative patient education for patient-controlled analgesia. *J Clin Anesth* 2001;13:465–469.

McDonald DD, Freeland M, Thomas G, Moore J: Testing a preoperative pain management intervention for elders. *Res Nurs Health* 2001;24:402–409.

Pellino T, Tluczek A, Collins M, et al: Increasing self-efficacy through empowerment: preoperative education for orthopaedic patients. *Orthop Nurs* 1998;17:48–51, 54–59.

Watt-Watson J, Stevens B, Costello J, et al: Impact of preoperative education on pain managment outcomes after coronary artery bypass graft surgery: a pilot. *Can J Nurs Res* 2000;31:41–56.

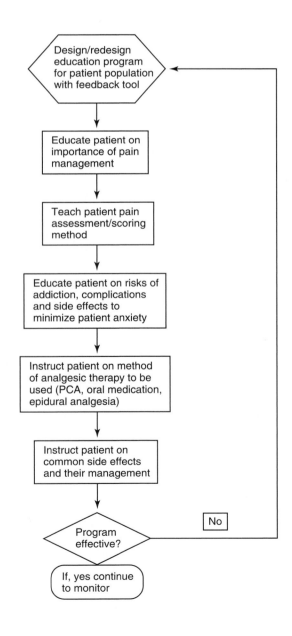

Medical Management of Cancer Pain

TED GINGRICH

Cancer pain should be treated aggressively and immediately. The benefits of timely treatment include facilitation of the diagnostic workup and treatment, improved functional status, better quality of life, and possibly better survival rates. Most cancer pain can be effectively relieved with oral analgesics. Despite this, cancer pain is undertreated for a variety of reasons. A comprehensive medical management team that includes oncologists, pain specialists, physical therapists, mental health providers, social workers, and hospice workers can provide optimal care.

A. Cancer can produce any type of pain in any location. Evaluation should include pain characterization, including the intensity of the pain, its location, its pattern of radiation, temporal factors (onset, duration, frequency), provocative and remitting factors, and the effect of previous control measures. Cancer pain syndromes vary by tumor type and are related to patterns of tumor growth and metastasis. The pain can be classified broadly as somatic (well localized) visceral (not well localized), or neuropathic (burning, lancinating). All pain in the cancer patient is not necessarily from the cancer. This fact must be considered whenever the pain changes character or breaks through a previously effective regimen. When choosing a regimen, consider the patient's social status, health care access, comorbidities, and life expectancy as well as the individual's desires and expectations.

B. About 90% of patients with cancer can have their pain adequately managed with oral medications, which is certainly the most convenient route of administration. Oral therapy should be viewed as an integral part of the spectrum of strategies available, which include radiotherapy, chemotherapy, surgery, physiotherapy, anesthetic blocks, and transcutaneous nerve stimulation, among others. It is important to (1) tailor pharmacologic analgesia to the individuals needs, (2) choose the appropriate drugs, (3) titrate the agent carefully, and (4) frequently reassess therapy and adjust it as necessary.

C. The World Health Organization proposed a three-step analgesic ladder that provides a logical basis for the pharmacologic treatment of cancer pain. It has three points of entry, depending on the severity of pain, and allows progression between the various steps. Due to patient variability in the response to the various opioid agonists, sequential trials (or "opioid rotation"), help identify the medication with the more favorable balance between the analgesic effects and the side effects.

1. Step 1 begins with the use of no-opioid analgesics such as acetaminophen, aspirin, and nonsteroidal antiinflammatory drugs (NSAIDs). NSAIDs are potent analgesics and effectively alleviate mild cancer pain. They should be considered as an addition at any step in the analgesic ladder for bone pain, soft tissue infiltration, pressure sores, and any pain with an inflammatory component. These nonopioid analgesics are associated with ceiling effects, and exceeding the maximum dose range can result in organ toxicity.

2. Step 2 progresses to acetaminophen and "weak" opioids (e.g., codeine, hydrocodone, oxycodone, propoxyphene). Combination medications may provide better analgesia than a drug alone. These short-duration medications should be given on a scheduled basis if a continuous baseline pain is present.

3. Step 3 introduces the potent opioids (e.g., morphine, hydromorphone, methadone, fentanyl). No strong evidence speaks for the superiority of one opioid over another. However, unique pharmacologic profiles play a role in tailoring the analgesic regimen. Examples include transdermal fentanyl for patients unable to swallow or who are prone to constipation, methadone for patients with a neuropathic pain component, and hydromorphone with its nonactive metabolites for patients with impaired metabolism and clearance. Sustained-release formulations can be extremely effective. Remember to provide for both baseline and breakthrough pain.

D. Adjuvant analgesics typically have primary indications other than cancer pain (Table 1), but they provide analgesia in many situations and may reduce the systemic opioid requirement. They should therefore be considered early in treatment. Agents given for other complaints are listed in Table 2.

E. Side effect management is an essential aspect of therapy assessment. Uncontrolled side effects negatively affect the quality of life. The key is to anticipate medication side effects and treat them promptly and aggressively.

F. Reassess the efficacy of therapy frequently. As the disease progresses, titrate medications appropriately. New-onset pain or breakthrough pain should direct the provider to look for new pathology or progression of the disease.

G. If standard oral therapy fails, whether due to inadequate analgesia or intolerable side effects, consider invasive therapies. They include neuroablative techniques, conduction blockade, and neuraxial analgesic delivery systems.

MEDICAL MANAGEMENT OF CANCER PAIN

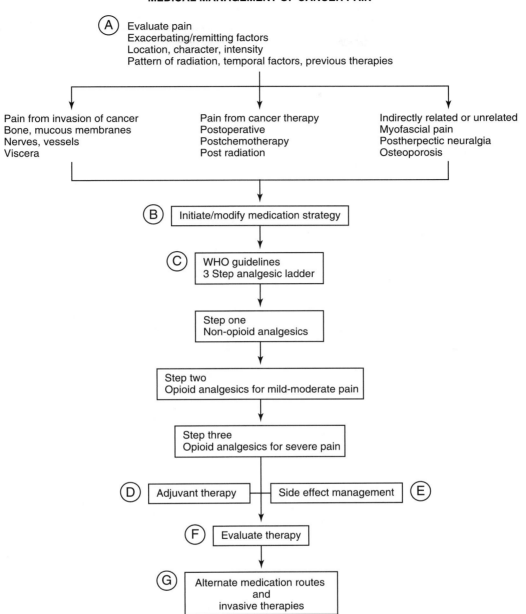

TABLE 1
Adjuvant Analgesics

General analgesia potentiation
  Corticosteroids (prednisone, dexamethasone)
  Anxiolytics and muscle relaxants (diazepam, baclofen)
  SSRIs (paroxetine)
  α_2-Agonists (tizanidine, clonidine)
  Topical agents (capsaicin, local anesthetics)

Neuropathic drugs
  TCAs (amitriptyline, desipramine)
  Anticonvulsants (gabapentin, lamotrigine, topiramate)
  Antidysrhythmics (mexilitine, tocainide)
  NMDA antagonists (ketamine, dextromethorphan)
  Miscellaneous: baclofen, calcitonin

Bone pain
  Bisphosphonates (pamidronate)
  Osteoclast inhibitors (calcitonin, radiopharmaceuticals)

NMDA, *N*-methyl-D-aspartate; SSRIs, selective serotonin reuptake inhibitor; TCAs, tricyclic antidepressants.

TABLE 2
Other Agents and Their Indications

Constipation
  Stimulating agents (docusate, senna bisacodyl)
  Osmotic agents (lactulose, magnesium citrate)
  Prokinetic agents (metaclopromide)
  Opioid antagonists (oral naloxone)
  Miscellaneous: octreotide, mestinon, hyoscine

Sedation
  Psychostimulants (methylphenidate, dextroamphetamine, caffeine)

Nausea
  Hydroxyzine, phenergan, ondansetron, halperidol, metaclopramide scopolamine, meclizine

Edema
  Diuretics

Insomnia
  Amitriptyline, hydroxyzine, trazadone

Pruritus
  Diphenhydramine, naloxone, nalbuphine, hydroxyzine

REFERENCES

Bonica JJ. Cancer pain. In: Bonica JJ (ed) *The Management of Pain*. Philadelphia, Lea & Febiger, 1990.

Payne R. Cancer pain: anatomy, physiology, and pharmacology. *Cancer* 1989;63:2266.

Portenoy RK: Cancer pain: epidemiology and syndromes. *Cancer* 1989;63:2298–2307.

Portenoy RK: Clinical strategies for the management of cancer pain poorly responsive to systemic opioid therapy: pain 2002—an updated review. In: Giamberardino MA (ed) *IASP Scientific Program Committee*. Seattle, IASP Press, 2002.

World Health Organization: *Cancer Pain Relief and Palliative Care*. Geneva, WHO, 1990.

Metastatic Cancer Pain

EULECHE ALANMANOU

It is estimated that 60% to 90% of patients with advanced cancer experience significant pain. Tragically, adequate cancer pain management remains a major health care problem. Minorities, women, and the elderly may be at even greater risk for undertreatment of pain. Experts agree that 90% of cancer pain can be managed using simple approaches.

A. Cancer pain may be classified as nociceptive (somatic or visceral) or neuropathic, although psychological factors play an important role in individual perception. Pain assessment is a systematic clinical evaluation that ends with a diagnosis that emphasizes the etiology and pathophysiology of the pain complaint. The medical history emphasizes pain characteristics (e.g., location, quality, duration, intensity, palliative or provocative factors), cancer history and treatment, and psychological factors such as depression, fear, anxiety, and anger. In addition, patients with advanced cancer may also have generalized weakness, fatigue, and delirium. These symptoms affect pain perception, pain reporting, and the overall quality of life. The clinician should perform a physical examination of the painful sites and of the various systems with special attention to the neurologic and musculoskeletal systems. This systematic approach helps identify the causes of pain in the cancer patient.

B. Cancer pain results from direct tumor invasion, anticancer therapies, or causes not related to the cancer. Common cancer pain syndromes, such as bone metastasis, visceral pain, neuropathic pain, and mucositis, among others, can be identified, as can an oncologic emergency (e.g., spinal cord compression, cardiac tamponade).

C. The involvement of specialists from multiple disciplines results in improved analgesia and other health outcomes. Discussing treatment decisions with the patient and family members is beneficial. Due to the lack of high quality evidence, optimally combining drug with nondrug therapies remains a challenge. Matching the options for optimal pain control depends on individual variations in needs, preferences, costs, and anticipated responses.

D. The best available evidence for cancer pain control is the effectiveness of the World Health Organization's analgesic ladder. The ladder recommends administration of oral agents (nonopioids, opioids, adjuvants) and relies primarily on pain intensity and to a lesser extent on the mechanism of the pain as determinants of therapy. The use of alternative routes of opioid administration (transdermal, transmucosal, parenteral delivery) depends on the patient's circumstances.

1. Opioids are titrated to effect; there should be no predetermined maximum dose. The correct dose of an opioid is that which effectively relieves pain without inducing unacceptable side effects. Opioids are administered around the clock, with additional doses available for breakthough pain.

2. Constipation is a common side effect in patients undergoing opioid therapy. These patients should receive prophylactic therapy with stool softener, often in combination with bulk agents, osmotic laxatives, or stimulant cathartics.

3. Other side effects of opioids, including tolerance, physical dependence, sedation, respiratory depression, nausea and vomiting, cognitive impairment, myoclonus, pruritus, and urinary retention should be treated when they occur. Prophylaxis is not indicated. When tolerance to an opioid develops, another opioid can be substituted to provide better analgesia because the cross-tolerance among opioids is incomplete. However, it is recommended that the calculated dose be reduced by 25% to 50% to account for that incomplete cross-tolerance when converting from one opioid to another. Addiction to opioids is rare in cancer pain patients.

4. Studies show variable results when physical or psychological treatments (acupuncture, relaxation, massage, heat or cold, music, exercise) are added to the management of cancer-related pain. The literature suggests that biphosphonates reduce pain due to bony metastases.

E. For patients who do not respond to simple techniques, high-tech approaches such as nerve blocks, neuroablative procedures, or implantation of drug delivery systems may be offered.

1. Neural blockade with local anesthetics may be helpful for treating pain in a defined anatomic location. The patient is made aware that effective pain relief with a diagnostic block does not guarantee pain relief after a neuroablative procedure. Neuroablation can be accomplished by chemical, thermal, or surgical means. Deafferentation pain after a neuroablative procedure may be worse than the initial pain, however. Unwanted motor weakness or bladder/bowel dysfunction is a concern. Neuroablation does not always lead to cessation of opioid administration, but the dosage of the opioid should be reduced to avoid respiratory depression in case of significant pain relief.

2. Drug delivery systems for chronic cancer pain management include epidural, spinal, and intraventricular systems. The spinal route for analgesia is widely employed. Evidence-based data regarding optimal patient selection and the selection of initial or secondary agents or combinations remain sparse.

F. The indication for neuraxial drug delivery and neuroablative procedures include inadequate pain relief with oral analgesics, intolerable side effects, and neuropathic pain. These high-tech modalities should be offered to the motivated, compliant patient in a setting that can provide follow-up around the clock.

REFERENCES

American Society of Anesthesiologists: Practice guidelines for cancer pain management. *Anesthesiology* 1996;84:1243–1257.

Cleeland CS, Gonin R, Hatfield AK, et al: Pain and its treatment in outpatients with metastatic cancer. *N Engl J Med* 1994;330: 592–596.

Management of Cancer Pain. Summary, Evidence Report/Technology Assessment: No. 35. AHRQ Publication 01-E033. Rockville, MD, Agency for Healthcare Research and Quality, January 2001 (http://www.ahrq.gov/clinic/epcsums/canpainsum.htm).

Zhukovsky DS, Gorowski E, Hausdorif J, et al: Unmet analgesic needs in cancer patients. *J Pain Symptoms Manage* 1995; 10:113–119.

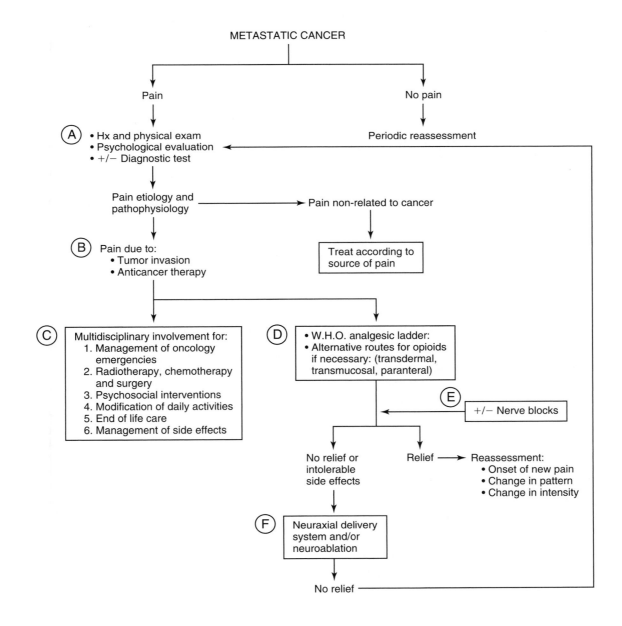

Neurolytic Blocks

JAY ELLIS

A panel of experts convened by the Agency for Healthcare Research and Quality noted that 90% of cancer pain is manageable with simple measures (Jacox et al. 1994). Current recommendations for cancer pain management stress the use of oral and parenteral analgesics for cancer pain. Unfortunately, some patients do not achieve effective pain relief with oral or parenteral medication, even when given large doses of parenteral opioids. It is for these patients that neurolytic blocks may be appropriate.

A. Most patients who require a neurolytic block fall into three general categories: The first, most common group includes those who have tried oral and parenteral therapy but failed to achieve adequate pain relief or failed to get pain relief without intolerable side effects. It should be noted that all side effects should be aggressively managed, including the use of stimulants for severe sedation, aggressive antinausea medication, and potent osmotic agents for constipation. The second group of patients requiring a neurolytic block are those who have incident pain. An example is the patient with bone metastases who is comfortable at rest but cannot ambulate because weight-bearing produces severe pain. These patients are unlikely to achieve adequate relief for ambulation with oral opioid therapy. The third group of candidates for a neurolytic block includes patients with neuropathic pain. Painful neuropathy often responds poorly to opioids, even at high doses. For patients who do not respond, a neurolytic block may provide pain relief, although the idea that pain relief derived from further damaging an already injured nerve seems incongruous.

B. Several neurolytic blocks have high utility. Neurolysis of the celiac plexus is extremely effective for alleviating pain due to pancreatic cancer or upper abdominal tumors. Some investigators believe that the celiac plexus block does not necessarily need to be reserved for those who fail opioid therapy. Moreover, because of the good side effect profile of the celiac plexus block and its relatively low risk of complications, it should be tried early in the course of this devastating malignancy (AHRQ 2001). The hypogastric plexus block is extremely useful for managing refractory pain due to a pelvic malignancy. Prospective studies done in women with severe, unremitting pain due to a pelvic malignancy found that the hypogastric plexus block provided a significant degree of pain relief in most patients. Complication rates for this procedure are low as well.

C. Not all patients with refractory cancer pain are candidates for a neurolytic block. An example is the patient with widely metastatic multiple myeloma in whom the large number of painful sites would greatly exceed the ability to anesthetize the affected area adequately. Neurolytic blocks are best used in patients who have a well defined anatomic location for their pain. In addition, there is a shortage of prospective, well controlled studies on the effectiveness of neurolytic blocks (AHRQ 2110). The exceptions to this lack of scientific evidence are the celiac plexus block and the hypogastric plexus block, for which there is some prospective evidence indicating their usefulness in specific patient populations (AHRQ 2001; Eisenberg et al. 1995; Plancarte et al. 1990).

D. Patients with pain on one side of the body at dermatomes between T4 and L1 may be candidates for an alcohol spinal block, which comprises percutaneous chemical rhizotomy of the posterior spinal rootlets. The keys to success here are as follows. (1) Choose a patient with unilateral pain in a restricted number of dermatomes. (2) Limit the volume of alcohol to 1 mL through any one needle, with no more than two needles placed during any one procedure on a given day. This practice dramatically limits the most-feared complication of the alcohol spinal block: bowel and bladder incontinence. Most cases of bowel and bladder incontinence associated with the alcohol spinal block have been due to large volumes of alcohol being used for the procedure, sometimes in excess of 5 mL or more, and use of alcohol to treat pain in the lower lumbar segments. This block may be most useful in patients with metastatic colon cancer, as these patients often have a diverting colostomy and ureterostomy, which makes the risk of bowel and bladder incontinence moot. The standard alcohol spinal block is performed with a hypobaric solution of alcohol. Alternatively, if the pain is in the sacral region, a hyperbaric procedure is done with subarachnoid phenol and glycerine. The alcohol spinal block is probably an underutilized procedure because of the fear of bowel and bladder incontinence, but it can be quite effective for patients with severe chest wall metastases, especially those not amenable to blockade by multiple intercostal nerve blocks.

E. Once the anatomic site has been chosen, diagnostic blocks using local anesthetics should precede all neurolytic blocks. The exception is the alcohol spinal block, for which there is no good diagnostic procedure. The practitioner should also understand the limitations of prognostic blocks. A successful prognostic block with local anesthetic does not guarantee pain relief with a neurolytic procedure. There are several reasons for this. First, local anesthetics produce more intense blockade of a nerve condition than does a neurolytic procedure. Second, local anesthetics generally allow use of a larger volume of solution than one would be able to use with a neurolytic procedure. Third, the difference in the mechanisms of action of the local anesthetics compared to neurolytic agents may provide pain relief through other mechanisms, such as muscle relaxation or systemic effects.

Patient requiring NEUROLYTIC BLOCKS

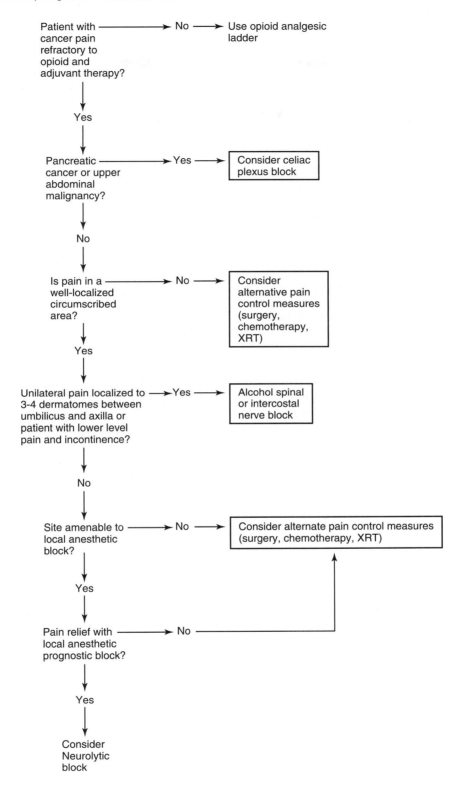

Patient with cancer pain refractory to opioid and adjuvant therapy? ——→ No ——→ Use opioid analgesic ladder

Yes

Pancreatic cancer or upper abdominal malignancy? ——→ Yes ——→ Consider celiac plexus block

No

Is pain in a well-localized circumscribed area? ——→ No ——→ Consider alternative pain control measures (surgery, chemotherapy, XRT)

Yes

Unilateral pain localized to 3-4 dermatomes between umbilicus and axilla or patient with lower level pain and incontinence? ——→ Yes ——→ Alcohol spinal or intercostal nerve block

No

Site amenable to local anesthetic block? ——→ No ——→ Consider alternate pain control measures (surgery, chemotherapy, XRT)

Yes

Pain relief with local anesthetic prognostic block? ——→ No

Yes

Consider Neurolytic block

Therefore the real value of prognostic blocks does not lie in identifying patients in whom success is guaranteed but in eliminating patients for whom the chance of success is negligible. In other words, a successful prognostic block does not guarantee pain relief, but an unsuccessful block can certainly identify patients for whom neurolytic blocks are *not* indicated.

F. Neurolysis of other peripheral nerves may be useful for pain control as well. Head and neck cancers may be responsive to neurolytic block of the branches of the trigeminal nerve. Isolated chest wall pain may respond to intercostal nerve blockade. This is a simple, easy procedure to perform, with a risk profile that is a little different from that of the intercostal nerve block with a local anesthetic. The advantage of blockade of the trigeminal and intercostal nerves is that, except for the third division of the trigeminal nerve, these nerves perform mostly sensory functions, so their block does not result in significant loss of motor function.

G. Blockade of other peripheral nerves is occasionally useful for pain control as well, but the degree of pain relief must be balanced against the loss of significant motor function. Neurolytic blockade of the brachial plexus would most often result in significant loss of motor function as well. This may be appropriate if the patient already has no function in these areas, but otherwise it may cause as much disability as the pain itself. Prognostic blocks would help answer this question and give the patient an idea of what the results of the neurolytic block might be. Patients may choose to have a somewhat painful, though functional extremity rather than have one that is numb and painless but totally nonfunctional.

H. Another caveat to remember when talking to patients about a neurolytic block is that it seldom results in total elimination of the need for opioid therapy. Most patients with cancer pain must continue their oral medication if for no other reason than to prevent an abstinence syndrome. However, most patients continue to have some pain for which oral analgesics are needed; and if there is progression of the tumor, pain may recur, reaffirming the need for oral analgesic therapy. Patients who are undergoing neurolytic blockade solely for the purpose of eliminating oral analgesics have unrealistic expectations as to the effectiveness of these procedures. Patients should experience improved effectiveness of their medication at reduced doses and thus should also experience reduced side effects. The patient should also be counseled that pain may recur within several weeks to months, and additional procedures may be needed.

REFERENCES

De Leon-Casasola OA, Kent E, Lema MJ: Neurolytic superior hypogastric plexus block for chronic pelvic pain associated with cancer. *Pain* 1993;54:145–151.

Eisenberg E, Carr DB, Chalmers TC: Neurolytic celiac plexus block for treatment of cancer pain: a meta-analysis. *Anesth Analg* 1995;80:290–295.

Jacox A, Carr DB, Payne R, et al: *Management of Cancer Pain. Clinical Practice Guideline No. 9* (AHCPR Publication No. 94-0592). Rockville, MD, Agency for Health Care Policy and Research, US Department of Health and Human Services, 1994.

Management of Cancer Pain. Summary, Evidence Report/Technology Assessment: No. 35. AHRQ Publication No. 01-E033. Rockville, MD, Agency for Healthcare Research and Quality, 2001 (http://www.ahrq.gov/clinic/epcsums/canpainsum.htm).

Mercadante S: Celiac plexus block versus analgesics in pancreatic cancer pain. *Pain* 1993;52:187–192.

Plancarte R, Amescua C, Patt RB, Aldrete JA: Superior hypogastric plexus block for pelvic cancer pain. *Anesthesiology* 1990;73:236–239.

Hospice Care and Palliative Care

AARON MALAKOFF AND SOMAYAJI RAMAMURTHY

A. Hospice. In the United States Hospice is a program that provides palliative care to terminally ill patients and supporting services to the patients and their families, 24 hours a day both at home and inpatient settings. Physical, social, spiritual, and emotional care is provided during the last stages of illness during the dying process and during bereavement by a medically directed interdisciplinary team consisting of patient/family, professionals, and volunteers.

Hospice in the United States is a reimbursement mechanism in which the patient must relinquish curative or life-prolonging therapy to qualify for the financial benefit. The provider agrees to direct all the treatment toward the relief of symptoms and forego life-prolonging and curative treatment. Admission to a hospice is limited to patients who have a diagnosis that if untreated would be fatal within 6 months. The patient must agree to forego curative treatment or other treatment in which the object of the treatment is to prolong life rather than alleviate symptoms. The duty of the hospice is to provide medical care regarding the terminal diagnosis. This includes provision of all durable and disposable medical equipment, medications related to terminal diagnosis, as well as visits by hospice professionals. The hospice is responsible for payment of all treatments including invasive interventions such as radiation therapy, palliative chemotherapy, and so forth but the hospice is reimbursed on a per diem basis. High-tech therapy can impose a severe financial burden on the hospice provider.

B. Palliative care. Palliative care embraces the hospice philosophy but is not confined by the regulations that define hospice programs in the United States. Palliative care seeks to prevent, relieve, and reduce the symptoms of disease or disorder without effecting a cure. Palliative care is not restricted to patients who are dying or those enrolled in hospice programs. It attends closely to the emotional, spiritual, and practical needs and goals of patients and those close to them. It affirms life and regards dying as a normal process. It neither hastens nor postpones death. It provides relief from pain and other symptoms and integrates psychological and spiritual care utilizing an interdisciplinary team and a support system for the family.

The goals of palliative care are to relieve suffering and improve the quality of life.

C. Palliative care service. The emphasis is on symptom control using a team approach, treating the patient/family as a unit of care and incorporating a continuity of settings. Palliative care service also provides the bereavement support for 1 year following the death of the patient.

D. Consultation and referral. The palliative care service is consulted when help is needed with symptom control.

Pain control is the most frequent cause of palliative care consultation. Other symptoms include dyspnea, fatigue, weakness, nausea and vomiting, abdominal distension, ascites, constipation, bowel obstruction, diarrhea, anorexia, cachexia, urinary retention, incontinence of the bowel and bladder, skin breakdowns, edema, anasarca, hiccups, depression, anxiety, delirium, and insomnia.

Consultation can be obtained only when recommendations are made. Consultation can also be made requesting the management of specific symptoms by the palliative care team. A referral is made when the patient is transferred to the palliative care or hospice service.

E. Team approach. Palliative care recognizes and treats all aspects of pain: physical, mental, or psychological, especially depression; social pain, especially communication with loved ones and attention to grief and bereavement; and spiritual pain, involving patients' and families' awareness of death, making peace, opportunity for growth, and find life's deepest meaning.

Since no one person has expertise in all aspects, the palliative care service treats patients using an interdisciplinary team that includes a physician, nurse, social worker, spiritual counselor such as a chaplain, and volunteers. Success is measured by relief of suffering, not by termination of the disease or even prolongation of life.

F. The physician attends to physical symptoms using both pharmacological and nonpharmacological modalities.

G. The nurse acts as the case manager and coordinates all the services, including the ongoing assessments, and acts as triage for the patient needs. The nursing team does the hands-on care of the patient and has the most intimate relationship with the patient and the family, training the family members to take care of the patient with regard to medication management, feeding, ostomy care, catheter care, wound care, and even management of parenteral medications.

H. The social worker assesses the social pain of the patient, addressing problems such as loss of the patient's role in the family and in the community. In addition to connecting patients and their families to community resources, social workers also provide counseling. They teach patients how to link to life work and provide information about advance directives and medical durable power of attorney.

I. The pastoral care given by the spiritual counselor assists in the relief of existential suffering and coordinates the bereavement support to the patient and the family while teaching them to cope.

J. Hospice volunteers assist the patient and family by providing companionship, assistance with errands and transportation, occasional caregiver respite, and

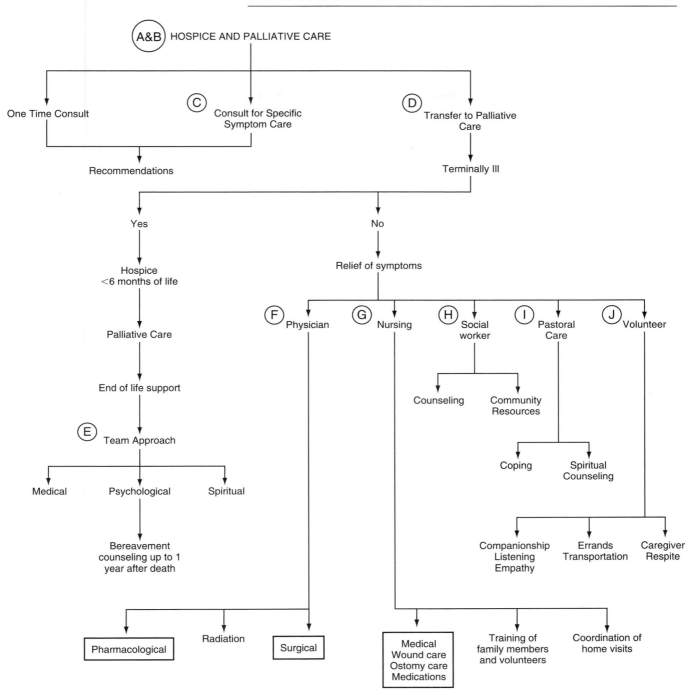

empathetic listening. Hospice volunteers undergo formal training before being involved with direct patient contact. A minimum ratio of voluntary to paid employee hours is mandated for hospice accreditation and thereby the third-party reimbursement.

REFERENCES

Bruera E, Higginson I, Neumann CM: Palliative care. In: Loeser JD (ed) *Bonica's Management of Pain,* 3rd ed. Philadelphia, Lippincott Williams & Wilkins, 2001, pp. 759–762.

Trent Hospice Audit Group: *Palliative Care Core Standards; A Multidisciplinary Approach. Trent Hospice Audit,* 1992. Derby, UK: Nightingal MacMillian Continuing Care Unit.

HEAD AND NECK PAIN

Head and Neck Pain

JEFFREY T. SUMMERS

In any given month, 10% of the adult population experience neck pain, with or without radiating symptoms. Although spontaneous improvement occurs in most cases, the diagnosis of persistent head and neck pain can be difficult because of the complex anatomy and referral patterns in this region.

A. Initial testing should include plain radiography, especially if there is any antecedent history of trauma. Magnetic resonance imaging (MRI) evaluation is also indicated if the patient has any systemic symptoms, such as fever, night sweats, or weight loss, that suggest an infectious process.

B. The presence of neurologic changes, myelopathic signs, or persistent pain despite treatment indicates a need for MRI, computed tomography (CT), or electromyography (EMG).

C. Surgical management is considered necessary if there is a surgical lesion with progressive motor or sensory loss or bladder/bowel dysfunction. Usually there is compressive pathology or gross instability. Treatment of a neoplasm or infection may or may not involve surgery.

D. Degenerative processes such as degenerative joint disease may lead to reactive bone spurs and result in compression. Mass lesions such as tumors or a syrinx usually start as poorly localized neck or radiating pain that is worse at night. Pain is almost always associated with a neurologic deficit involving sensory loss over the upper back and proximal extremities that may be subtle initially but can rapidly progress to upper extremity motor loss, gait disturbance, and signs of myelopathy. Pain from a syrinx usually becomes less prominent as the neurologic deficits progress. Cervical central canal stenosis can be congenital, or it may result from degenerative changes or disc bulging/ herniation. Stenosis presents with neck pain and increased reflexes, and it can progress to gait disturbance and extremity weakness. Epidural injection may be contraindicated at the level of the stenosis, depending on the canal diameter. Intervertebral disc herniation may cause direct nerve root compression, or it may result in inflammatory changes that lead to radiculitis; the latter usually is not associated with neurologic changes. Pain radiates in a dermatomal pattern, depending on the disc involved. In this instance, initial treatment is usually nonsurgical for the neuropathic pain and includes the use of epidural steroids.

E. Muscle contraction or tension headache is usually bilateral, wrapping around the head in a "band-like" ache or tightness. The pain is usually constant but may be worse in the early morning or the evening. Treatment usually avoids analgesics, particularly those with abuse potential, and centers on antidepressant medications, stress reduction, and physical therapy. Arthritic involvement of joints in the high cervical spine may present with a picture identical to that of tension headache.

F. Cervical pain involving the upper roots (C1 has no dermal sensory component) or upper facets may present as neck pain radiating into the posterior head, neck, or shoulder. Occipital neuralgia involves irritation of the occipital nerves, but similar pain can be caused by upper nerve root or facet involvement. Pharmacologic treatment for neurogenic pain is similar; but therapeutic joint, nerve root, or peripheral nerve blocks should be specific for the pain generator. Diagnostic injections can be invaluable for directing treatment.

G. Nonradiating neck pain may be due to a variety of factors, including disc, joint, soft tissue, or neurogenic pathology. Many of the same processes that cause radiating pain can produce nonradiating neck discomfort if the neural elements are spared. Therefore intraspinal pathology cannot be excluded based solely on the absence of neurologic changes or radiating pain. The workup proceeds similarly to that for nonradiating neck pain, although treatment differs if no neural elements are involved. Diagnostic injections are useful if the diagnosis is not apparent after obtaining the patient's history, performing a physical examination, and examining the imaging results.

H. Facet pain may be related to degenerative joint changes leading to inflammatory changes or instability. Arthritis may be evident on radiographic imaging, but the severity of the disease on imaging does not correlate with the severity of the pain. It may progress to involve compression or inflammation of neural tissue.

I. Myofascial neck pain presents as a deep aching that is poorly localized and may be referred to adjacent structures. It is diagnosed by the presence of trigger points that reproduce pain.

J. Intrinsic bone pain may result from osteoporotic fracture, bony tumor, or Paget's disease. Bony pathology often presents as a dull, aching pain that usually is not aggravated with neck movement. The patient is tender to palpation over the bone lesion.

K. Disc pain may be primary or cause pain due to compression or instability. It may be diagnosed by a physical examination or diagnostic injections.

L. Referred pain may be cardiac, myofascial, neoplastic, or visceral.

REFERENCES

Bogduk N: Medical *Management of Acute Cervical Radicular Pain: An Evidence-Based Approach.* Newcastle, Australian Acute Musculoskeletal Pain Guidelines Group, 1999, Chapters 5-7, 11, 13.

Raj PP: *Practical Management of Pain,* 2nd ed. St. Louis, Mosby Year Book, 1992, Chapter 17.

Tollison CD, Satterthwaite JR, Tollison JW: *Practical Pain Management,* 3rd ed. Philadelphia, Lippincott Williams & Wilkins, 2002, Chapter 26.

Patient with HEAD AND NECK PAIN

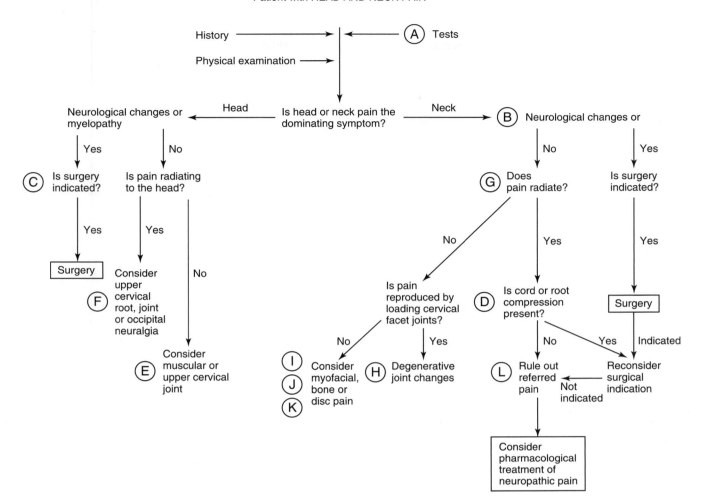

Approach to the Patient with Headache

RENEE BAILEY

A. When a patient presents with headache (HA), the most important question is whether the HA is due to a serious or potentially life-threatening condition. Features of the history suggestive of intracranial pathology include an acute "thunderclap" onset, occipitonuchal location, age over 55 years, HA that awakens the patient from sleep, focal neurologic symptoms, diplopia, episodic visual loss lasting seconds, personality or mental status changes, position-dependent HA, and increasing HA frequency. Physical examination features that suggest a serious etiology include fever, significant hypertension, papilledema, anisocoria, meningismus, and an abnormal neurologic or mental status examination.

B. Any of the above signs or symptoms warrant computed tomography examination of the head and further neurologic investigation. In this setting imaging should be performed prior to considering a lumbar puncture. Magnetic resonance imaging is usually not necessary for the investigation of acute HA but may be useful in the setting of chronic HA. The addition of contrast enhancement should be considered to evaluate possible meningitis or mass lesions.

C. Patients over age 50 with unilateral frontotemporal HA should be screened for temporal arteritis with an erythrocyte sedimentation rate or a C-reactive protein assay. Fever, vision loss, myalgias, scalp tenderness, and jaw claudication are other associated signs and symptoms. Temporal arteritis is rare in patients under age 50.

D. Further diagnostic evaluation of the HA usually is unnecessary if the patient is free of the above features that indicate a serious etiology.

E. Lumbar puncture should be performed only if there is no blood or mass on neuroimaging. It is done to evaluate the patient for possible meningitis, subarachnoid hemorrhage, or pseudotumor cerebri. An accurate opening pressure should always be measured as part of the routine cerebrospinal fluid evaluation, along with cell counts, glucose, protein, and Gram stain/culture.

F. Tension HAs are often characterized by diffuse pressure-like pain throughout the head, and many are described in a "hatband" distribution around the forehead, temples, and occiput. The HAs may be associated with neck or shoulder pain and tension, and they are often worsened by social stress.

G. The use of nonsteroidal antiinflammatory drugs (NSAIDs) is usually sufficient acute abortive treatment of the HA. Muscle relaxants, such as methocarbamol, may be useful for patients complaining of neck or shoulder pain.

H. Preventive treatment for HAs occurring more frequently than twice per week and for many hours each day and for HAs that significantly limit the patient's activities includes amitriptyline, selective serotonin reuptake inhibitors for patients with symptoms suggestive of underlying depression, and stress reduction, which might include regular exercise or biofeedback.

I. Dental and sinus disorders, overuse of analgesic medications ("rebound" HAs), and ocular disease may manifest as an acute or chronic HA, although these HAs occur less commonly than tension or migraine HAs. Many patients who report sinus HAs or who abuse analgesics are found to have tension or migraine HAs when a more thorough history is available.

REFERENCES

Ramirez-Lassespas M, Espinosa CE, Cicero JJ, et al: Predictors of intracranial pathologic findings in patients who seek emergency care because of headache. *Arch Neurol* 1997;54:1506–1509.

Silberstein SD, U.S. Headache Consortium: Practice parameter: evidence-based guidelines for migraine headache (an evidence-based review). *Neurology* 2000:55;754–762.

Silberstein SD, Lipton RB, Goadsby PJ (eds): *Headache in Clinical Practice.* Oxford, Isis Medical Media, 1998.

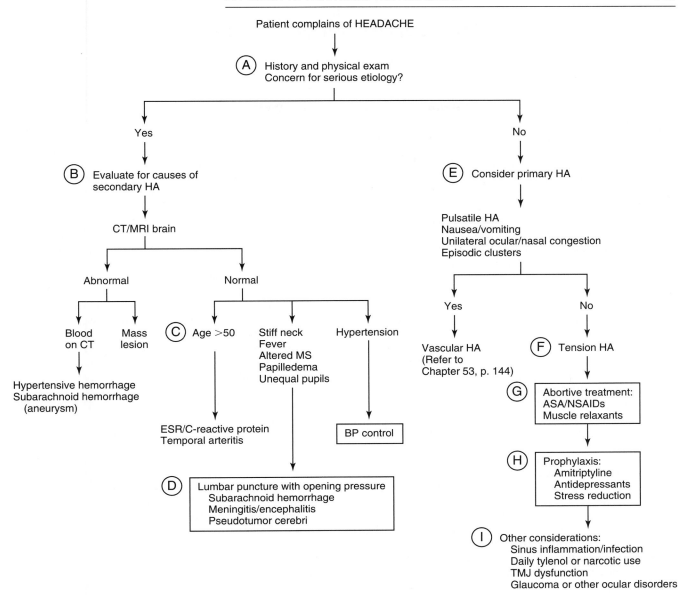

Vascular Headache

RENEE BAILEY

Among vascular headaches (HAs), the migraine HA is extremely common, occurring in about 20% of women and 6% of men. Cluster HAs are rarer, with an estimated prevalence of less than 0.5%. The onset of vascular headaches is between the first and third decades of life. Other diagnoses should be pursued in patients over the age of 40 who have no known history of vascular HAs.

A. Migraine HAs are characterized by pulsatile pain, usually with a unilateral onset or focus. These HAs are often associated with nausea, vomiting, and sensitivity to light or sound. Migraine sufferers often seek out a dark, quiet room; and most report alleviation or resolution with sleep. Many patients have a family history of migraine, or "sick" HAs.

B. The migraine HA is now classified by the presence or absence of an aura, or prodrome. This aura most often manifests as a visual phenomenon preceding or accompanying the HA. The visual symptoms are described as an area of sparkling or flashing lights with an associated region of visual loss; however, this prodrome may consist of any transient neurologic symptoms, including somatic sensory, motor, or brain stem disturbances.

C. Acute treatment of migraine HA consists of both nonpharmacologic and pharmacologic therapy. Nonpharmacologic treatments include sleep, resting in a dark, quiet area, and cool compresses on the forehead. Pharmacologic treatments are many, and the smallest effective dose should be employed. Combinations of agents are often used, including analgesics, caffeine, and antiemetics. For mild to moderate HAs, the abortive agents include nonsteroidal antiinflammatory drugs (NSAIDs), analgesic combinations containing caffeine, and isomeheptene-containing agents (Midrin). Oral antiemetics are used for nausea and as adjunctive agents for pain.

D. For moderate to severe migraine or for milder HAs that have not responded to more conservative measures, acute treatment includes ergotamine preparations (oral or rectal); intranasal, intramuscular, intravenous, or subcutaneous dihydroergotamine (DHE); and the "triptans" (naratriptan, rizatriptan, sumatriptan, zolmitriptan). Intravenous, intramuscular, and per rectum antiemetics are useful in patients with severe migraine to control nausea and pain. Opiates and sedatives should be avoided but may be considered if abuse potential and sedation risk are low. Intravenous corticosteroids may also be considered for rescue therapy in patients with status migrainosus.

E. Preventive measures for migraine HA are used in individuals with three or more severe HAs each month to decrease HA frequency and severity. There is grade A evidence supporting the use of propranolol, timolol, amitriptyline, and verapamil. Propranolol and verapamil may be used at a maximum of 240 mg/day. Amitriptyline is titrated to a dose of 100 to 150 mg/day. These agents should be taken daily and at the highest tolerated dose for at least 6 to 8 weeks before the agent is deemed ineffective. Patients should be monitored for bradycardia and hypotension when the drugs are initiated. Behavior modification is also a useful, nonpharmacologic means of HA prevention.

F. Cluster HAs are characterized by sharp, boring, unilateral, temporal or periorbital pain associated with unilateral tearing, nasal congestion or rhinorrhea, and Horner's syndrome. Men are affected more frequently than women. Attacks last for up to 3 hours and occur almost daily—sometimes even multiple times each day—for days to months, often with a remission of weeks to years. Compared to migraine sufferers, these patients are restless and may engage in head-banging or other activities as a means of distraction.

G. Acute treatment of individual attacks includes 100% oxygen, sumatriptan, intramuscular, intravenous, or intranasal DHE, and intranasal lidocaine. Intranasal agents are used in the nostril ipsilateral to the HA.

H. Preventive treatment may help decrease attack duration and frequency. Useful daily agents include oral ergotamine preparations, lithium, valproic acid, verapamil, and prednisone (short term to induce remission). These agents should be continued until the patient is HA-free for at least 2 weeks and then slowly tapered. Preventive therapy should resume at the onset of the next attack.

REFERENCES

Silberstein SD, for the US Headache Consortium: Practice parameter: evidence-based guidelines for migraine headache (an evidence-based review). *Neurology* 2000:55;754–762.

Silberstein SD, Lipton RB, Goadsby PJ (eds): *Headache in Clinical Practice.* Oxford, Isis Medical Media, 1998.

Swanson JW, Dodick DW, Capobianco DJ: Headache and other craniofacial pain. In: Bradley WG, Daroff RB, Fenichel GM, Marsden CD (eds) *Neurology in Clinical Practice,* 3rd ed. Boston, Butterworth-Heinemann, 2000.

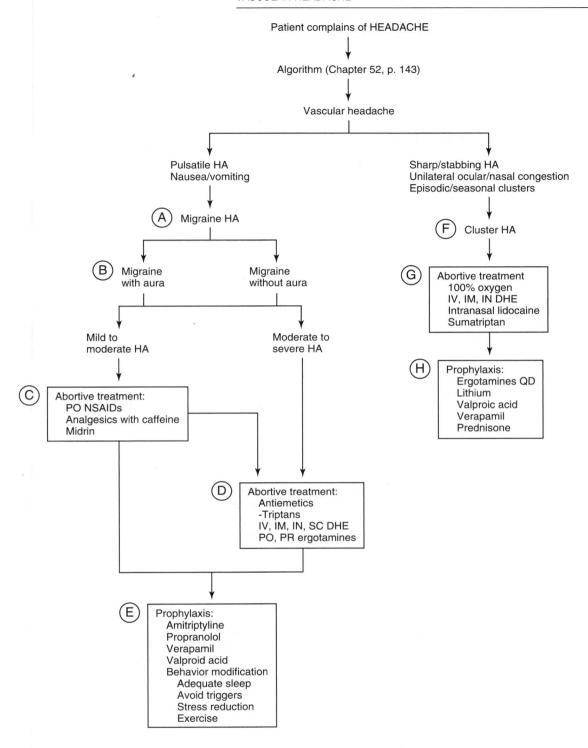

Patient complains of HEADACHE

Algorithm (Chapter 52, p. 143)

Vascular headache

Pulsatile HA
Nausea/vomiting

(A) Migraine HA

(B) Migraine
with aura

Migraine
without aura

Mild to
moderate HA

Moderate to
severe HA

(C) Abortive treatment:
PO NSAIDs
Analgesics with caffeine
Midrin

(D) Abortive treatment:
Antiemetics
-Triptans
IV, IM, IN, SC DHE
PO, PR ergotamines

(E) Prophylaxis:
Amitriptyline
Propranolol
Verapamil
Valproid acid
Behavior modification
Adequate sleep
Avoid triggers
Stress reduction
Exercise

Sharp/stabbing HA
Unilateral ocular/nasal congestion
Episodic/seasonal clusters

(F) Cluster HA

(G) Abortive treatment
100% oxygen
IV, IM, IN DHE
Intranasal lidocaine
Sumatriptan

(H) Prophylaxis:
Ergotamines QD
Lithium
Valproic acid
Verapamil
Prednisone

Trigeminal Neuralgia

RICHARD BAROHN

Facial pain due to trigeminal neuralgia (TN), also known as tic douloureux, has the following features: (1) brief, paroxysmal, intense, lancinating, or shock-like pain; (2) unilateral; (3) confined to the distribution of the fifth cranial nerve (CN-V), with the mandibular and maxillary divisions affected more often than the ophthalmic; and (4) provocation by minimal stimuli (chewing, talking, brushing teeth, cold wind on face). TN occurs most often in the sixth and seventh decades. The etiology is unknown although some physicians, principally led by Jeanetta, believe that the cause is external compression of the trigeminal nerves in the posterior fossa by arteries or veins.

A. Patients with TN do not complain of numbness, and examination of all cranial nerves including CN-V is normal, as is the entire neurologic examination. If these are abnormal, TN is unlikely, and a search for a mass lesion (intrinsic to the pons, cerebellopontine angle, or cavernous sinus) or chronic meningitis should be conducted. MRI of the brain and posterior fossa is indicated, followed by lumbar puncture if the MRI is normal.

B. Occasionally patients with connective tissue disease (Sjögren's disease, systemic lupus erythematosus, scleroderma) can present with trigeminal neuropathy. Usually the serum antinuclear antibody assay (ANA) is positive.

C. Patients with continuous unilateral aching pain are often diagnosed with atypical facial pain. If all possible causes have been eliminated (including dental and temporomandibular joint disease), treatment is difficult; occasionally tricyclic antidepressants can be useful. Herpes zoster can involve CN-V, usually in the ophthalmic division. The characteristic rash will eventually erupt. The pain is burning and constant and can persist after the rash has resolved (postherpetic neuralgia).

D. If TN occurs in a patient 20 to 40 years old and the pain is bilateral the possibility of multiple sclerosis should be considered.

E. Medical therapy for TN consists of the following options: (1) carbamazepine (CARB) and oxcarbamazepine, (2) gabapentin (Neurontin), (3) lamotrigine (Lamictal), or (4) baclofen. Each drug should be tried for at least two to three weeks before it is considered ineffective.

F. CARB is the drug of choice for TN; however the drug dose needs to be increased gradually to avoid unpleasant side effects (nausea, ataxia, confusion). Begin with 200 mg daily and increase by 200 mg every 2 to 3 days (in three divided doses). A dose adequate to relieve pain may not be reached for 4 to 7 days.

G. If the patient is in so much pain that the delay needed to reach an effective CARB dose is not advisable, phenytoin can be administered IV at the same time that oral CARB therapy is begun. The phenytoin IV dose (18 mg/kg) must be given slowly (50 mg/kg), and the blood pressure and the heart rate need to be closely monitored while the drug is being administered. Pain relief often is immediate and may last for several days until oral CARB becomes effective.

H. If all of the medical therapies fail, consider more invasive interventions. The following approaches may relieve pain in 80% to 90% of patients: (1) retrogasserian glycerol injection as described by Hakanson, (2) percutaneous radiofrequency rhizotomy of the trigeminal ganglion, and (3) microvascular decompression by a posterior craniotomy. Unfortunately, about 8% of patients develop a dysesthetic pain syndrome (anesthesia dolorosa) following percutaneous rhizotomy. Microvascular decompression, the third option, has a surgical morbidity and mortality rate of 7% and 1%, respectively. Recently Gamma Knife has been used effectively. The invasive procedure of choice varies from institution to institution. We employ retrogasserian glycerol injection or percutaneous rhizotomy initially as it is less invasive and has a very good success rate in medically refractory TN. If this fails or pain recurs the more invasive microvascular decompression is done.

REFERENCES

Carrazana E, Mikoshiba I: Rationale and evidence for the use of oxcarbazepine in neuropathic Pain. *J Pain Symp Manage* 2003;(Suppl 1) 25:S31–35.

Hagen NA, Stevens JC, Michet CJ Jr: Trigeminal sensory neuropathy associated with connective tissue diseases. *Neurology* 1990;40:891.

Hakanson S: Retrogasserian injection of glycerol in the treatment of trigeminal neuralgia and other facial pains. *Neurosurgery* 1982;10:300.

Janetta PJ: Microsurgical management of trigeminal neuralgia. *Arch Neurol* 1985;42:800.

Morley TP: Case against microvascular decompression in the treatment of trigeminal neuralgia. *Arch Neurol* 1985;42:801.

Sindrup SH, Jensen TS: Pharmacotherapy of trigeminal neuralgia. *Clin J Pain* 2002;18:22–27.

Sweet WH: The treatment of trigeminal neuralgia (tic douloureux). *N Engl J Med* 1986;315:174.

Sweet WH: Percutaneous methods for the treatment of trigeminal neuralgia and other faciocephalic pain: comparison with microvascular decompression. *Semin Neurol* 1988;8:272.

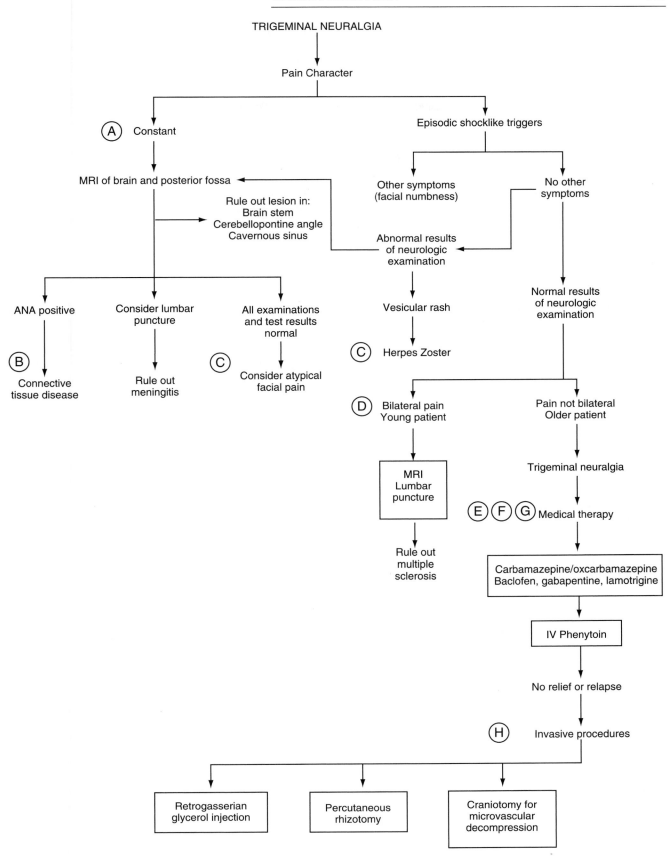

Temporomandibular Disorders

STEPHEN B. MILAM

Temporomandibular disorder (TMD) is a term that refers to a variety of painful derangements of the temporomandibular joint (TMJ) and masticatory musculature. Because of the complex pain referral patterns, these disorders are commonly misdiagnosed. For example, masticatory myalgias can mimic odontalgias. In fact, many patients have undergone unnecessary endodontic therapy, or even dental extractions, as a result of misdiagnosed TMDs. Likewise, patients often seek treatment by otolaryngologists for TMDs that refer pain to the ear. Adding to the confusion, TMDs are commonly associated with subjective auditory symptoms (i.e., tinnitus, subtle hearing impairment), even though audiometric studies are typically normal.

The TMDs can be mimicked by other derangements of the head and neck. For example, patients suffering from cervical flexion-extension injuries often complain of pain in the preauricular and periorbital areas. Because common TMDs also refer pain to these areas, these patients may be misdiagnosed. For this reason, many clinicians believe that cervical flexion-extension injuries contribute to TMDs, although recent studies suggest that this is unlikely. It is interesting to note that the TMJ receives sensory innervation from the trigeminal nerve and from branches of cervical nerves (C2-5 in rodents).

Epidemiologic data indicate a female preponderance for common TMDs. In fact, some clinical reports indicate as high as a 9:1 female/male preponderance. Studies have implicated estrogens in the pathogenesis of some TMDs, although their significance has not been firmly established. For example, nerve growth factor (NGF), a neurotrophin involved in sensory and sympathetic nerve development, has been implicated in the genesis of some myalgias. The primary receptor for NGF is termed trkA. The trkA gene is positively regulated by an estrogen-response element. Clinical trials suggest that women are more susceptible to NGF-induced myalgias, presumably owing to the abundance of trkA relative to their male counterparts.

Some TMDs are exacerbated by psychological stress. Clinical studies have provided evidence that jaw clenching increases in subjects subjected to stressful conditions. Most experts believe that this parafunctional behavior contributes to some TMDs by overuse of some masticatory muscles and by increasing or sustaining mechanical loads to the TMJs. However, another mechanism is suggested from studies that have confirmed that NGF is released from cellular stores, predominantly mast cells, in response to psychological stress.

The patient typically presents with pain felt in the preauricular, temporal, periorbital, masseteric, or posterior cervical regions and the ear. The pain may vary in quality from a protracted aching sensation to an intermittent sharp, stabbing sensation. Patients may also complain of tinnitus, vertigo, or subtle hearing impairments that are typically not detected by audiometric studies. Pain from TMDs is commonly intermittent, with the intensity varying

from day to day. Often patients experience periods of remission that can last days to weeks before recurrence. Patients suffering from TMDs may rarely report nausea with severe episodes of pain. Vomiting is extremely unusual. Scotomas and photophobia are not typically associated with TMDs.

Patients suffering from TMD or severe masticatory myalgias exhibit a reduction in the range of jaw movement. The maximum interincisal distance (MID), measured in millimeters from the incisal edges of the maxillary and mandibular central incisors at maximum opening, is commonly used to assess jaw movement. A normal MID for adults ranges from 45 to 60 mm. Recordings of 40 mm or less are viewed as abnormal in most cases. In addition, some derangements of the TMJ (e.g., articular disc displacement, mass lesions) can interfere with the normal translational (i.e., forward) movements of the joint, resulting in jaw deviations that are clinically evident. Under normal conditions, the jaw opens and closes in a straight vertical movement observed in the frontal plane. However, TMJ derangements that restrict joint movement result in deviation of the jaw toward the affected side.

Some TMJ disorders (e.g., osteoarthritis, rheumatoid arthritis, synovial chondromatosis) can result in irregular articular surfaces that may produce pops or clicks with jaw movements. These are easily detected with auscultation of the affected joint. In addition, articular disc interference can produce pops or clicks with jaw movements.

Laboratory tests, including creatine kinase assay, erythrocyte sedimentation rate, and C-reactive protein assay, typically are normal for usual TMDs. Magnetic resonance imaging and computed tomography of the TMJ can delineate a variety of joint diseases.

Manual palpation of involved masticatory muscles (i.e., masseter, temporalis, medial pterygoid, and lateral pterygoid muscles) produces pain similar in quality and distribution to that described by the patient as the chief complaint. Injection of a small volume (< 0.25 ml) of a dilute solution of local anesthetic into the affected muscle site provides temporary pain relief. Patients with TMDs who have undergone previous TMJ surgery may experience secondary pain, including sympathetically mediated pain (i.e., complex regional syndrome). These patients typically complain of burning pain in the preauricular region of the operated joint and exhibit marked mechanical allodynia to light touch of this region.

Treatment protocols for common TMDs include tricyclic antidepressants (i.e., mixed serotonin-norepinephrine reuptake inhibitors, e.g., amitriptyline). Ironically, selective serotonin reuptake inhibitors (SSRIs), commonly administered to manage depression, can exacerbate some TMDs by inducing nocturnal bruxism. Drug-induced bruxism is observed in approximately 1% to 5% of patients taking SSRIs. Other treatments, including nonsteroidal anti-inflammatory drugs (for inflammatory joint derangements only), benzodiazepines (e.g., clonazepam, diazepam), muscle relaxants (*e.g.*, cyclobenzaprine), opiates, trigger-point injections with local anesthetics or botulinum toxin, bite splints, or TMJ surgery may be indicated. Appropriate treatment protocols for managing sympathetically maintained pain is indicated in some patients.

REFERENCES

Bays RA, Quinn PD: Temporomandibular disorders. In: Fonseca RA (ed) *Oral and Maxillofacial Surgery*, vol 4. Philadelphia, Saunders, 2000.

Kaplan AS, Assael LA (eds): Temporomandibular Disorders: Diagnosis and Treatment. Philadelphia, Saunders, 1991.

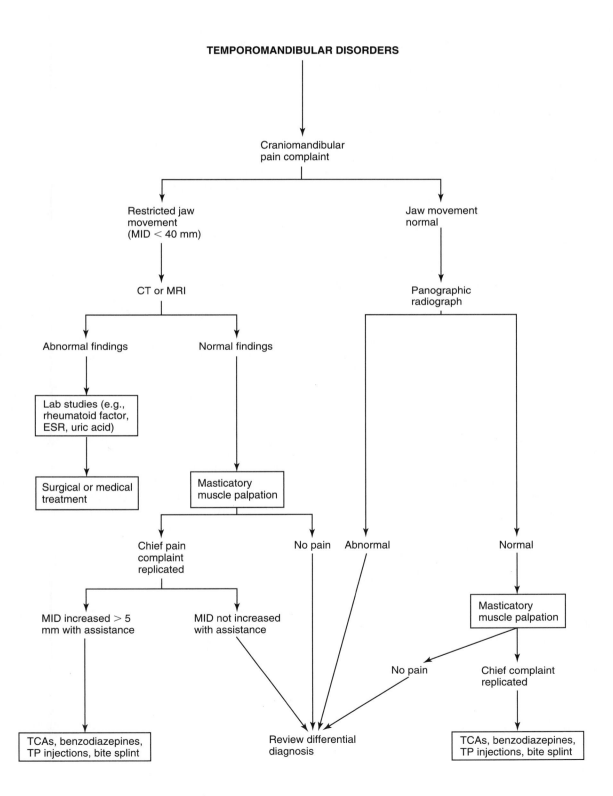

Orofacial Pain

JEFFREY T. SUMMERS

Generally, the diagnosis of orofacial pain conditions can be readily determined with an appropriate history and physical examination. However, the presentations of many pain syndromes overlap and also can be mimicked by pathologic processes involving the primary pain generator, such as when tumor or infection invades nerve tissue and presents as neuralgia.

A. Testing may include radiography and, where indicated, computed tomography, magnetic resonance imaging, magnetic resonance angiography, or brain scans. An infectious etiology workup may include a complete blood count, erythrocyte sedimentation rate, and C-reactive protein studies. Psychological testing is recommended for individuals with chronic or recalcitrant pain.

B. Dental or odontogenic pain is the most common form of orofacial pain. Tooth-related pain is the most common form, but others include pain arising from the pulp or periodontal structures. In such cases, the patient is referred to a dentist.

C. Orofacial cancer does not typically present as pain at its onset or during the early phases of the disease. If neurologic changes such as sensory loss are present in addition to the pain, there is increased likelihood of a destructive process such as malignancy or infection.

D. Temporomandibular joint (TMJ) disorders may have intraarticular or extraarticular origins. Pain is often a deep, aching pain involving the frontal or temporal head, preauricular region, or mandible.

E. Trigeminal neuralgia typically presents as a lancinating pain in the distribution of one or more branches of the trigeminal (V) nerve. The pain lasts seconds to minutes and is frequently unilateral. The pain usually involves a trigger stimulus such as talking, eating, chewing, or oral hygiene. It more commonly affects women and typically occurs after age 40. Earlier onset suggests possible multiple sclerosis.

F. Trigeminal neuropathic pain may result from acute herpes zoster (HZ). The pain is usually of a burning, tingling, or lancinating nature and may precede skin lesions by 2 to 3 days. If the pain persists for 1 month after the onset of skin lesions, the diagnosis becomes postherpetic neuralgia (PHN). This pain may be perceived as burning, tearing, or itching with a superimposed lancinating component. Sympathetic blocks (stellate ganglion) may alleviate the pain and, if employed early, may prevent or attenuate the PHN.

G. The complex regional pain syndrome manifests as superficial burning or aching pain in a diffuse nondermatomal pattern. Hyperpathia and allodynia are usually present along with possible vasomotor, sudomotor, and trophic changes.

H. Glossopharyngeal neuralgia involves episodic bursts of pain in the posterior tongue, pharynx, or soft palate. There may be trigger zones in these areas or posterior to the mandibular ramus. It is described as a stabbing pain precipitated by tongue movement, yawning, or coughing. The pain lasts about 30 seconds followed by a burning sensation that persists 2 to 3 minutes. It may be associated with bradycardia, syncope, or seizures due to involvement of the vagus nerve. The neuralgia may be diagnosed and the symptoms relieved by a local injection of anesthesia into the lateral pharyngeal wall.

I. Sphenopalatine ganglion neuralgia presents as a unilateral, constant boring pain in the lower half of the face below the eyebrows sometimes precipitated by sneezing. It is occasionally associated with rhinorrhea, lacrimation, conjunctival injection, and salivation. It may respond to sphenopalatine ganglion blocks (injected, topical).

J. Vidian neuralgia is similar to sphenopalatine neuralgia except it presents as severe paroxysmal attacks of pain involving the nose, face, eye, ear, head, neck, and shoulder; it often occurs at night. If an infection of the sphenoid sinus is present, see that it is treated, with an appropriate referral.

K. Ciliary neuralgia is a form of migraine caused by middle meningeal artery spasm. It presents as paroxysmal pain in one eye and the ipsilateral face, with accompanying rhinorrhea, nasal congestion, iritis, and keratitis. Immediate relief of ocular pain and keratitis/iritis may be obtained with cocainization of the anterior half of the lateral wall of the affected nostril (anterior ethmoidal nerve).

L. Atypical facial pain is a diagnosis of exclusion and may involve significant psychological factors. Patient denial of possible psychogenic factors and excessive use of the health care system are common. The pain may be bilateral and migratory. It is often perceived as a sensory loss but nondermatomal. Invasive treatments are usually avoided because of their poor success rates and the possibility of increasing the pain. Treatment should include psychological testing and intervention.

M. Orofacial pain of myofascial origin presents as persistent, deep, aching, poorly localized pain that involves facial muscles, often the muscles of mastication. The diagnosis is based on the presence of trigger points that reproduce the pain.

N. Pharmacologic treatment of orofacial pain of neurogenic origin is similar to that for other neuropathic pain states. Anticonvulsants, antidepressants, opioids, and in some cases muscle relaxants (baclofen) are the most common medications used. Diagnostic and therapeutic nerve blocks are of limited utility.

REFERENCES

Haasis JC: Alternative therapies. In: Tollison CD, Satterthwaite JR, Tollison JW (eds) *Practical Pain Management*, 3rd ed. Philadelphia, Lippincott Williams & Wilkins, 2001, pp 209–215.

Hsu FPK, Israel ZH, Burgess JA, Burchiel KJ: Orofacial Pain: Differential diagnosis and treatment. In: Tollison CD, Satterthwaite JR, Tollison JW (eds) *Practical Pain Management*, 3rd ed. Philadelphia, Lippincott Williams & Wilkins, 2001, pp 359–373.

Loeser JD: Cranial neuralgias. In: Bonica JJ (ed) *The Management of Pain*, 2nd ed. Philadelphia, Lea & Febiger, 1990, pp 676–686.

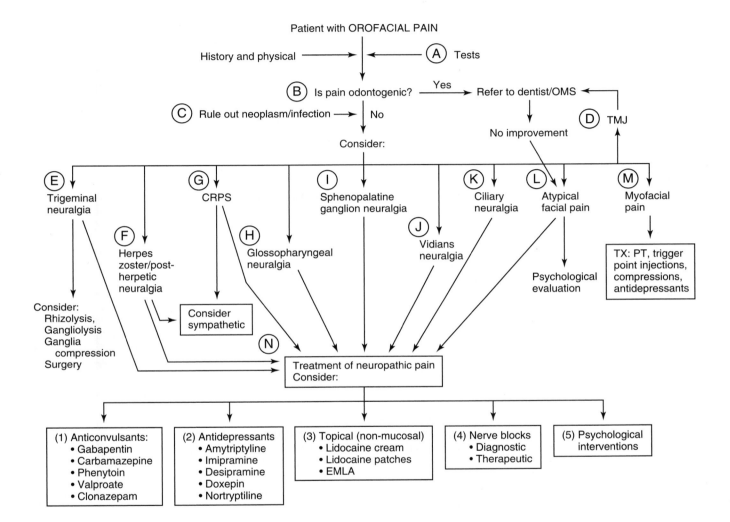

Cervical Zygapophyseal Joint Pain

NIKOLAI BOGDUK

The cervical zygapophyseal joints (Z joints) are paired, synovial joints located along the back of the neck between consecutive vertebrae from the C2-3 level to C6-7. They are one of the structures in the neck most commonly injured by whiplash, and cervical Z joint pain is the single, most common basis of chronic neck pain after whiplash injury. Its prevalence in patients with nontraumatic neck pain is not known.

A. Cervical Z joint pain, which may occur in isolation or concurrently with discogenic pain, is not related to neurologic signs. It may persist or occur behind and despite an anterior cervical fusion. However, there are no clinical features that are even suggestive, let alone diagnostic, of cervical Z joint pain. There are no radiographic, computed tomography, or magnetic resonance imaging features that implicate or refute the Z joints as a source of neck pain. Cervical Z joint pain cannot be diagnosed in patients who suffer acute neck pain, as it cannot be distinguished from any other cause of acute neck pain by clinical examination or medical imaging. Moreover, because many of these patients recover spontaneously or after empirical therapy, there is no justification for implementing invasive investigations during the acute phase in pursuit of the etiology of Z joint pain. Patients who prove to have cervical Z joint pain emerge from an inception cohort of patients with undifferentiated neck pain. These patients already have been screened for major traumatic, neurologic, and systemic disorders using conventional algorithms. Investigations for putative Z joint pain should be planned during the second or third month of unremitting acute neck pain and implemented by the third or fourth month if the pain does not diminish. This schedule allows natural resolution but minimizes the risk of psychosocial deterioration due to chronic pain.

B. Pain maps may be used to deduce the likely segmental location of a painful Z joint, but these maps are not diagnostic of Z joint pain; the same pattern of referred pain can be caused by discogenic pain at the same segment. Pain from C2-3 is typically experienced over the upper cervical region and occiput, and it may radiate into the forehead or orbit. Pain from C3-4 typically starts high in the neck but embraces the entire length of the posterolateral aspect of the neck. C4-5 pain is focused over the angle between the neck and the top of the shoulder girdle. Pain from C5-6 spreads to cover the supraspinous and deltoid regions of the shoulder. C6-7 pain radiates over the blade of the scapula. Because cervical Z joint pain is common, it should be suspected in any patient with such distribution of pain, and a provisional diagnosis of Z joint pain can be entertained on epidemiologic grounds alone. The pain maps serve only to direct where definitive investigations should commence.

C. Controlled, diagnostic blocks under fluoroscopic guidance are the only means of establishing a diagnosis of cervical Z joint pain. These joints can be anesthetized by blocking the nerves that innervate them. At levels C3-4 to C6-7, each joint is innervated from above and below by medial branches of the dorsal rami that bear the same segmental number as the joint. These nerves cross the middle of the ipsisegmental articular pillars, which provide radiographically recognizable landmarks for diagnostic blocks. Each nerve can be anesthetized with as little as 0.3 mL of local anesthetic. Larger volumes risk compromising the target specificity of the block. The C2-3 joint is innervated by the third occipital nerve, which crosses the lateral aspect of the joint. This nerve can be blocked by a series of three injections of 0.3 mL of local anesthetic deposited across the course of the nerve. Blocks are initiated at the segmental level suggested by the patient's pain map. If the first block is negative, investigations are resumed at the next joint above or below it until all joints that sensibly might be a possible source of the patient's pain have been tested. Thereafter investigations for other sources of neck pain may be undertaken. However, if at any time patients report relief of the pain following a Z joint block, they must return for controlled blocks to confirm the diagnosis.

D. Diagnostic blocks must be controlled lest a false diagnosis be made. The false-positive rate of single diagnostic blocks is at least 28%. Controls must be used for each and every patient. Placebo controls pose ethical and logistic problems and require a series of three injections to be valid. A practical, valid alternative is to use comparative local anesthetic blocks. On each of two occasions the patient undergoes a diagnostic block but using a different local anesthetic agent, such as lignocaine 2% or bupivacaine 0.5%. A positive response is one in which the patient obtains complete relief of the pain on each occasion but longer-lasting relief when the long-acting agent is used and shorter-lasting relief when the short-acting agent is used. Such blocks can be performed on a double-blind basis to optimize their validity. No diagnosis is entertained until the patient completes both blocks and the code is broken.

E. There is no evidence that any form of conservative therapy relieves cervical Z joint pain. The use of physiotherapy, manipulative therapy, nonsteroidal antiinflammatory drugs (NSAIDs), or trigger point injections is entirely speculative. The use of intraarticular steroids has been discredited as a valid option, as few patients respond for longer than a few days, and just as many benefit from an intraarticular local anesthetic as from steroids. The one definitive, proven therapy for cervical Z joint pain is percutaneous radiofrequency medial branch neurotomy. The power of this therapy has been demonstrated in open trials, and its validity has been established in a placebo-controlled, double-blind trial. The operation involves coagulating the medial branches of the

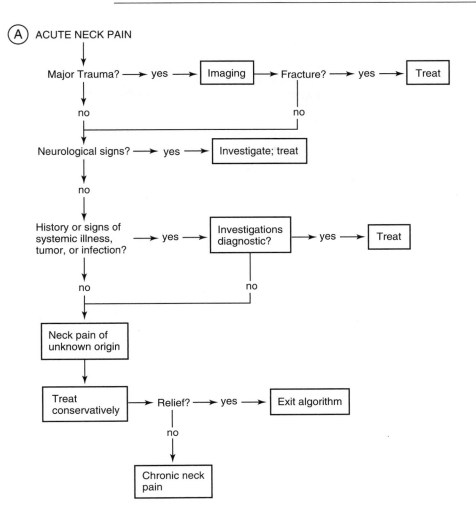

dorsal rami that innervate the painful joint. For this reason, the diagnostic protocol to locate a painful joint must involve medial branch blocks instead of intra-articular blocks. Medial branch blocks are thereby not only diagnostic but prognostic of a response to radiofrequency neurotomy. Cervical medial branch neurotomy is not an easy procedure. When performed correctly, it requires 3 hours to complete, and even then it is associated with technical failures. The lesions made by radiofrequency exposure are barely 2 mm in radius; the medial branches are less than 1 mm in diameter, and the tiny, target nerves may escape coagulation. This does not impugn the patient. Technical failure impugns the surgeon.

REFERENCES

Barnsley L, Lord S, Bogduk N: Comparative local anaesthetic blocks in the diagnosis of cervical zygapophyseal joints pain. *Pain* 1993;55:99–106.

Barnsley L, Lord S, Wallis B, Bogduk N: False-positive rates of cervical zygapophyseal joint blocks. *Clin J Pain* 1993;9:124–130.

Barnsley L, Lord SM, Wallis BJ, Bogduk N: Lack of effect of intraarticular corticosteroids for chronic pain in the cervical zygapophyseal joints. *N Engl J Med* 1994;330:1047–1050.

Bogduk N: International Spinal Injection Society guidelines for the performance of spinal injection procedures. I. Zygapophyseal joint blocks. *Clin J Pain* 1997;13:285–302.

Bogduk N, Aprill C: On the nature of neck pain, discography and cervical zygapophyseal joint pain. *Pain* 1993;54:213–217.

Dwyer A, Aprill C, Bogduk N: Cervical zygapophyseal joint pain patterns. I. A study in normal volunteers. *Spine* 1990;15:453-457.

Jónsson H, Bring G, Rauschning W, Sahlstedt B: Hidden cervical spine injuries in traffic accident victims with skull fractures. *J Spinal Dis* 1991;4:251-263.

Lord SM, Barnsley L, Bogduk N: The utility of comparative local anaesthetic blocks versus placebo-controlled blocks for the diagnosis of cervical zygapophyseal joint pain. *Clin J Pain* 1995;11:208–213.

Lord S, Barnsley L, Wallis BJ, Bogduk N: Chronic cervical zygapophyseal joint pain after whiplash: a placebo-controlled prevalence study. *Spine* 1996;21:1737–1745.

Lord S, Barnsley L, Wallis B, Bogduk N: Third occipital nerve headache: a prevalence study. *J Neurol Neurosurg Psychiatry* 1994;57:1187–1190.

Lord S, Barnsley L, Wallis BJ, et al: Percutaneous radio-frequency neurotomy for chronic cervical zygapophyseal joint pain. *N Engl J Med* 1996;335:1721–1726.

Spitzer WO, Skovron ML, Salmi LR, et al: Scientific monograph of the Quebec task force on whiplash-associated disorders: redefining "whiplash" and its management. *Spine* 1995;20:1S–73S.

Taylor JR, Twomey LT: Acute injuries to cervical joints: an autopsy study of neck sprain. *Spine* 1993;18:1115-1122.

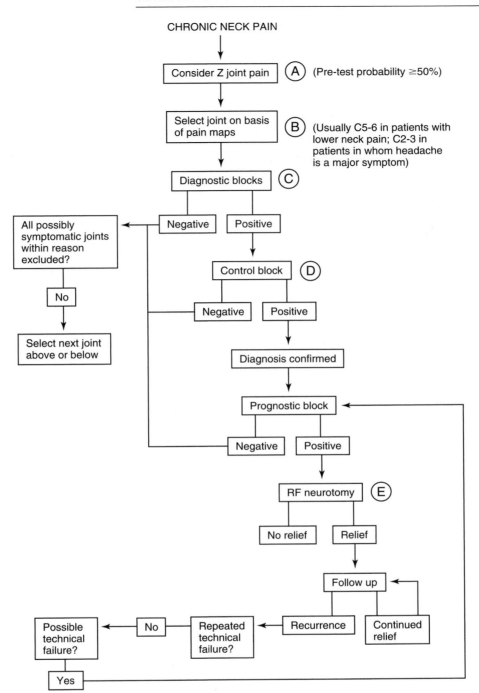

Cervical Radiculopathies

SOMAYAJI RAMAMURTHY

Radiculopathy in the cervical region is usually caused by cervical spondylosis and herniation of the cervical intervertebral disc. Pain is caused by the irritation and compression of the cervical nerve root, producing radicular symptoms and signs in the upper extremity. Severe trauma such as a whiplash following an automobile accident can also lead to a herniated disc and radicular symptoms. Pain due to cervical radiculopathy usually begins in the middle of the neck and radiates to the shoulder and the arm in the distribution of the involved nerve root. Pain with the movement of the neck and a positive Spurling's sign indicate radicular involvement. In-line traction to decrease the pain and compression of the head to reproduce the patient's pain aid in diagnosis. The radicular pain may be associated with sensory motor and reflex changes in the upper extremity corresponding to the involved nerve root as shown in Table 1.

A. *Differential diagnosis.* Pain originating from the neck muscles, facet joints, cervical disc, involvement of the brachial plexus due to inflammation or malignancy of the lung, referred visceral pain from the thorax and the neck, and so forth. It is essential therefore to obtain a thorough history and perform neurologic examination not only of the upper extremity but also the lower extremity because cervical spondylosis and disc herniation are frequently associated with the compression of the spinal cord. Spinal cord compression from other causes such as vertebral disease (tuberculosis, secondary malignancy, and syrinx) can produce cervicobrachial pain.

B. *Diagnostic studies.* Imaging studies such as plain X-ray film, magnetic resonance imaging (MRI), and bone scan can be very valuable in determining the nature and the level of the pathology. Significant degenerative changes are very common even among asymptomatic individuals. Thus it is very important to correlate results of the imaging studies to the clinical findings.

Electrodiagnostic studies such as electromyography (EMG) and nerve conduction velocity studies are of great value, especially when positive. They will help to correlate functional changes to the anatomical changes observed in the imaging studies. Electrodiagnostic studies are also helpful in differentiating cervical radiculopathy from other upper extremity entrapment syndromes.

C. *Treatment.* Ninety-five percent of the acute pain usually resolves in 6 to 8 weeks. Use of a neck collar, nonsteroidal antiinflammatory drugs (NSAIDs), transcutaneous electrical nerve stimulation (TENS) and other conservative measures are beneficial. If the radicular pain continues and if there is no involvement of the spinal cord, epidural steroid injections can be very effective in relieving the symptoms in 65% of patients. The epidural steroids can be administered either through the interlaminar foramen or through the intervertebral foramen (Transforaminal). This procedure should be performed by experienced physicians because of the potential for serious complications such as spinal cord injury caused by needle trauma or injection of particulate matter into the radicular artery during Transforaminal epidural injection. An epidural catheter advanced from an upper thoracic level can be selectively placed at the involved root level under fluoroscopy and may be a very safe and effective technique. If the patient obtains only temporary benefit from epidural steroid injections and if he or she is not a candidate for surgery, radiofrequency lesion of the cervical dorsal root ganglion may provide long-term pain relief.

D. *Surgical approach.* Surgical procedures are indicated if conservative therapy is not successful and the imaging studies indicate clear-cut etiology or if there is significant spinal cord compression. Anterior cervical discectomy with fusion is commonly performed. But if multiple levels are involved or if posterior compression is causing the problem, posterior laminectomy is more likely to be beneficial.

TABLE 1
Manifestations of cervical root lesions

Nerve Root	Pain Radiation and Sensory Changes	Muscle Weakness	Affected Reflex
C5	Over the deltoid muscle	Deltoid, supraspinatus	Biceps
C6	Upper lateral arm, lateral forearm thumb, and index finger	Biceps, brachioradialis	Biceps
C7	Posterolateral arm and forearm index and middle fingers	Triceps	Triceps
C8	Medial arm and forearm	Triceps, extensors of digits and wrist	Biceps, fourth and fifth digits

REFERENCES

Rowlingson JC: Epidural analgesic technique in the management of cervical pain. *Anesth Analg* 1986;65:938–942.

Van Kleef M, Liem L, Lousberg R, et al: Radiofrequency lesion adjacent to the dorsal root ganglia and for cervicobrachial pain: a prospective double-blind randomized study. *Neurosurgery* 1996;38:1127–1132.

Warfield C, Biber M, Crews D, Nath DGK: Epidural steroid injection as a treatment for cervical radiculitis. *Clin J Pain* 1987;3:13–15.

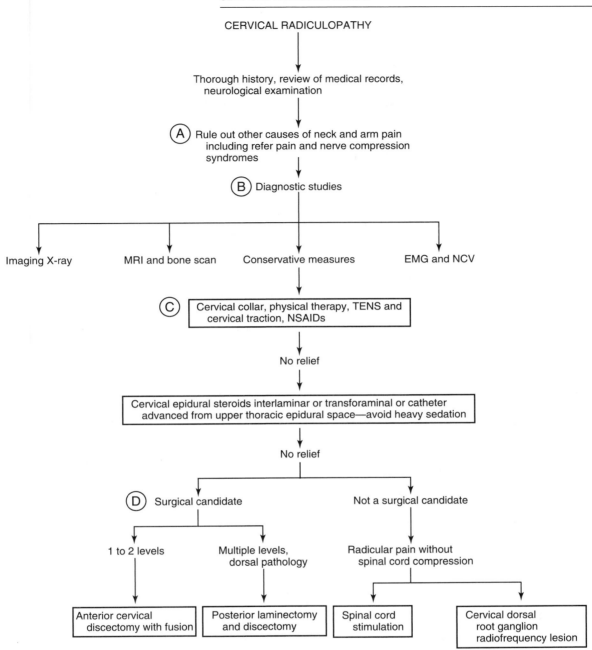

CERVICAL RADICULOPATHY

Thorough history, review of medical records,
neurological examination

(A) Rule out other causes of neck and arm pain
including refer pain and nerve compression
syndromes

(B) Diagnostic studies

Imaging X-ray   MRI and bone scan   Conservative measures   EMG and NCV

(C) Cervical collar, physical therapy, TENS and
cervical traction, NSAIDs

No relief

Cervical epidural steroids interlaminar or transforaminal or catheter
advanced from upper thoracic epidural space—avoid heavy sedation

No relief

(D) Surgical candidate   Not a surgical candidate

1 to 2 levels   Multiple levels,
dorsal pathology   Radicular pain without
spinal cord compression

Anterior cervical
discectomy with fusion   Posterior laminectomy
and discectomy   Spinal cord
stimulation   Cervical dorsal
root ganglion
radiofrequency lesion

UPPER EXTREMITY PAIN

SHOULDER PAIN

SHOULDER-HAND SYNDROME

ENTRAPMENT SYNDROMES: UPPER
EXTREMITIES

TENDONITIS: UPPER EXTREMITIES

BURSITIS

Shoulder Pain

T.R. CHRISTIAN REUTTER

When formulating any treatment plan for a patient with pain in the shoulder region, it is important to conduct a precise, comprehensive evaluation of the current signs and symptoms and how they existed at the onset of the pain. Shoulder pain may originate from the cervical spine, chest, or visceral structures; or it may be caused by intrinsic disease of the shoulder joints or pathology of the periarticular structures. This chapter discusses musculoskeletal shoulder pain.

A. The following information is useful when evaluating the patient: age, dominant hand, sport or work activity, the mechanism of the injury, provoking and relieving factors, duration of the pain, muscle spasm, deformity, bruising, wasting, paresthesia or numbness, weakness or heaviness of the limb, and signs indicating nerve injury. The possibility of referred or radiated pain should be excluded. Neck pain and pain radiating below the elbow are often subtle signs of a cervical spine disorder that is mistaken for a shoulder problem. Pneumonia, peptic ulcer disease, and cardiac ischemia can also present with shoulder pain. In patients with a history of malignancy, metastatic disease should be considered.

1. A physical examination includes inspection and palpation, assessment of range of motion and strength, and provocative shoulder testing for possible impingement problems. Swelling, asymmetry, muscle atrophy, scars, ecchymosis, and any venous distension should be noted. Palpation includes examination of the acromioclavicular and sternoclavicular joints, cervical spine, and biceps tendon. The anterior glenohumeral joint, coracoid process, acromion, and scapula are palpated for any tenderness or deformity.

2. The affected extremity is compared with the unaffected side to determine the patient's normal range of motion. Active and passive ranges are assessed. For example, the loss of active motion alone is more likely due to the weakness of the affected muscles, rather than joint disease. True weakness is distinguished from weakness caused by pain.

3. Provocative testing, which is performed after a complete history and physical examination have been undertaken, provides a more focused evaluation of specific problems. Provocative tests used to evaluate the shoulder include the Apley scratch test, Neer's sign, Hawkin's test, drop-arm test, cross-arm test, Spurling's test, apprehension test, relocation test, sulcus sign, Yergason test, Speed's maneuver, and the "clunk" sign.

B. Shoulder pain can be divided into acute and chronic disorders. Acute disorders include fractures of the humerus, scapula, and clavicle; dislocation of the humerus; sprains of the acromioclavicular and sternoclavicular joints; and injury of the rotator cuff. Chronic disorders fall into one of the following categories: impingement syndrome, frozen shoulder syndrome, biceps tendonitis, rotator cuff tendonitis/bursitis, labral injury, and osteoarthritis of the glenohumeral or acromioclavicular joint.

C. The presentation of shoulder pain varies according to the etiology. Clavicular fractures are relatively easy to diagnose, as palpation reveals point tenderness or an obvious deformity. Proximal humeral fractures exhibit crepitus at the fracture site and often present with ecchymosis 24 to 48 hours after the injury. With scapular fractures, the patient has tenderness at the fracture site and pain during arm abduction. Patients presenting with a glenohumeral dislocation hold the affected arm in external rotation and abduction. The humeral head is palpable anteriorly, and the diagnosis is confirmed by locating a dimple in the skin underneath the acromium. Acromioclavicular (AC) joint sprain shows well localized swelling and tenderness over the AC joint. A palpable "stepped" deformity between the acromium and the clavicle indicates more severe injury, possibly a complete dislocation. The patient with a sternoclavicular joint injury complains of pain, particularly with shoulder adduction. With a rotator cuff tear, the resulting muscular atrophy often limits the patient's ability to perform necessary diagnostic maneuvers.

D. Pain related to an impingement syndrome occurs over the anterolateral aspect of the shoulder, often with some radiation to, but not usually beyond, the elbow. Typically, the pain with an impingement syndrome is aggravated by overhead activity; it is worse at night, and patients often report a clicking or popping sensation in the affected shoulder. The patient with adhesive capsulitis has discomfort localized near the deltoid insertion and is unable to sleep on the affected side; moreover, glenohumeral elevation and external rotation are restricted. Patients with biceps tendonitis present with painful arm flexion. A labral injury is common in throwing athletes, who present with a painful shoulder and a positive "clunk" test. In patients with glenohumeral arthritis, pain with activity, loss of passive motion, stiffness, and nighttime pain are common findings.

E. Diagnostic tests for shoulder pain include plain films, magnetic resonance imaging (MRI), and ultrasonography. Anteroposterior (AP) and lateral radiographs show a fracture of the humerus, glenohumeral dislocation, scapular fracture, degenerative changes, and AC joint sprain. An axillary view is included if the patient is able to perform the necessary maneuvers. The axillary view is most appropriate for diagnosing dislocations or subtle scapular fractures. The Y view (scapular lateral view) is useful if the patient is unable

SHOULDER PAIN

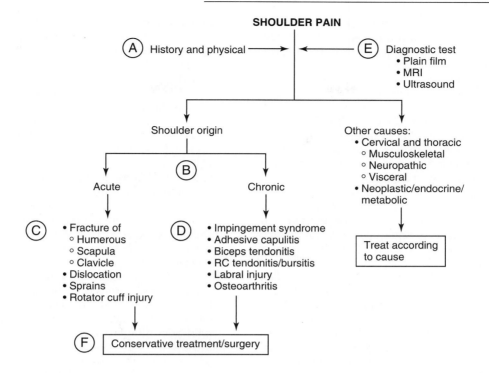

(A) History and physical ⟶ ⟵ (E) Diagnostic test
• Plain film
• MRI
• Ultrasound

Shoulder origin

(B)

Acute

Chronic

Other causes:
• Cervical and thoracic
  ○ Musculoskeletal
  ○ Neuropathic
  ○ Visceral
• Neoplastic/endocrine/
  metabolic

(C) • Fracture of
    ○ Humerous
    ○ Scapula
    ○ Clavicle
  • Dislocation
  • Sprains
  • Rotator cuff injury

(D) • Impingement syndrome
  • Adhesive capulitis
  • Biceps tendonitis
  • RC tendonitis/bursitis
  • Labral injury
  • Osteoarthritis

Treat according
to cause

(F) Conservative treatment/surgery

to abduct the arm. Fractures of the greater tuberosity may be best visualized with an axillary or a Y view. Additional AP views with the humerus in internal and external rotation are sometimes necessary. MRI has 95% sensitivity and specificity for detecting complete rotator cuff tears, cuff degeneration, chronic tendonitis, and partial cuff tears. Ultrasonography can accurately diagnose complete rotator cuff tears, although it is less useful for identifying partial cuff tears. It should be noted that shoulder radiography is thought to be unnecessary unless the pain causes severe restriction, atypical features such as weight loss or general malaise exist, or the initial treatment is unsuccessful.

F. A number of modalities are used to treat shoulder pain, depending on the etiology. The treatment of most fractures consists of immobilization, commencement of range-of-motion (ROM) exercises as soon as the acute pain resolves (usually within 2 weeks), and nonsteroidal antiinflammatory drugs (NSAIDs). Orthopedic referral is indicated for patients with fractures that are unstable or involve the articular site. The humeral head can dislocate anteriorly, posteriorly, or inferiorly in relation to the glenoid fossa, with most dislocations being anterior. Shoulder dislocations are treated with relocation of the humerus and immobilization to allow capsular healing. Mobilization of the shoulder and the elbow can usually be resumed within 7 to 10 days following treatment. AC joint sprain (also known as shoulder separation grades 1 and 2) and sternoclavicular (SC) joint sprains can be treated conservatively with slings or a figure-of-eight appliance and progressive ROM exercises. Patients with grade 3 or higher AC sprains or acute SC dislocations should be referred to an orthopedist for possible operative repair. Rotator cuff tear treatment consists of surgical repair and rehabilitation in young and selected older patients and rehabilitation alone in others. Repair within 3 weeks of the injury is recommended to avoid tendon retraction, reinjury, tendon degeneration, and muscle atrophy. Initial treatment of most patients with impingement syndrome (primary and secondary) is conservative, especially during the acute phase of the pain. Rest, NSAIDs, icing, and abstention from aggravating activities are recommended. After most of the pain has resolved, a rotator cuff strengthening program is instituted. A corticosteroid injection can be therapeutic and diagnostic in patients with impingement syndrome. If the diagnosis is uncertain, lidocaine, bupivicaine, or both can be injected into the subacromial space. A decrease in pain after the injection increases the certainty that impingement is the primary process. Treatment for adhesive capsulitis includes physical therapy (weighted pendulum exercises and passive stretch exercises in abduction and external rotation), a course of NSAIDs, and occasionally subacromial injection with a corticosteroid. Management of biceps tendonitis includes ice applied over the anterior shoulder, restrictions of lifting, an oral NSAID for 2 to 3 weeks, and eventual biceps curls to restore full elbow flexion strength after more than 50% of the pain and inflammation has subsided. Labral injuries are treated with rest, analgesics, and physical therapy, although arthroscopic or open surgical repair are sometimes indicated. Glenohumeral arthritis treatment is initially conservative, using heat and ice, NSAIDs, ROM exercises, and corticosteroid injections.

REFERENCES

Anderson B: *House Officers Guide to Arthrocentesis and Soft Tissue Injection*. Portland, JJ&R Medical Publishing, 1997, pp 12–24, 27.

Magee D: *Orthopedic Physical Assessment*, 3rd ed. Philadelphia, Saunders, 1997, pp 175–233.

Shipley M: Managing the painful shoulder. *Practitioner* 1999;243: 880–885.

Woodward T: The painful shoulder. Parts I and II. *Am Fam Physician* 2000;61:3079–3088, 3291–3299.

Shoulder-Hand Syndrome

MARK E. ROMANOFF

Shoulder-hand syndrome (SHS) was first described by Steinbrocker in 1947, but the term was coined by Freyberg in the same article. It appears to be a form of chronic regional pain syndrome, and it has been associated with many factors, which are listed in Table 1.

A. Three stages of SHS have been identified. Stage 1 lasts approximately 3 to 6 months. Initial symptoms include shoulder, hand, and finger pain and tenderness. Shoulder disability and osteoporosis of the shoulder, humeral head, and wrist are evident. Vasomotor and skin changes are also seen. Hand and finger hyperesthesia and swelling are noted. The second stage lasts 3 to 6 months. Muscles atrophy, and early dystrophy may occur. The pain and disability may either continue or lessen during this period. Vasodilation and swelling usually abate, and the resulting vasospasm causes atrophic changes in the hair, nails, and skin. Osteoporosis continues into the third stage, which can last years and is characterized by less pain but more disability. Dystrophic changes and contractures occur in the shoulder, hand, and fingers. Ultimately a "frozen shoulder" may be evident. As these dystrophic changes occur, they appear irreversible. SHS is unilateral in 75% of cases. Elbow involvement is rare. The syndrome is seen more frequently in women and in patients over 50 years of age.

B. A wide range of syndromes should be considered in the differential diagnosis. Referred visceral pain should be excluded early in the course. Abdominal visceral pain can be referred to the shoulder. Myocardial ischemic pain may also be referred to the shoulder (right or left) and may not be associated with the chest pain. History taking, physical examination, and electrocardiography should be performed to rule out this entity in the population at risk. Initially, the inflammatory symptoms predominate, so arthritis, tendonitis, and bursitis may be mistaken for SHS. Laboratory studies, including tests for rheumatoid factor levels or the presence of uric acid crystals in a joint effusion, can help differentiate these entities from SHS. A myofascial pain syndrome should be assessed by careful palpation. Most commonly, the scalene, deltoid, sternocleidomastoid, and suprascapular muscles are involved. Scalenus anterior or thoracic outlet syndromes may cause vasomotor changes and can be identified by palpation, checking pulses with the arms abducted, and radiography to identify a cervical rib. Evidence of cervical disk disease (extremity weakness, numbness, paresthesias) can be evaluated by computed tomography, magnetic resonance imaging, or myelography as needed. The diagnosis of SHS can be confirmed when the pain is relieved by a diagnostic stellate ganglion block.

C. Initiate treatment immediately after diagnosis to avoid irreversible musculoskeletal changes. Recent treatment has concentrated on analgesics, physical therapy, and sympathetic blocks.

D. The early use of physical therapy (PT), including passive and active exercises of the shoulder and hand, has proved effective alone or in combination with stellate ganglion blocks or steroid therapy. There is one reported caveat: Avoid orthopedic manipulation under anesthesia. Whether this includes PT after brachial plexus, suprascapular, or dorsal scapular nerve blocks has not been determined.

E. Nonsteroidal anti-inflammatory drugs (NSAIDs) should be begun promptly because the early phase of this syndrome involves inflammation. Analgesia is also necessary to allow the patient to participate more fully in PT. If NSAIDs are not effective, opioids can be added temporarily for adequate pain control.

F. Stellate ganglion blocks have been advocated for the treatment of SHS since its discovery. Early studies have shown good to excellent improvement in more than 80% of patients treated with PT and stellate ganglion blocks. Coordination of PT and the blocks is important. Performing these blocks before PT decreases pain during therapy and enhances progress. Usually a series of three to five blocks at 2- to 7-day intervals is necessary. The injections should be continued if deemed appropriate; a patient in one study required a series of 14 blocks for effective pain relief. Brachial plexus continuous catheter techniques can provide prolonged sympathetic blockage, allowing aggressive PT.

G. Trigger point injections (TPIs) have been recommended to treat SHS itself or associated myofascial pain syndrome. Anecdotal reports suggest that TPIs alone are not particularly effective. Combination of other therapy with adjunctive treatment of a myofascial pain syndrome has a higher success rate. The use of steroids in TPIs has been suggested, but their efficacy compared to that of local anesthetic injections has not been studied.

H. High-dose oral steroid therapy (prednisone 40 to 60 mg/day) has been proposed for treatment of this syndrome since 1947. Two more recent reports confirmed the effectiveness of this treatment. One study in patients with SHS after a cerebrovascular accident described a 100% "cure" rate within 1 week of treatment; a 10% remission rate was also noted.

I. Prophylaxis should focus on PT and should be started early after the occurrence of a clinical entity associated with SHS (Table 1). This may help prevent the later stages of SHS. The use of prophylactic stellate ganglion blocks has not been evaluated and is not recommended at this time.

TABLE 1
Factors Associated with Shoulder-Hand Syndrome

Cardiovascular factors
  Myocardial infarction
Neurologic factors
  Cerebrovascular accident
  Intracranial/extracranial tumor
  Epilepsy
  Parkinson's disease
  Herpes zoster
Musculoskeletal factors
  Trauma
  Arthritis
  Cervical disk degeneration
Idiopathic factors
Miscellaneous factors
  Barbiturate use
  Laparoscopic surgery
  Pulmonary tuberculosis
  Neoplasms
  Diabetes mellitus

REFERENCES

Davis SW, Petrillo CR, Eichberg RD, Chu DS: Shoulder-hand syndrome in a hemiplegic population: a 5 year retrospective study. *Arch Phys Med Rehabil* 1977;58:353.

Russek HI: Shoulder-hand syndrome following myocardial infarction. *Med Clin North Am* 1958;42:1555.

Steinbrocker O: Painful homolateral disability of shoulder and hand with swelling and atrophy of hand. *Ann Rheum Dis* 1947;6:80.

Steinbrocker O, Argyros TG: The shoulder-hand syndrome: present status as a diagnostic and therapeutic entity. *Med Clin North Am* 1958;42:1533.

Van der Korst JK, Colenbrander H, Cats A: Phenobarbital and the shoulder-hand syndrome. *Ann Rheum Dis* 1966;25:553.

Walker J, Belsole R, Germain B: Shoulder-hand syndrome in patients with intracranial neoplasms. *Hand* 1983;15:347.

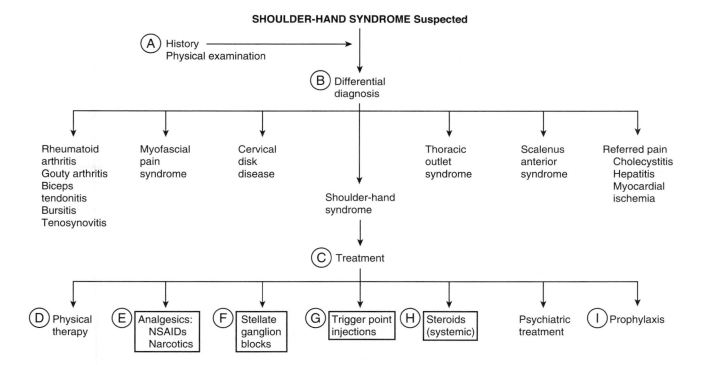

Entrapment Syndromes: Upper Extremities

NIKESH BATRA

Entrapment syndromes are conditions where focal chronic compression of a peripheral nerve by anatomic structures causes neuropathy. Usually, these patients present with typical clinical features, pain being the most common symptom; they also complain of paresthesias and weakness usually in the distribution of the affected nerve. Signs on physical examination include a sensory abnormality, with or without motor deficit, in an identifiable peripheral nerve distribution. Lower motor neuron signs such as muscle atrophy, fasciculation, or depressed deep tendon reflexes may be present. The presence of upper motor neuron signs may prompt a search for a more central cause of the patient's symptoms.

For diagnostic purposes, a thorough neurologic examination remains the most important modality in the physician's arsenal. Electrophysiologic testing [e.g., electromyography/nerve conduction velocity (EMG/NCV) testing, searching for focal slowing or a conduction block] may be helpful in identifying other underlying conditions that cause a focal neuropathy, such as metabolic conditions and inflammatory or immunologic processes. Magnetic resonance imaging (MRI) or computed tomography (CT) may reveal physical structures such as fibrous bands or tumors that can cause the compressive lesion and may be amenable to surgical correction.

A. *Median nerve entrapment.* The medial and lateral chords of the brachial plexus form the median nerve. It has contributions from the C5, C6, C7, C8, and T1 nerve roots. There are three entrapment syndromes that involve the median nerve: carpal tunnel syndrome, anterior interosseus syndrome, and pronator teres syndrome.

1. *Carpal tunnel syndrome.* The patient feels tingling or burning in the first two fingers and thumb. On physical examination there is a sensory deficit in the distal palm and motor deficits in hand muscles supplied by the median nerve. Tinel's and Phalen's signs may be present. If they are present bilaterally, systemic causes should be sought, including overuse syndromes where pain may be caused by tendonitis or fibrositis. These patients may be treated conservatively or by surgical decompression. Conservative methods include the use of splints (neutral position splint is preferred over the traditional cock-up splint), nonsteroidal anti-inflammatory drugs (NSAIDs) and steroid injections. The median nerve can be blocked at this location. The patient is asked to make a fist and flex her wrist to make the palmaris longus tendon prominent. A 25-gauge 5/8-inch needle is inserted lateral to the tendon and at the proximal wrist crease; it is advanced until the tip is just beyond the tendon.

Local anesthetic (3 ml) with or without steroid is injected after negative aspiration.

Conservative measures have a success rate of 60% in patients who have only one risk factor (age >50 years, Phalen's test at 30 seconds, symptoms for more than 10 months, constant paresthesias, associated trigger fingers). Those patients who have three risk factors have a failure rate of 93%, and those with four or more have a 100% failure rate. In patients who have thenar softening atrophy or whose symptoms persist for at least 6 months despite conservative measures, surgery should be considered.

2. *Anterior interosseous syndrome.* There is weakness in the flexor pollicis longus and sometimes weakness of the flexor digitorum profundus to the index finger. Usually there is no sensory deficit. The syndrome, which may present as an acute pain in the proximal forearm, may be related to vigorous exercise or repetitive motions such as using an ice pick. These individuals usually respond well to conservative treatment in the absence of trauma.

3. *Pronator teres syndrome.* The median nerve can be trapped under the pronator teres muscle or its anterior interosseous branches distal to the elbow. The patients have forearm pain, hand paresthesias, and weakness; on examination they have forearm tenderness and sensory deficit in the median nerve distribution. Many present with thenar weakness. Symptoms are worse with forearm pronation and deep palpation of the pronator teres muscle. The flexor digitorum superficialis stress test (long finger) is positive, and there is tenderness of the median nerve at the point of compression. Electromyographic abnormalities usually spare the pronator teres, the first and second flexor digitorum profundus, and the flexor pollicis longus.

The median nerve can be blocked at this location by a 25-gauge 1.5-inch needle that is advanced just medial to the brachial artery at the elbow crease until a paresthesia is elicited. Alternatively, a nerve stimulator can be utilized. After negative aspiration 5 to 7 ml of local anesthetic may be injected.

B. *Radial nerve entrapment.* The radial nerve is a continuation of the posterior cord of the brachial plexus and receives fibers from C5 to C8 cervical roots. There are two major syndromes associated with radial nerve entrapment: posterior interosseus nerve syndrome and radial tunnel syndrome.

ENTRAPMENT SYNDROMES

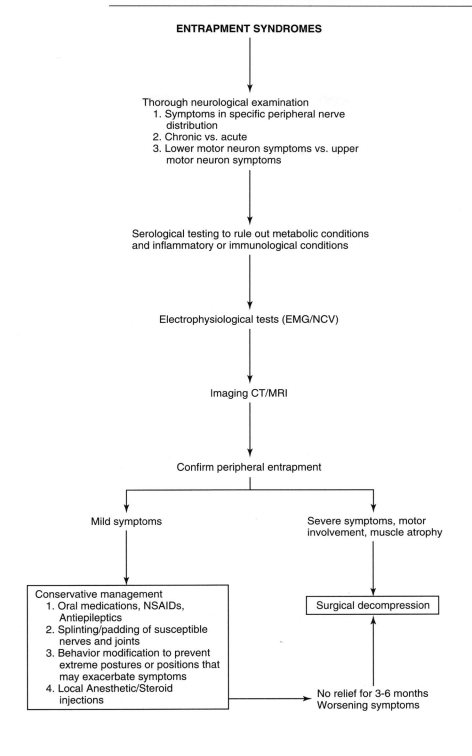

Thorough neurological examination
1. Symptoms in specific peripheral nerve distribution
2. Chronic vs. acute
3. Lower motor neuron symptoms vs. upper motor neuron symptoms

Serological testing to rule out metabolic conditions and inflammatory or immunological conditions

Electrophysiological tests (EMG/NCV)

Imaging CT/MRI

Confirm peripheral entrapment

Mild symptoms

Severe symptoms, motor involvement, muscle atrophy

Conservative management
1. Oral medications, NSAIDs, Antiepileptics
2. Splinting/padding of susceptible nerves and joints
3. Behavior modification to prevent extreme postures or positions that may exacerbate symptoms
4. Local Anesthetic/Steroid injections

Surgical decompression

No relief for 3-6 months
Worsening symptoms

1. *Posterior interosseus nerve syndrome.* The common causes of this syndrome are anatomic variants, usually at the arcade of Frohse, which is a fibrous band at the origin of the supinator, the leash of Henry (an arcade of vessels), a tendinous origin of the extensor carpi radialis brevis, and a fibrous band from the radiocapitellar joint. Mass lesions such as rheumatoid synovitis emerging from the lateral elbow joint or bicipital tendon bursitis may also cause this syndrome. This condition can coexist with lateral epicondylitis, or tennis elbow.

2. *Radial tunnel syndrome.* This syndrome can produce pain without muscle weakness. Usually there is pain just below the lateral epicondyl of the humerus. There are four places where compression occurs in radial tunnel syndrome: the fibrous edge of the extensor carpi radialis brevis, fibrous bands of the radiohumeral joint, the leash of Henry, and the arcade of Frohse. Unless there is loss of motor function, treatment is conservative during the initial period. It includes rest, avoidance of aggravating motions, splinting, and NSAIDs. A wrist extension splint with the elbow flexed and supinated provides maximal relief in patients with the radial tunnel syndrome. Surgical exploration is indicated if conservative measures fail after 3 to 6 months. The radial nerve is blocked in this location by identifying the musculospiral groove by deep palpation between the heads of the triceps muscle at a point approximately 3 inches above the lateral epicondyl of the humerus.

C. *Ulnar nerve entrapment.* The ulnar nerve is the continuation of the medial cord of the brachial plexus. It is derived from the C7, C8, and T1 nerve roots. There are two sites where the ulnar nerve may be entrapped. The first is at the wrist in Guyon's canal and the second is the cubital tunnel. Entrapment of the ulnar nerve at the elbow occurs at least 10 times more frequently than at the wrist.

1. *Guyon's canal.* The ulnar nerve may be entrapped in Guyon's canal, where patients develop numbness of the little finger and medial aspect of the hand. Tinel's sign may be positive on examination, and there may be a sensory deficit in the ulnar distribution along with weakness of the hypothenar and interosseus muscles. Among other causes, scarring after injury, a lipoma, or a ganglion usually causes this deficit. The dorsal ulnar cutaneous nerve is generally spared. If the deep terminal branch of the ulnar nerve is affected the syndrome is purely motor, whereas if the superficial terminal branch of the ulnar nerve is affected the syndrome is purely sensory at the distal palm. The ulnar nerve may be blocked in this location by having the patient make a fist and flex the wrist to make the flexor carpi ulnaris tendon prominent. A 25-gauge 5/8-inch needle is inserted on the radial side of the tendon proximal to the wrist crease at a 30° angle. The needle is advanced until the tip is just beyond the tendon. Local anesthetic (3 ml) is then injected at this spot after negative aspiration.

2. *Cubital tunnel.* The other site of entrapment of the ulnar canal is the cubital tunnel, where the ulnar nerve passes between the heads of the flexor carpi ulnaris. There is pain near the elbow (which may spread proximally or distally) and paresthesias in the fourth and fifth fingers along with weakness. The patient may have a positive Tinel's sign and usually has weakness of the ulnar musculature, atrophy, and a claw hand. Similar symptoms can be seen with position injuries to the ulnar nerve during compression in the ulnar groove at the medial epicondyle. The ulnar nerve is blocked at this level by inserting a 25-gauge 5/8-inch needle just proximal to the ulnar nerve sulcus between the olecranon process and the medial epicondyle of the humerus and injecting 5 to 7 ml of a local anesthetic/methylprednisolone mixture.

D. *Entrapment of the C8-T1 roots or the lower brachial plexus trunk.* This syndrome, which is more common in female patients, especially those with droopy shoulders and long necks, is commonly referred to as the thoracic outlet syndrome. There is a fibrous band from the C7 transverse process to the first rib, also seen in the cervical rib or a large C7 transverse process. The syndrome is characterized by pain and parasthesias in the medial arm and hand as well as the neck, shoulder, and chest. On examination, weakness is noted in the thenar musculature, and Tinel's sign is positive over the brachial plexus at the supraclavicular fossa. Upward or downward arm traction worsens the pain, whereas shoulder elevation and turning the neck toward the symptomatic arm relieves it. EMG/NCV testing along with MRI are the keys to the diagnosis.

E. *Suprascapular nerve entrapment.* The suprascapular nerve originates from the upper trunk at Erb's point from C5 and C6 nerve roots. Suprascapular nerve entrapment syndrome results from injury to the nerve as it passes below the transverse scapular ligament through the suprascapular notch. This results in denervation of both the supraspinatus and infraspinatus muscles, with resultant atrophy, pain, and muscle weakness. Anomalies resulting in entrapment at this point include narrow notch, bifid transverse scapular ligament, calcified ligament, and fractures. Injuries occurring in the spinoglenoid notch result in isolated infraspinatus muscle atrophy or weakness. Repetitive motion injury can also cause suprascapular neuropathy. The least common entrapment is caused by a traction injury at its origin at Erb's point. On physical examination, the patients have weak external rotation and abduction, atrophy of the supraspinatus and infraspinatus muscles, but normal sensation and intact deltoid muscle function, with point tenderness over the area of nerve compression. Provocative testing can be achieved with cross-body adduction, which brings the nerve into maximal tension. The diagnosis is facilitated by notch-view radiographs, EMG, MRI to identify muscle atrophy, and a diagnostic lidocaine injection into the area of the nerve impingement.

Traction injuries at the nerve's origin generally recover well. Lesions at the suprascapular notch or spinoglenoid notch respond to conservative measures, including rest, activity modification, NSAIDs, corticosteroid injections, or a combination of these measures. Rotator cuff strengthening and scapular stabilization exercises are prescribed. Surgical exploration should be reserved for patients who fail to respond to conservative measures.

REFERENCES

Aldridge JW, Bruno RJ, Strauch RJ, Rosenwasser MP: Nerve entrapment in athletes. *Clin Sports Med* 2001;20:95–122.

Levine BP, Jones JA, Burton RI: Nerve entrapments of the upper extremity: a surgical perspective. *Neurol Clin* 1999;17:549–565.

Waldman SD: *Atlas of Interventional Pain Management*. Philadelphia, Saunders, 1998.

Williams VB, Pappagallo M: Entrapment neuropathies. In: *Essentials of Pain Medicine and Regional Anesthesia*. New York, Churchill Livingstone, 1999, p. 295.

Tendonitis: Upper Extremities

ERIK SHAW

Tendonitis is a common condition usually caused by overuse of a muscle or muscle group. Inflammation is thought to be a contributing factor to the pain and limited motion caused by this problem. One study showed no inflammatory cells but, rather, mucoid degeneration of the collagen structure of the tendon. In the upper extremity, several locations are subject to this condition due to certain activities or anatomic structures.

A. Several anatomic locations are common locations for tendonitis because of certain stresses placed on them during activities.

1. In the rotator cuff the supraspinatus and subscapularis tendons are commonly inflamed by repetitive overhead motion such as throwing and swimming. These situations can be exacerbated by a hooked acromion (type 3), a narrowed subacromial space, or an imbalance or tear in the rotator cuff muscles. Impingement testing and pain upon internal and external rotation can often indicate tendonitis. Pain can be worse at night and aggravated by overhead movements.

2. Bicipital tendonitis occurs also with frequent overhead motions and lifting. It can be exquisitely painful. The pain is located anterior in the groove where the long head of the biceps tendon inserts into the superior aspect of the glenoid. Resisted flexion of the supinated arm (Speed's test) or resisted supination of the flexed elbow (Yergason's test) can help define this condition.

3. Triceps tendonitis is relatively uncommon but does occur with frequent lifting; and it can be quite painful. It may be associated with olecranon bursitis.

4. Golfer's elbow (medial epicondylitis) is a common painful condition noted in the medial aspect of the elbow. It is associated with overuse of the common musculotendinous flexors (flexor carpi radialis) of the anterior compartment of the antebrachium. Care must be taken to ensure that the ulnar nerve is not responsible for the pain. A forearm strap can diffuse the strain placed on the tendinous insertion, helping to prevent recurrence.

5. Tennis elbow (lateral epicondylitis) is similar to medial epicondylitis and can be caused by playing tennis and other activities that require forceful extension of the forearm extensors. The extensor carpi radialis brevis and extensor digitorum communis tendons are the most common culprits. Tests of resisted extension of the hand radially or of the middle finger can be painful in this condition.

6. DeQuervain's tenosynovitis is the most common tendonitis of the wrist. It involves the tendon sheath of the abductor pollicis longus and extensor pollicis brevis near the radial styloid. Finkelstein's test is positive. Rheumatoid arthritis should be considered.

7. Evaluation shows tenderness over the involved area and frequently weakness of the affected muscle group. Inquiry as to activity level, exercise routine, and work-related activities can help pinpoint the causative factors. Education and conservative treatment comprise the mainstays of treatment. Preventing reinjury begins with a steady course of conservative treatment and activity reduction.

8. Muscular imbalance is frequently the cause of tendonitis. Weakness of the rotator cuff muscles allows the humeral head to affect the acromion, leading to tendonitis. An imbalance of the forearm flexors and extensors can lead to abnormal forces placed on the tendinous insertions, leading to tendonitis. Additionally, overuse of these muscle groups can lead to this inflammatory process.

B. Begin with a course of nonsteroidal anti-inflammatory drugs (NSAIDs), which can be highly effective along with rest. Alternating ice and heat can also be useful adjuncts to treatment. NSAIDs have known gastrointestinal (GI) side effects. These effects can be limited by concomitant use of an H_2-blocker or a proton pump inhibitor. Cyclooxygenase-2 inhibitors have significantly fewer GI side effects and can be useful for daily pharmacologic therapy. Rarely, opioids are useful in severe cases.

C. Therapeutic exercise begins with gentle range of motion exercises and stretching. Gentle strengthening of agonists and antagonists together help maintain proper balance of the tendinous insertion. The patient should gradually increase resistance and resume activity slowly and in a controlled manner. Ultrasonography and diathermy can also be helpful for rehabilitation.

D. In recalcitrant cases, corticosteroid injection may be helpful. Care must be taken to not inject the tendon directly, as it could substantially weaken the collagenous structure of the tendon, potentially causing rupture. This is especially likely with tendonitis.

E. In extremely severe cases, surgical consultation may be necessary. Acromioplasty, for instance, can relieve irritation on the supraspinatus and subscapularis tendons from a narrowed subacromial space due to a type III acromion. With de Quervain's tendinitis, release of the tendons is often helpful.

REFERENCES

Bracker MD: *The 5-Minute Sports Medicine Consult.* Philadelphia, Lippincott Williams & Wilkins, 2001.

Braddom RL: *Physical Medicine and Rehabilitation.* Philadelphia, Saunders, 1996.

Buschbacher RM, Braddom R: *Sports Medicine and Rehabilitation: A Sports Specific Approach.* St. Louis, Hanley & Belfus, 1994.

Choi H, Sugar R, Shatzer M, et al: *Physical Medicine and Rehabilitation Pocketpedia.* Philadelphia, Lippincott Williams & Wilkins, 2003.

Khan KM, Coo JL, Bonar F, et al: Histopathology of common overuse tendon conditions: update and implications for clinical management. *Sports Med* 1999;27:393–408.

Mellion MB: *Sport Injuries and Athletic Problems.* St. Louis, Hanley & Belfus, 1988.

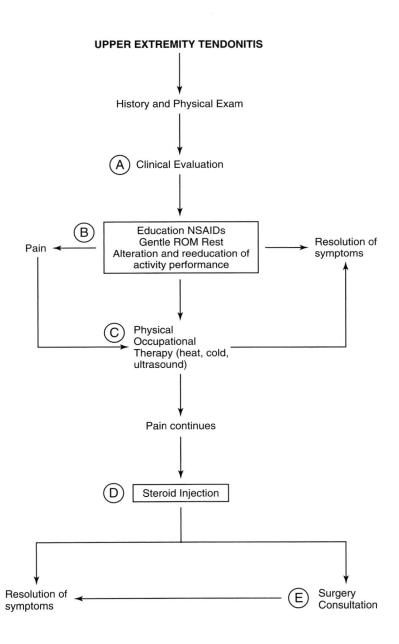

Bursitis

BERT BLACKWELL

Upper extremity bursitis is a common cause of pain. Injury may occur from trauma, repetitive overuse, or pathologic entities such as autoimmune disorders. The three most commonly affected bursae in the upper extremity are the subacromial (which extends to become the subdeltoid), the olecranon, and the subscapular. Careful evaluation of the nature of the underlying pathology affecting the bursa is critical not only to adequately treat pain, but also to recognize potentially serious causes of morbidity and mortality associated with a septic joint.

A. Subacromial bursitis may be primary (autoimmune disorders or crystal deposition) or, more commonly, secondary to rotator cuff pathology. Subacromial bursitis is most commonly associated with supraspinatus tendon injury. On examination the most painful arc of motion is between 70 and 120 degrees of shoulder abduction. Physical maneuvers such as the Neer and Hawkins impingement tests as well as supraspinatus muscle testing can localize injury. Radiographs may show a curved or hooked acromial process, humeral/acromial margin of 5 mm or less, or even humeral head osteopenia and calcification of the supraspinatus tendon. Magnetic resonance imaging (MRI) yields little additional information but may be helpful in demonstration of a rotator cuff tear or a septic bursitis. Diagnostic injection with anesthetic can be used to confirm the clinical diagnosis.

B. Aspiration of the subacromial bursa may be performed if there is a clinical suspicion of infection. Infection of the subacromial bursa is relatively rare without prior history of penetrating trauma.

C. Rotator cuff tears or exuberant fibrosis may result in the need for repair or débridement. It is worth noting, however, that even with these conditions, many patients may still get pain relief from conservative treatment.

D. Olecranon bursitis usually presents with tenderness and swelling about the elbow. The differentiation between infection within the joint and simple inflammation is relatively difficult. An overlying skin lesion, abrupt onset of symptoms, or fever is indicative of septic bursitis. In contrast to subacromial bursitis, diagnosis usually does require aspiration of fluid. Physical and radiographic findings are relatively nonspecific.

E. Septic bursitis is a serious cause of morbidity and its early recognition and treatment are of paramount importance. Treatment consists of antibiotic therapy directed at the causative organism. Repeat aspiration is often necessary to allow adequate penetration. Surgical drainage may be required.

F. Subscapular bursitis is a relatively rare disorder. Inflammation usually results from exostoses or abnormal gliding of the scapula over the chest wall. Scapular "snapping" is a common, often painless sequela and often precedes bursitis. The most common cause of

exostoses in this location is the presence of osteochondromas. Although scapular osteochondromas are usually benign, malignant transformation can be seen. Radiographs are indispensable to the diagnosis in this case.

G. Exostoses and osteochondromas can be surgically resected. This is somewhat drastic and usually unnecessary. Conservative treatment can usually alleviate pain. Scapular "snapping" can be minimized by shoulder girdle strengthening.

H. Conservative treatment for bursitis follows a common algorithm. Relative rest of the affected joint is important to prevent further exacerbation of pain and swelling. Application of cold decreases enzymatic activity associated with proteolysis and may provide some analgesia. Heat should be avoided initially as it may exacerbate swelling and inflammation. Heat application may be useful in resolving bursitis to make surrounding structures more flexible. Nonsteroidal antiinflammatory drugs (NSAIDs) administered on a regular basis curtail the ongoing inflammatory cascade. Acetaminophen may also be helpful. Although the subacromial and subscapular bursae are difficult to compress, compression is particularly useful in olecranon bursitis to prevent fluid reaccumulation. Exercise should begin after acute inflammation has been treated and should initially consist of range-of-motion exercises to maintain and regain joint flexibility. Once normal range of motion is restored, strengthening of muscles crossing and stabilizing the joint is used in an attempt to prevent recurrence.

I. Corticosteroid injections may be employed when conservative therapy fails, or early on in evaluation to terminate inflammation. There is a risk in that such use may decrease the local immunologic response and exacerbate a smoldering septic bursitis. Simply piercing the skin may also seed a compromised joint with a sufficient number of organisms to precipitate infection. Since bursa are so superficial, overlying skin atrophy and cutaneous fistulas are possible.

REFERENCES

Braddom RL: *Physical Medicine and Rehabilitation*. Philadelphia, WB Saunders, 1996.

Green A: Arthroscopic treatment of impingement syndrome. *Orthop Clin North Am* 1995;26:631.

O'Meara PM, Bartal E: Septic arthritis: process, etiology, treatment outcome. A literature review. *Orthopedics* 1988;11:623.

Salzman KL, Lillegard WA, Butcher JD: Upper extremity bursitis. *Am Fam Physician* 1997;56:1797.

Santavirta S, Korittinen YT, Antti-Poika I, Nordstrom D: Inflammation of the subacromial bursa in chronic shoulder pain. *Arch Orthop Trauma Surg* 1992;111:336.

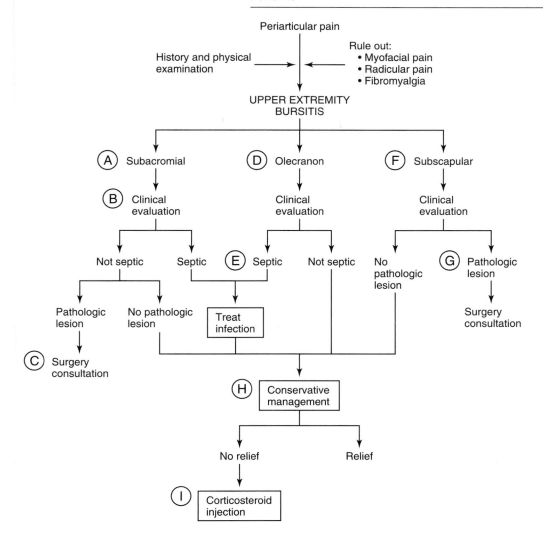

Periarticular pain

History and physical examination → ← Rule out:
• Myofacial pain
• Radicular pain
• Fibromyalgia

UPPER EXTREMITY BURSITIS

Ⓐ Subacromial   Ⓓ Olecranon   Ⓕ Subscapular

Ⓑ Clinical evaluation   Clinical evaluation   Clinical evaluation

Not septic   Septic   Ⓔ Septic   Not septic   No pathologic lesion   Ⓖ Pathologic lesion

Pathologic lesion   No pathologic lesion   Treat infection   Surgery consultation

Ⓒ Surgery consultation

Ⓗ Conservative management

No relief   Relief

Ⓘ Corticosteroid injection

THORACIC PAIN

CHRONIC CHEST WALL PAIN
POSTMASTECTOMY PAIN
CHRONIC VERTEBRAL PAIN
RIB DYSFUNCTION

Chronic Chest Wall Pain

SOMAYAJI RAMAMURTHY

A. Chronic chest wall pain is a multidimensional pain syndrome. The pain can result from multiple etiologic factors including referred pain from thoracic viscera such as the heart, lungs, and esophagus. The pain results most commonly from thoracotomy scar, postherpetic neuralgia, intercostal neuralgia, myofascial pain, rib, costochondral joints, and primary or secondary malignancy originating from the vertebral bodies or the ribs.

B. A thorough history, physical examination, laboratory tests and imaging studies should be completed to rule out serious visceral disease or malignancy. The history and physical examination is very helpful in determining the etiologic factors responsible for pain production.

C. Scar pain. Palpation by picking up the scar between two fingers can localize the pain to the scar and neuromas can be found. Usually there is decreased sensation to pinprick distal to the scar, together with allodynia and/or hyperpathia.

Treatment consists of desensitization, topical local anesthetics, transcutaneous electrical nerve stimulation (TENS), antineuropathic drugs, and injection of the scar with local anesthetic and steroids. Cryo- or radiofrequency lesion provides long-term relief. We do not recommend injection of alcohol or phenol because of the potential for skin breakdown and neuritis with increased pain. Postherpetic neuralgia is characterized by healed herpetic scars, allodynia, and hyperpathia.

D. Myofascial pain is characterized by the reproduction of pain on palpation of the muscular trigger points, most commonly in the pectoralis major and minor, serratus anterior, trapezius, and latissimus dorsi muscles. Stretching of the muscles reproduces the patient's pain and injection of the trigger points relieves the pain. Injection of *Botulinum* toxin may be beneficial if physical therapy and exercises do not produce long-term pain relief.

E. Rib pain. The most common cause of rib pain is rib dysfunction with the involvement of the thoracic facet joints. The syndrome is characterized by tenderness over the rib anteriorly, laterally, and posteriorly and over the corresponding thoracic facet joints. Pain is associated with deep breathing. The physical examination also reveals decreased motion of the rib with breathing, on the affected side. Mobilization of the ribs with manual methods followed by physical therapy and exercises is likely to relieve the pain. Paravertebral local anesthetic blocks may be necessary to provide analgesia for mobilization. If the patient gets only short-term relief and if diagnostic thoracic medial branch blocks provide pain relief, long-term pain relief may be obtained by radiofrequency lesioning of the medial branches.

Pain due to costochondritis (Tietze's syndrome) is usually felt over the anterior chest over the costochondral junction. Arthritis and swelling of the sternochondral joints can also cause chest wall pain. Palpation of the joints reproduces the patient's pain. Pain is relieved by intrarticular injection of local anesthetic and steroids.

Pain associated with slipping rib syndrome is usually seen among young people between 20 and 40 years of age who complain of lower rib pain. The diagnosis is made by pulling up the lower edge of the rib cage and reproducing the clicking and the patient's pain. Patients usually respond to physical therapy and occasionally injection of local anesthetic and steroids. If the pain does not respond to conservative therapy, surgical resection of the ends of the ribs can be helpful.

F. Malignancy. Pain secondary to malignancy is managed with opioids, adjuvants, radiation therapy, and surgical decompression as required. If the pain continues, neurolytic blocks may be beneficial.

Secondary malignancy of the ribs with or without fracture can produce severe pain. Localized rib pain distal to the angle of the ribs can be relieved temporarily with local anesthetic blocks and on a long-term basis with neurolytic blocks using phenol, alcohol, or radiofrequency or cryoablation techniques. Neurolytic blocks are employed less frequently because of the pain relief provided by intravertebral opioids. Primary or secondary malignancy involving the visceral structures in the thoracic cage or the vertebral canal or the vertebral bodies or the ribs medial to the angle can produce pain over the chest wall. Local anesthetic paravertebral blocks may be beneficial. Phenol or alcohol neurolytic blocks should be avoided in the paravertebral area because of the possible spread to the epidural and subarachnoid space, resulting in serious complications including paralysis. Intrathecal phenol or alcohol is very effective in relieving pain confined to an area of fewer than three to four segments.

If the pleural cavity is intact, interpleural injection of local anesthetic followed by the injection of 5% to 10% phenol in water or glycerin can provide significant long-term pain relief.

REFERENCE

Bonica JJ, Graney DO: General considerations of pain in the chest. In: Loeser JD (ed) *Bonica's Management of Pain,* 3rd ed. Philadelphia, Lippincott Williams & Wilkins, 2001, pp. 1113–1148.

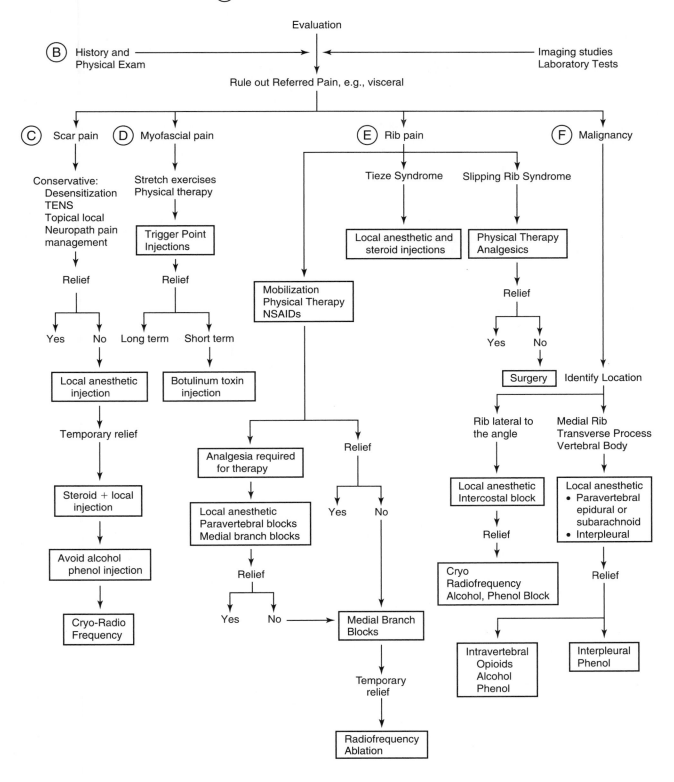

Postmastectomy Pain

LINDA TINGLE

Postmastectomy pain syndrome (PMPS) is a known complication of the surgical treatment of breast cancer. It is a neuropathic pain condition that arises from damage to the axillary, intercostal, or intercostobrachial nerves during surgery. It is characterized as a sharp, burning, aching pain accompanied by lancinating pain in the distribution supplied by the injured nerve. It is aggravated by movement in 94% of women. The prevalence of PMPS ranges from 4% to 40%. Hyperesthesia, hyperalgesia, and hypoesthesia are present. A palpable neuroma may be present.

A. Medical management includes a trial of oral analgesics, tricyclic antidepressants, and anticonvulsants used for neuropathic pain. Capsaicin cream has few side effects and may provide improvement (Watson et al. 1989).

B. Physical modalities such as transcutaneous nerve stimulation (TENS), myofascial release (Crawford et al. 1996), thoracic facet joint or rib mobilization (or both), and stretching exercises may benefit if indicated.

C. Surgical excision of palpable neuromas can result in complete pain relief (Wong 2001).

D. A successful intercostal block with local anesthetic may be followed by pulsed radiofrequency lesioning or cryoablation of the intercostal nerve. Paravertebral blocks, epidural blocks, or interpleural blocks provide analgesia for desensitization techniques and mobilization. Spinal cord stimulation may be considered when more conservative interventions are unsuccessful.

REFERENCES

Crawford JS, Simpson J, Crawford P: Myofascial release provides symptomatic relief from chest wall tenderness occasionally seen following lumpectomy and radiation in breast cancer patients. *International Journal of Radiation Oncology, Biology, Physics* 34(5):1188-9,1996,

Sloan P, Carpenter J, Andrykowski M: Post-mastectomy pain syndrome in women treated for breast cancer. *Anesthesiology* 1997;87:751A.

Watson CP, Evans RJ, Watt VR: The post-mastectomy pain syndrome and the effect of topical capsaicin. *Pain* 1989;38:177–186.

Wong L: Intercostal neuromas: a treatable cause of postoperative breast surgery pain. *Ann Plast Surg* 2001;46:481–484.

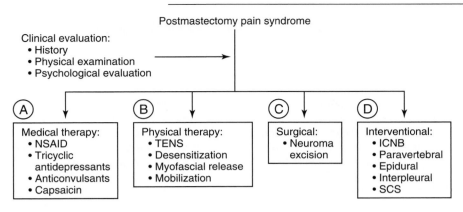

Chronic Vertebral Pain

SOMAYAJI RAMAMURTHY

A. Patients in whom a physical examination and imaging reveals radicular pain, mechanical pain such as facet joint syndrome, internal disk disruption, sacroiliac joint disease, and myofascial pain should be managed as outlined in corresponding chapters.

B. Osteoporosis. Elderly patients, especially women with a history of osteoporosis and patients who develop secondary osteoporosis following treatment with steroids for the management of asthma, rheumatologic diseases, and autoimmune disorders, can develop severe chronic pain with or without fractures. Bone density studies are helpful in the diagnosis and follow-up. Patients without fractures are managed conservatively with bracing, education, physical therapy, extension exercises, analgesics, bisphosphonates (Fosamax), calcitonin, and calcium.

Patients who have compression fractures secondary to osteoporosis are treated with bracing, heat, and analgesics. In patients with fracture of less than 3 months, vertebroplasty and/or kyphoplasty is beneficial. For chronic vertebral fracture pain of longer than 3 months duration, medial branch, and/or rami communicantes, local anesthetic blocks may provide temporary pain relief. Long-term relief may be obtained with radiofrequency lesioning of these nerves.

C. Metastasis. Patients with metastasis in the vertebrae secondary most commonly to lung, prostate, and breast cancers should be evaluated using imaging, especially magnetic resonance imaging (MRI), to ascertain epidural and spinal cord involvement. If there is evidence of neurologic compromise due to the compression of spinal cord, spine surgical and radiotherapy consult should be requested. Patients with neurologic compromise obtain excellent results if decompression and stabilization by spinal surgery is followed by radiation therapy.

In the absence of epidural and spinal cord involvement patients are likely to obtain significant pain relief with radiation therapy. These patients should be followed with conservative therapy including analgesics and should be followed up for recurrence and possible adverse effects of radiation therapy on the spinal cord. Patients with radicular pain may obtain significant relief following epidural steroid injection. Intrathecal alcohol, epidural phenol, alcohol, intravertebral opioids, and analgesics should be considered in suitable patients.

Hospice and palliative therapy should be considered in patients who have significant impairment secondary to the neurologic deficits.

REFERENCE

Loeser JD (ed): *Bonica's Management of Pain*, 3rd ed. Philadelphia, Lippincott Williams & Wilkins, 2001.

VERTEBRAL PAIN-CHRONIC

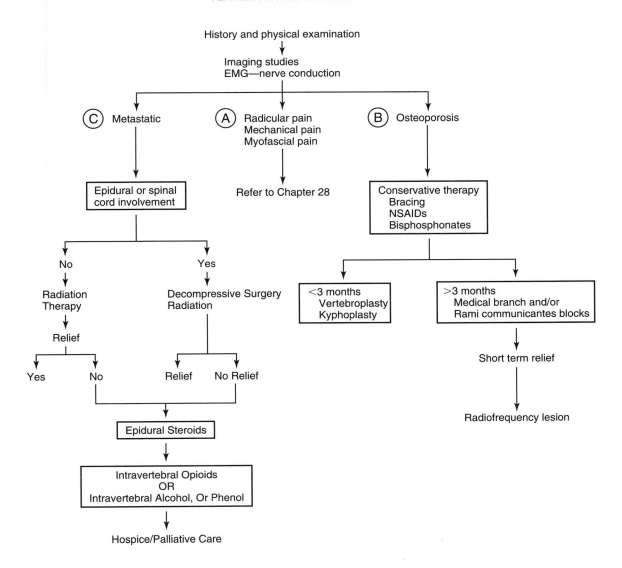

Rib Dysfunction

JAMES G. GRIFFIN

Patients presenting with thoracic pain, rib cage pain, flank pain, or abdominal pain may have one of a variety of conditions, including trauma resulting in rib fractures, diseases of the ribs, or medical conditions that refer pain to the rib cage or abdomen. The latter include, but are not limited to, visceral tumors, pain of cardiac origin, aortic dissection, esophageal disorders, tracheobronchial pain, cholecystitis, peptic ulcer disease, renal disease, postherpetic neuralgia, and intercostal neuralgia.

Patients may have a primary mechanical rib problem that produces pain in the above-mentioned areas for which no medical disorder or disease can be found to be responsible. Workups reported for chest pain have included hospitalization, electrocardiography, radiography, isotopic/perfusion lung scans, pulmonary angiography, echocardiography, and bone scans. Diagnostic workups reported for patients with abdominal pain due to rib dysfunction include barium meals, barium enemas, ultrasound scanning, intravenous urography, laparotomy, and noncurative cholecystectomy.

A. Rib fractures secondary to trauma are more common in adults than children. They may be secondary to trauma or a result of metastatic disease. Pain on inspiration is a common complaint. Coughing may produce a fracture in individuals with a disease process of the ribs or osteoporosis. The physical examination may reveal ecchymosis, tenderness, and a palpable defect on palpation. Radiographs are indicated to rule out pneumothorax, hemithorax, and pleural effusion. Treatment may include intercostal nerve block, an intrapleural catheter, oral medication, transcutaneous electrical nerve stimulation (TENS), a rib binder or belt, and relative rest to avoid painful activities during healing.

B. Stress fractures are not uncommon in active or athletic individuals. Stress fracture of the first rib has been confused with lytic lesions on magnetic resonance imaging examination. Stress fractures of the first rib seem to occur more often in the weight lifting and throwing population, whereas those of the lower ribs seem to occur more frequently in athletes who are "swingers" (i.e., golfers and tennis players). Lower rib fractures are found in elite competitive rowers. Cases of stress fractures in swimmers have also been reported. Treatment consists of oral medication for acute symptoms, TENS, rest (relative in an athletic population), and alteration of sport-specific mechanics.

C. Mechanical dysfunction of the rib is often unrecognized as a source of chest or abdominal pain. Rib dysfunction is easily diagnosed by exactly reproducing the patient's pain complaint by palpating the ribs along their course from the costovertebral region to the costosternal border. The patient's history may reveal pain that is relieved or exacerbated by certain activities or positions or by respiration. Pain may have begun after a relatively benign injury or activity.

Rib dysfunction is commonly seen after thoracotomy. Sweating, nausea, and other systemic effects may be attributed to the proximity of the intercostal nerves to sympathetic afferent fibers.

Treatment of primary rib pain of mechanical origin may begin conservatively by mobilizing the restricted segments. The diagnosis and treatment of joint restriction is described in various texts devoted to manual medicine. This may be the only intervention necessary. Chronic, painful thoracic and rib dysfunction may require medical intervention in the form of facet blocks, paravertebral blocks, rib blocks, or continuous epidural or intrapleural blockade to assist with mechanical treatment. Associated soft tissue problems must also be addressed, and the patient often requires a home exercise or stretching program. Neurolytic blockade of the facet joint and intercostal nerve is sometimes necessary in resistant cases.

D. Mechanical dysfunction of the first rib has been associated with upper extremity conditions such as thoracic outlet syndrome and reflex sympathetic dystrophy. Radiographic motion pictures have shown a lack of normal motion with respiration on the involved side. Clinical studies emphasizing restoration of first rib motion have demonstrated significant improvement in upper extremity symptoms.

E. The twelfth rib appears to have a unique connection of its subcostal nerve to the L1 nerve, which may explain the referral of pain to the lower abdomen, groin, and thigh in the "twelfth rib syndrome." This rib is also an attachment for the costodiaphragmatic recess of the pleura and several muscles of the back and flank. This syndrome is diagnosed by reproducing the patient's exact pain by palpating the twelfth rib. The diagnosis is confirmed when pain relief is achieved by subcostal nerve blockade (although the relief may be temporary). Permanent relief has been achieved with blockade using a local anesthetic and a steroid, or cryoablation, or surgical excision of the painful rib.

F. "Slipping rib syndrome" is more common in adults than children. This problem is caused by inadequacy or rupture of the medial fibrous attachments of the eighth, ninth, or tenth ribs, allowing the cartilage tip to impinge on the intervening intercostal nerve. This situation can produce somatic as well as visceral complaints. The diagnosis is confirmed by "hooking" the lowest costal cartilage and pulling it forward, which then elicits a clicking sensation and reproduces the patient's symptoms. Diagnosis and transient relief is reported with intercostal blocks. Postural changes and avoidance of provocative motion is advocated in the elderly. Subperichondral resection of the involved cartilages is the treatment for those in whom nonsurgical management fails.

REFERENCES

Abbou S, Herman J: Slipping rib syndrome. *Postgrad Med* 1989; 86:75–78.

Arroyo JF, Jolliet P, Junod AF: Costovertebral joint dysfunction: another misdiagnosed cause of atypical chest pain. *Postgrad Med J* 1992; 68:655–659.

Cranfield KA, Buist RJ, Nandi PR, Baranowski AP: The twelfth rib syndrome. *J Pain Symp Manage* 1997;13:172–175.

Flynn TW: *The Thoracic Spine and Rib Cage: Musculoskeletal Evaluation and Treatment.* Boston, Butterworth-Heinemann, 1996.

Gamble JG, Comstock C, Rinsky LA: Erroneous interpretation of magnetic resonance images of a fracture of the fist rib with non-union: two case reports. *J Bone Joint Surg Am* 1995;77:1883–1887.

Jalovaaro P, Ramo J, Lindholm R: Twelfth rib syndrome simulating intra-abdominal disease. *Acta Chir Scand* 1988;154:407–408.

Karlson KA: Rib stress fractures in elite rowers: a case series and proposed mechanism. *Am J Sports Med* 1998;26:516–519.

Lindgren KA, Leino E: Subluxation of the first rib: a possible thoracic outlet syndrome mechanism. *Arch Phys Med Rehabil* 1988;69: 692–695.

Mooney DP, Shorter NA: Slipping rib syndrome in childhood. *J Pediatr Surg* 1997;32:1081–1082.

Roberge RJ, Morgenstern MJ, Osborn H: Cough fracture of the ribs. *Am J Emerg Med* 1984;2:513–517.

Scott EM, Scott BB: Painful rib syndrome: a review of 76 cases. *Gut* 1993;34:1006–1008.

Sinha HK, Kaeding CC, Wadley GM: Upper extremity stress fractures in athletes: clinical symptoms in 44 cases. *Clin J Sports Med* 1999; 9:199–202.

Taimela S, Kujala UM, Oravs S: Two consecutive rib stress fractures in a female competitive swimmer. *Clin J Sports Med* 1995;5:254–257.

RIB PAIN

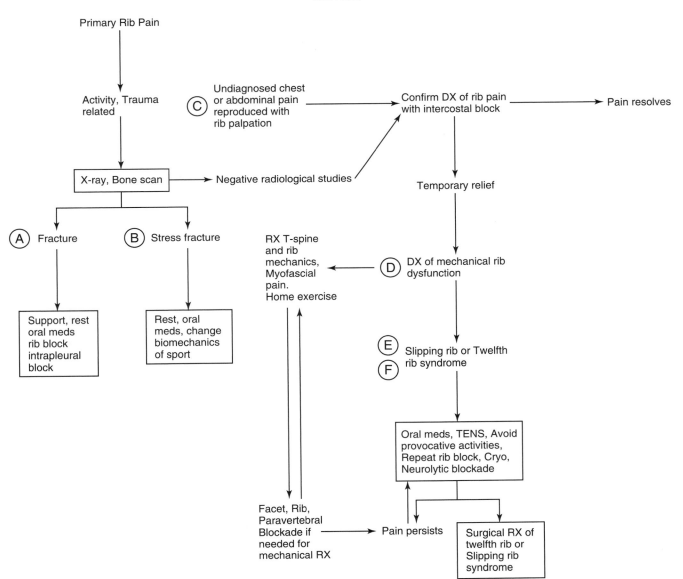

BACK PAIN

Acute Low Back Pain
Chronic Low Back Pain
Lumbosacral Radiculopathy
Spinal Stenosis
Ankylosing Spondylitis
Failed Laminectomy Syndrome
Facet Joint Syndrome
Sacroiliac Joint Pain

Acute Low Back Pain

JONATHAN P. LESTER

Acute low back pain is one of the most common medical disorders in industrialized societies. Most cases are self-limited and may be treated conservatively. In most cases it can be accurately diagnosed by a detailed history and physical examination. Laboratory studies, radiologic imaging, and electrodiagnostic testing are used to confirm the diagnosis or the pathology in difficult cases. Treatment strategies utilize pain control measures, physical therapy, and patient education. Early return to functional activities is achieved in most cases. Serious disease or pathology mandating immediate surgical intervention is uncommon.

A. Back pain resulting from a high energy injury or impact or the sudden onset of back pain in osteoporotic or elderly individuals must be evaluated for spinal fracture. Compression fractures with less than 50% loss of anterior column height, transverse process fractures, or spinous process fractures can be managed conservatively. Compression fractures with loss of more than 50% of anterior column height, or burst fractures, may be unstable and should be referred to a surgeon. Back pain that develops following lifting or flexion-rotation injuries may result from disruption or a tear of the disc annulus fibrosis or acute herniated nucleus pulposus (HNP). Back pain radiating into the lower extremity with or without neurologic loss may indicate acute lumbosacral radiculopathy secondary to acute HNP or spinal stenosis. Acute bowel or bladder dysfunction with or without saddle anesthesia or radicular symptoms suggest cauda equina compromise and should be evaluated emergently with magnetic resonance imaging (MRI) or computed tomography (CT). Back pain resulting from repetitive stress or sudden overload of the spine in neutral position or extension may be due to injury of the posterior elements, including the zygapophyseal (facet) joints or the pars interarticularis. Facet joint pain is often aggravated by standing or spinal extension. Low back pain following a shear injury to the pelvis or lower extremities may indicate an insult to the sacroiliac joint.

B. Back pain associated with constitutional symptoms, weight loss, changes in genitourinary or gastrointestinal function, abdominal or pelvic pain, night pain, or profound morning stiffness suggest a medical disorder and demand appropriate evaluation with laboratory, imaging, or diagnostic studies. Common medical causes of low back pain include pancreatic disease, gallbladder disease, hepatitis, the presence of diverticuli, colorectal cancer, kidney stones, pyelonephritis, endometriosis, pelvic inflammatory disease, cervical or uterine malignancy, pregnancy, aortic aneurysm, spinal neoplasm, prostatitis, prostate cancer, or inflammatory arthropathy.

C. A history of radicular pain associated with the presence of dural tension signs (straight leg raise, Lasegue's sign, bowstring sign) suggests acute lumbosacral radiculopathy secondary to HNP or spinal stenosis.

Conservative care consists of medications—nonsteroidal antiinflammatory drugs (NSAIDs), narcotic and nonnarcotic analgesics, muscle relaxants, oral corticosteroids epidural steroid injections—and physical therapy modalities (superficial heat, ultrasound application, electrical stimulation) are used to control pain and reactive muscle spasm and to decrease inflammation. Specific low back exercise protocols are implemented to strengthen the spinal musculature and stability. Spinal manipulation and massage benefits some patients. Home exercise programs and patient education in spinal biomechanics and lifestyle factors help prevent future episodes of back pain. Imaging studies (CT or MRI) and electrodiagnostic examination can be used to clarify the pathology in patients unresponsive to conservative care. Patients with intractable pain or progressive neurologic deficits should be referred for surgical management.

D. Acute low back pain not associated with traumatic onset, systemic symptoms, or features of discogenic or posterior element injury or dysfunction suggests an isolated soft tissue disorder. Myofascial pain is indicated by the presence of discrete trigger points in affected muscle groups. Fibromyalgia is identified by the presence of multiple tender points in classic joint, bursa, or articular locations. In some patients the physical examination and secondary diagnostic studies are unremarkable, and the patient is given the nonspecific diagnosis of acute lumbosacral strain. Conservative therapies are successful in resolving or controlling symptoms in most cases.

E. A bone scan can differentiate acute pars interarticularis fracture from isthmic spondylolysis. Acute pars injuries are managed with a spinal immobilization orthosis. Mild or moderate back pain associated with low grade spondylolisthesis can be treated conservatively. Those with severe refractory back pain or radiculopathy and patients with high grade spondylolisthesis should be referred for surgical management.

REFERENCES

Berhard T, Kirkaldy-Willis W: Recognizing specific characteristics of nonspecific low back pain. Clin Orthop 1987;217:266.

Lester J, Derebery J: Discogenic low back pain. In: Derebery J, Anderson J (eds) Low Back Pain: An Evidence-Based, Biopsychosocial Model for Clinical Management. Beverly Farms, MA, OEM Press, 2002, p 125.

Lyman M, Fitko J, Horton G: Medical causes of low back pain. In: Derebery J. Anderson J (eds) Low Back Pain: An Evidence-Based, Biopsychosocial Model for Clinical Management. Beverly Farms, MA, OEM Press, 2002.

McGill S: Low back exercises: evidence for improving exercise regimens. Phys Ther 1998;7:754.

Saal JA, Saal JS: Nonoperative treatment of herniated intervertebral disc with radiculopathy: an outcomes study. Spine 1989;14:431.

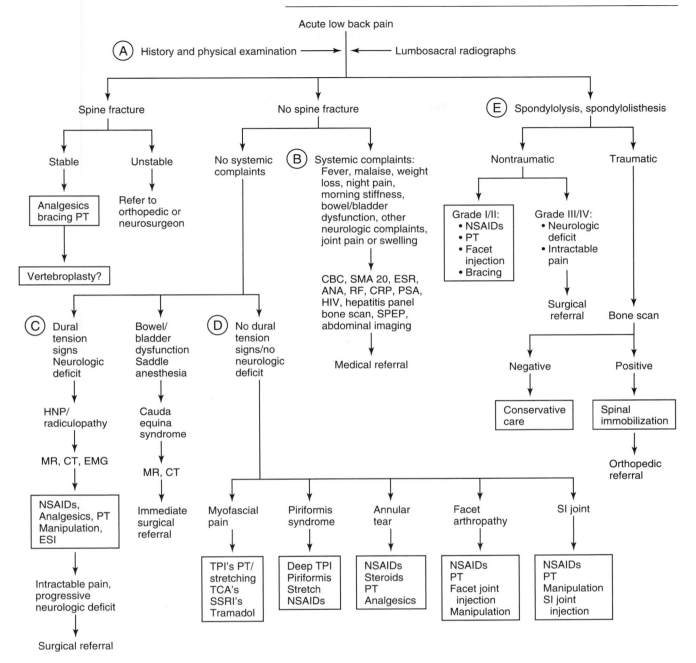

Chronic Low Back Pain

JOHN C. KING

Evaluation of the chronic low back pain patient must be thorough to rule out reversible causes, even though many of these patients do not have disease amenable to pharmacologic or surgical interventions alone. The chronicity of the pain leads to physical, social, and psychological adaptations that may manifest in illness behavior, which is reinforced. Such learned behavior can be "unlearned" with appropriate reinforcers for improved function and healthy living. Frequently, a team approach is required to deal with the physical, psychological, and social factors that impede performance and add to the suffering of these patients.

A. Narcotics and tranquilizing muscle relaxants offer effective short-term benefits but are controversial adjuncts to chronic low back pain management because of their limited effectiveness secondary to tolerance, the creation of medical dependence, and their adverse effects on mood and cognition. These medications are easily withdrawn during inpatient programs over a 2- to 3-week period, usually without any increase in the pain pattern or intensity. Outpatient withdrawal is more difficult, typically requiring 6 to 8 weeks in motivated, cooperative patients.

B. With chronic pain syndrome, the patient experiences pain for more than 6 months (occasionally less), which has led to disability and problems in physical, psychological, social, and vocational areas. This is a learned dysfunctional adjustment pattern that requires behavioral intervention to restore optimal functioning in all spheres of life, which helps reverse suffering.

C. Tricyclic antidepressants, anticonvulsants, and occasionally phenothiazines, with or without nonsteroidal anti-inflammatory drugs (NSAIDs), may be useful chronic pain medications, but all require some monitoring. If benefit is uncertain, the trial should be stopped (usually by tapering off over 2 weeks) every 6 months. If pain is exacerbated, the medication is likely benefiting the patient; if it does not and the trial dosing was adequate, the medication should be discontinued and its failure documented. Other medications that have less clear chronic effects but occasionally are found to be beneficial include mexilitine and alprazolam (difficult from which to wean the patient, even if not helpful for the pain).

D. Treatment should not include passive modalities such as hot packs, massage, or ultrasonography but should involve active therapies that increase self-reliance and self-management: exercises, stretching, self-pacing, and paced planning of work, rest, and recreation. If no actively or progressively destructive process (e.g., cancer) is found, the pain should not be interpreted as a signal to stop activities or to withdraw from life. The functional perspective, or rehabilitation model in which the impairments caused by the pain are treated, becomes the most beneficial approach to decreasing the patient's suffering. The goals include increased activity (which counterintuitively consistently decreases chronic pain), decreased medication, and no increased pain. The ability to do more, without necessarily hurting more, helps decrease suffering. Suffering aspects can also be minimized by concurrent cognitive therapies, such as cognitive rationale emotive therapy, which examines alarming destructive self-talk.

E. Reassuring patients who have a chronically painful condition requires significant time for exhaustive evaluation, review of records, and patient education. Many pain patients state that, "No one has ever really listened to me." The thorough initial evaluation helps build trust. Treat both the mind and the body.

F. Pure psychogenic pain is rarely encountered. The absence of clinical signs along with normal laboratory and imaging studies do not rule out all causes of physical pain (e.g., chronic bursitis, early osteoarthritis, fibromyalgia). When there is a suggestive neurophysiologic pain pattern, surreptitious testing, or observation, the possibility of purely psychogenic causes or motivational issues should be pursued. Most chronic pain patients have both a physical problem and secondary psychosocial changes with variable premorbid psychological strengths.

G. If no suggestive psychogenic causes are found and there is no likely physical cause, malingering and secondary gain issues may be related to the decreased function. Unless there is a severe antisocial personality, dementia, or uncontrolled schizophrenia, behavior modification inpatient programs may still be effective in improving function and restoring abilities that may be lost simply due to disuse deconditioning.

H. Inpatient programs should not be dualistic: "It's all in your mind" or "It's all in your body." They should deal with all aspects of the pain problem: physical, psychological, social, family, and vocational and nonvocational aspects of the disabling pain.

I. If patients are reasonably screened, it is rare for medical problems to preclude progression to the patient's premorbid capabilities. The patient's usual pattern of pain is not a reason to end a rehabilitation program that is increasing the patient's physical abilities.

J. A home program is best and ideally consists of fewer than seven exercises that require less than 45 minutes to complete. Such regimens enhance compliance.

K. Follow-up should occur every 3 to 13 months to evaluate the long-term effectiveness of the interventions, enhance compliance, and minimize "doctor shopping," which increases the risk of unnecessary invasive procedures. Initially, as-needed follow-up is allowed to alleviate any anxiety associated with the initial transition back to a full, active lifestyle, but this should become progressively less frequent. Having comprehensively

MANAGEMENT OF LOW BACK PAIN

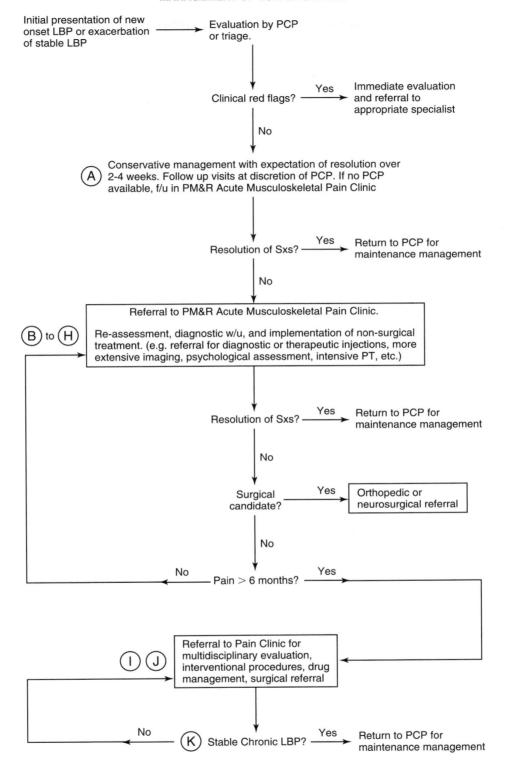

evaluated and followed the patient, you are in the best position to evaluate any new pain complaints. For routine follow-ups, Fordyce's ten steps to help chronic pain patients offers practical suggestions.

1. Accept patients' pain as real. Find out *why* they hurt, not *whether* they hurt.
2. Protect patients from unnecessary invasive procedures.
3. Set realistic goals. Expect to manage rather than cure.
4. Evaluate chronic pain in terms of what patients do—not what they say.
5. Let patients know that *you* are the expert on medications and procedures.
6. Shift patients to oral, time-contingent medications (not "as needed").
7. Prescribe exercises to start at easily achieved levels, but increase at a preset rate.
8. Educate patients' families to encourage increased activity.
9. Focus your attention on the patient's activities rather than on the pain. Ask not how patients feel but what they have done.
10. Help patients get involved in pleasurable activities. Remember, people who have something better to do do not hurt as much.

REFERENCES

Abramowicz M: Alprazolam for panic disorder. *Med Lett* 1991;33:3.

Bowsher D: Assessment of the chronic pain sufferer. *Surg Rounds Orthop* 1989;3:70.

Fordyce WE, Fowler RS, Lehman JF, DeLateur BJ: Ten steps to help patients with chronic pain. *Patient Care* 1978;12:263.

Hildebrandt J, Pfingsten M, Saur P, et al: Prediction of success from a multidisciplinary treatment program for chronic low back pain. *Spine* 1997;22:990.

King JC: Chronic pain. In: Grabois M, Garrison SJ, Lehmkuhl D, Hartt S (eds) *Physical Medicine and Rehabilitation*. New York, Blackwell, 1999.

King JC, Kelleher WJ: The chronic pain syndrome. *Phys Med Rehabil* 1991;5:168.

Lipman RS: Pharmacotherapy of anxiety and depression. *Psychopharmacol Bull* 1981;171:91.

Loeser JO, Eyar KJ (eds): *Managing the Chronic Pain Patient*. New York, Raven, 1989.

Mayer TG, Polatin P, Smith B, et al: Contemporary concepts in spine care: spine rehabilitation. *Spine* 1995;20:2060.

Vlok GJ, Hendrix MRG: The lumbar disc: evaluation the causes of pain. *Orthopaedics* 1991;14:419.

Lumbosacral Radiculopathy

JONATHAN P. LESTER

Lumbosacral (LS) radiculopathy is suggested by complaints of pain, sensory disturbance, weakness, or reflex asymmetry in the distribution of a distinct lumbosacral nerve root. Most LS radiculopathies involve the L5 or S1 root. Imaging modalities can suggest the anatomic cause of root compromise, and electrodiagnostic studies can assess the severity and specificity of root injury. Most causes of LS radiculopathy can be managed with conservative care.

A. The evaluation of LS radiculopathy should begin with a complete history, physical examination, and in some cases a complete set of LS spine radiographs.

B. A history of sudden onset of symptoms following high-energy spinal trauma suggests a spinal fracture or ligamentous disruption with radicular, cauda equina, or spinal cord injury. If this type of injury is suspected, the patient should be immobilized and LS radiographs or computed tomography (CT) scans obtained.

C. Acute LS radiculopathy following a flexion-rotation or lifting injury is most often due to acute herniated nucleus pulposus (HNP). Progressive failure of disc annular fibers leads to the formation of a posterior or posterolateral radial fissure with extravasation of nuclear contents. HNP can cause root injury by direct mechanical compression or inflammatory insult triggered by the release of cytokines or proinflammatory mediators from the nuclear material. Most cases can be managed conservatively with analgesic and anti-inflammatory medications, physical therapy emphasizing specific exercise programs, and epidural steroid injections. Patients with intractable pain or progressive neurologic deficit are referred for surgical care.

D. Spinal stenosis is a common cause of monoradicular or polyradicular disease. Stenosis may compromise the central spinal canal with polyradicular or cauda equina compromise or the lateral canal and neuroforamina with monoradicular compromise. Symptoms are usually exacerbated by standing or walking. LS spine radiographs often reveal sclerotic hypertrophy of the vertebral endplates and facet joints as well as narrowing of the interlaminar space. The severity of spinal narrowing can be assessed with CT or magnetic resonance imaging. Electrodiagnostic testing can define the extent of radicular compromise. Conservative care can manage or resolve symptoms for extended periods, but surgical decompression is often necessary to address the fixed bony lesion.

E. Peripheral entrapment neuropathies of the lower extremity may mimic the presentation of LS radiculopathy. Lesions of the peroneal nerve at the fibular head, the tibial nerve at the tarsal tunnel, the sciatic nerve at the piriformis muscle, the lateral femoral cutaneous nerve at the ilioinguinal ligament, and the saphenous nerve at Hunter's canal are common causes of radicular symptoms. Electrodiagnostic studies can be used to differentiate radicular from peripheral nerve compromise.

F. Isthmic or degenerative spondylolisthesis may cause lateral spinal or neuroforaminal stenosis with radiculopathy. LS spine radiographs reveal the pathology. Electrodiagnostic testing reveals the severity of nerve root insult. Conservative care can be effective with low degrees of listhesis, but surgical decompression and fusion is indicated in refractory cases or those with a high degree of slippage.

G. Inflammatory or infectious radiculopathy may occur, particularly in association with human immunodeficiency virus infection, hepatitis C, or Guillain-Barré syndrome. Common infectious agents include *Cryptococcus*, *Mycobacterium tuberculosis*, syphilis, Lyme disease, or borreliosis.

H. Metabolic radiculopathy or polyneuropathy is most often seen in association with diabetes mellitus. Toxicity from abnormal glucose metabolism may predispose one to nerve root or peripheral nerve injury at common points of compromise. In addition, diabetic polyneuropathy may present with a localized mononeuritis (most often the femoral nerve). Electrodiagnostic studies are used to diagnose diabetic polyneuropathy and to delineate the location and extent of radicular or peripheral nerve compromise. Some improvement may be achieved with better glucose control and medications for neuropathic pain (tricyclic antidepressants, neuroleptic drugs, capsacin).

I. Primary or metastatic tumors of the spine may first present with radiculopathy. Night pain, or pain unrelieved with rest in the supine position should alert the physician and prompt him or her to order appropriate imaging or laboratory studies.

J. Metabolic bone disorders such as Paget's disease may cause radicular pain if bony remodeling cause spinal stenosis. LS radiographs reveal hyperostotic vertebrae. A skeletal survey reveals tibial bowing and increased skull size.

REFERENCES

Couldwell W, Weiss M: Leg radicular pain and sensory disturbance: the differential diagnosis. In: *Spine State of the Art Reviews*, vol 2. Philadelphia, Hanley & Belfus, 1988, p 669.

Dumitru D: *Electrodiagnostic Medicine*. Philadelphia, Hanley & Belfus, 1995;453.

Gordon SL, Weinstein JN: A review of basic science issues in low back pain. *Phys Med Rehabil Clin N Am* 1998;9:323–342.

Lester J, Derebery J: Discogenic low back pain. In: Derebery J, Anderson J (eds) *Low Back Pain: An Evidence-Based, Biopsychosocial Model for Clinical Management*. Beverly Farms, MA, OEM Press, 2002, pp 125–142.

Saal J, Dillingham A, Gamburd R, Fanton G: The pseudoradicular syndrome: lower extremity peripheral entrapment masquerading as lumbar radiculopathy. Spine 1988;13:926.

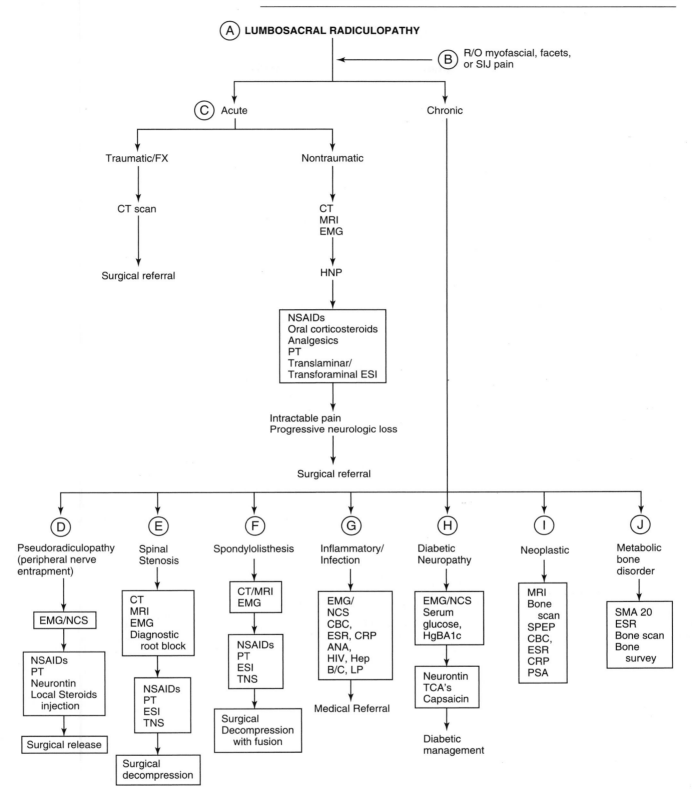

Spinal Stenosis

SUSAN J. DREYER

Spinal stenosis is the narrowing of the spinal canal in either the lateral (apophyseal) or anteroposterior (AP) (laminar) direction, resulting in nerve compression of the spinal roots laterally and of the cauda equina anteroposteriorly. This narrowing can occur anywhere along the spinal column, from occiput to sacrum, but there may be asymptomatic radiographic evidence. The origin of the stenosis can be congenital or acquired, although most cases are caused by degenerative arthritis. Typical onset is during the fifth decade, although individuals with absolute stenosis (AP diameter of the spinal canal < 10 mm) may show spinal stenosis as early as the third decade. Much controversy still exists regarding treatment, especially surgical timing and technique. The current literature indicates that degenerative lumbar stenosis is not as ubiquitous as had been originally thought.

A. Classic symptoms include low back and leg pain, especially when standing, walking, or hyperextending. The lower extremity pain and paresthesias are relieved by flexing the spine. Unlike vascular claudication, this pseudoclaudication is less predictable in onset, slower to subside, and not relieved simply by standing. Physical examination shows strong peripheral pulses (unless concomitant vascular disease exists) and minimal static tension signs such as straight-leg raises. Presenting symptoms of cervical stenosis may be those of myelopathy, with weakness, atrophy, hyperreflexia, and spasticity.

B. Plain radiographs usually demonstrate spondylosis with loss of disc height, osteophytes, and sclerosis of the facet joints. Computed tomography, myelography, and magnetic resonance imaging can further delineate the lesion, although far lateral stenosis is often missed with myelography. Degenerative lumbar stenosis most frequently involves the L4-5 facet joint. In the neck, the C5-6 level is most commonly involved. Clinical diagnosis cannot be based on isolated radiographic findings. Each radiographic examination has its limitations; for example, false-negative rates of 10% to 25% have been reported with myelography. Electrodiagnostic studies such as electromyography and somatosensory evoked potentials also aid in localization.

C. Much of the discomfort is believed to stem from concomitant soft tissue disorders, which should be treated aggressively.

D. Identify the cause of spinal stenosis as well as the region involved to better choose the form of treatment. Spinal stenosis secondary to Paget's disease responds to calcitonin, whereas other types of spinal stenosis do not. Surgical procedures are dictated by the underlying disorder.

E. Most patients deserve a trial of aggressive conservative therapy, including modalities such as stretching, going to back school, and the use of nonsteroidal anti-inflammatory drugs. The best results are achieved with a multidisciplinary team focused on returning the patients to productivity.

F. Epidural blocks with or without steroids help delay the need for surgery, especially in older patients with radicular pain.

G. Selective nerve blocks aid in diagnosing the symptomatic level(s), as multilevel stenosis is commonly seen on radiographs. Limiting surgical decompression to the symptomatic levels minimizes iatrogenic instability.

H. Surgery is indicated in patients who have significant neurologic involvement, such as marked or progressive muscle weakness. A neurogenic bowel or bladder requires emergent decompression of the cauda equina to prevent irreversible damage. Consider surgery in patients who have failed to achieve pain relief through conservative treatment. The basic goals of surgery for spinal stenosis are to achieve adequate decompression and adequate stability.

REFERENCES

Hopp E (ed): *Spine: State of the Art Reviews:* Vol 2: *Spinal Stenosis,* no. 3. Philadelphia, Hanley & Belfus, 1987.

Lispon SJ, Branch WT: Low back pain. In: Branch W (ed) *Office Practice of Medicine,* 2nd ed. Philadelphia, Saunders, 1987, p 875.

Loeser JD, Bigos SJ, Fordyce WE, Volinn EP: Low back pain. In: Bonica JJ (ed) *The Management of Pain,* 2nd ed. Philadelphia, Lea & Febiger, 1990, p 1468.

Wood GW: Other disorders of the spine. In: Creshaw AH (ed) *Campbell's Operative Orthopaedics.* St. Louis, Mosby, 1987, p 3347.

PATIENT WITH SPINAL STENOSIS

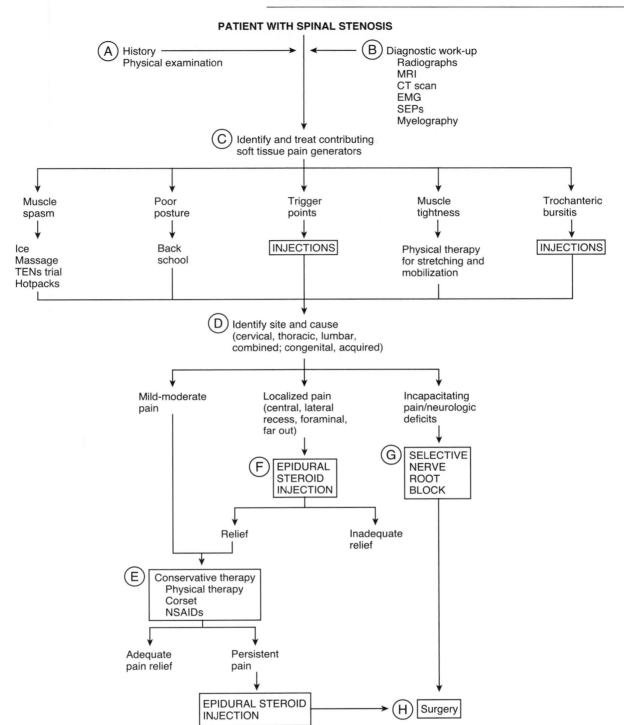

Ankylosing Spondylitis

ELLEN LEONARD AND BERT BLACKWELL

Ninety percent of persons with ankylosing spondylitis (Marie-Strümpell disease), a seronegative spondyloarthropathy that predominantly affects young men, are found to be positive for the HLA-B27 antigen.

A. Patients younger than 40 years of age who complain of back pain of insidious onset, which is worse in the morning, should be considered for a diagnosis of spondyloarthropathy. A careful history should be taken, with particular attention paid to family history of psoriasis; past medical history of uveitis and prostatitis; and symptoms of weight loss, fatigue, malaise, morning stiffness, and anterior chest pain. Complete a detailed physical examination, paying special attention to flexibility of the spine (Schober's test), pain in sacroiliac joints, and chest expansion.

B. Laboratory data should include sedimentation rate and presence or absence of HLA-B27. The sedimentation rate may or may not be increased, but HLA-B27 is found in 90% of patients with this disease. Radiography is essential. Findings can range from "blurring" of the sacroiliac joints to "bamboo" spine.

C. Three stages of pain occur in progression of the disease:

Stage I. Early sacroiliac inflammation is described as hip pain and is often mislabeled as sciatica. The pain awakens the patient at night and abates after he or she gets up and moves around.

Stage II. The chronic middle phase of the disease is characterized by morning stiffness that improves by afternoon. Many patients also experience anterior chest pain of mechanical origin.

Stage III. Late in the disease, patients have no morning stiffness and pain at rest but continue to have nagging interscapular neck and low back pain. By this stage, patients have rigid spines and dorsal kyphosis. If these patients have severe focal pain, a pseudoarthrosis should be suspected.

D. The treatment of ankylosing spondylitis pain is twofold: decrease the pain and deformity, and maintain function. Radiotherapy is no longer used because of the risk of leukemia. Pharmacology treatment consists of the administration of nonsteroidal antiinflammatory drugs (NSAIDs). The first choice is indomethacin, 25 to 50 mg, three or four times per day. The other traditional choice, phenbutazone, carries the risk of marrow aplasia. Other NSAIDs such as sulindac, 150 to 200 mg twice a day, may be used. The second prong of treatment is physical therapy and education. Instruct patients to sleep on a firm mattress with no pillow. Exercises are aimed at preventing kyphosis and maintaining flexibility, range of motion, and pulmonary function. Instruct patients in extension exercises, morning warm-up exercises, and flexibility exercises. Have patients perform chest expansion exercises to prevent restrictive lung disease, and encourage general endurance activities.

E. In the late stages of the disease, patients may develop painful pseudoarthroses, which should be treated with immobilization. Instruct patients in rest and positioning to decrease the strain on neck muscles. Surgery for vertebral wedge osteotomy may be indicated in some patients.

REFERENCES

Calliet R: *Low Back Pain Syndrome.* Philadelphia, FA Davis, 1986, p. 197.

Delisa J (ed): *Rehabilitation Medicine: Principles and practice.* Philadelphia: JB Lippincott, 1988, p. 726.

Good A: The pain of ankylosing spondylitis. *Am J Med* 1984;80:118

Kottke F, Lehmann JF: *Krusen's Handbook of Physical Medicine and Rehabilitation,* 4th ed. Philadelphia, WB Saunders, 1990, p. 631.

Rodnan G: *Primer on the Rheumatic Diseases.* Atlanta, Arthritis Foundation, 1983, p. 84.

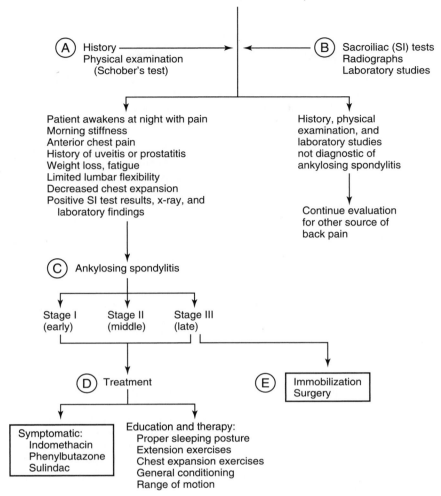

Patient with SACROILIAC PAIN;
ANKYLOSING SPONDYLITIS Suspected

(A) History
Physical examination
(Schober's test)

(B) Sacroiliac (SI) tests
Radiographs
Laboratory studies

Patient awakens at night with pain
Morning stiffness
Anterior chest pain
History of uveitis or prostatitis
Weight loss, fatigue
Limited lumbar flexibility
Decreased chest expansion
Positive SI test results, x-ray, and
    laboratory findings

History, physical
examination, and
laboratory studies
not diagnostic of
ankylosing spondylitis

Continue evaluation
for other source of
back pain

(C) Ankylosing spondylitis

Stage I   Stage II   Stage III
(early)   (middle)   (late)

(D) Treatment

(E) Immobilization
Surgery

Symptomatic:
  Indomethacin
  Phenylbutazone
  Sulindac

Education and therapy:
  Proper sleeping posture
  Extension exercises
  Chest expansion exercises
  General conditioning
  Range of motion

Failed Laminectomy Syndrome

MARK E. ROMANOFF

The failed laminectomy syndrome (FLS) is not a single entity. Bony abnormalities (spondylolisthesis, pseudarthrosis), joint problems (facet arthropathy, degenerative joint disease), muscular changes (myofascial pain syndrome, atrophy), neural disorders (nerve root impingement, arachnoiditis, deafferentation), and psychological difficulties (depression, compensation/litigation) may all play roles in this difficult-to-treat syndrome. Signs and symptoms vary, depending on which factor is prominent. A 40% failure rate for laminectomy surgery has been quoted when the preoperative diagnosis is in doubt. A failure rate of 10% to 15% with resultant pain and compromised mobility is more commonly observed.

Treatment for FLS must be individualized and creative. Success rates are poor and in most studies do not approach 50%. FLS is produced by inappropriate surgery, surgical complications, and patient factors. Strict guidelines concerning the indications for back surgery have been approved by the American Academy of Orthopedic Surgeons and the Association of Neurological Surgeons to help prevent inappropriate surgery.

A. A complete history, including previous surgical diagnosis, the number and types of previous surgery, medication use, and the extent of disability, is necessary. The work and home environment should be evaluated. Psychological screening should be performed. A comprehensive treatment plan taking into account all these factors is required for a good outcome. A thorough physical examination, including a detailed neurologic examination, should help confirm or refute preliminary diagnostic suspicions and may be used to follow progress. Provocative tests to elicit discomfort (straight-leg raise; sitting root test; Lasègue; palpation of muscles, ligaments, and joints) are important aspects of the physical examination. It can reveal valuable information, and also reassure patients that you are actively looking for the cause of their problem. An extensive search should be made for a myofascial pain syndrome (MFPS), which usually coexists with almost all FLS diagnoses. Early treatment may alleviate many symptoms and allow therapy to progress more rapidly. A differential spinal block and/or thiopental testing can help determine the source of pain.

B. Diagnostic studies focus on mechanical causes for pain in these patients, but other pathologic conditions should not be overlooked. The history, physical examination, laboratory studies, and radiographic procedures should be used to rule out important diagnoses such as osteomyelitis; spinal cord neoplasm; Paget's disease; hemachromatosis; and referred pain from the kidney, pancreas, or abdominal aorta.

C. Conservative treatment should begin soon after the initial history taking and physical examination.

Most patients have tried or are taking nonsteroidal antiinflammatory drugs (NSAIDs) at the time of evaluation. NSAIDs should be given an adequate trial of at least 8 weeks before changing or discontinuing medications. If one class of NSAIDs fails, one from another class should be substituted. Antidepressant medications can lessen depressive symptoms and sleep disturbances and affect pain thresholds. The choice of antidepressant should be made with the drug's side effects and the patient's medical profile and psychological state in mind. Narcotic medications usually are not helpful and should be discontinued. Physical and/or occupational therapy (PT/OT) should be started. Increasing activity levels may help reverse learned patient behavior as well as improve muscular tone and flexibility. Transcutaneous electrical nerve stimulation (TENS) is often effective in decreasing pain in MFPS, degenerative joint disease, and nerve root irritation. TENS has often been tried in the past and deemed ineffective by the patients. A TENS trial should be repeated. Psychological interventions may also help manage the pain.

D. Imaging techniques during the initial phase of therapy should be limited to patients with suspected surgical disease (radicular symptoms on physical examination), those with new symptoms, or those whose response to conservative treatment has not been optimal. An enhanced magnetic resonance imaging (MRI) or computed tomography (CT) scan can aid in the diagnosis of epidural fibrosis versus retained disk material. MRI produces sharper images of soft tissues, but CT is more effective in imaging bony abnormalities. Patients with metal appliances should not undergo MRI.

E. Repeat operations should be performed only if there is overwhelming evidence of a surgically correctable lesion. Examples include retained disk material or a recurrent disk at the site of previous surgery; a new herniated nucleus pulposus; or instability or a pseudarthrosis at the site of a previous fusion (this may be diagnosed by CT/MRI but requires confirmation by lateral flexion–extension radiography, as motion may be found but is not always the cause of pain); or spinal stenosis. One study that evaluated repeat operations in patients with FLS found that >79% of 67 patients had some pain relief and 43% discontinued narcotic use. However, only 12% of these patients experienced good relief of pain, and a 13% complication rate was also noted. Approximately 50% of patients with epidural fibrosis showed a poor result after repeat surgery. The best outcomes after repeat surgery were associated with four factors: (1) a pain-free interval of more than 1 year after the initial surgery, (2) a complete myelographic block, (3) a true disk herniation, and (4) evidence of instability.

Patient with FAILED LAMINECTOMY SYNDROME

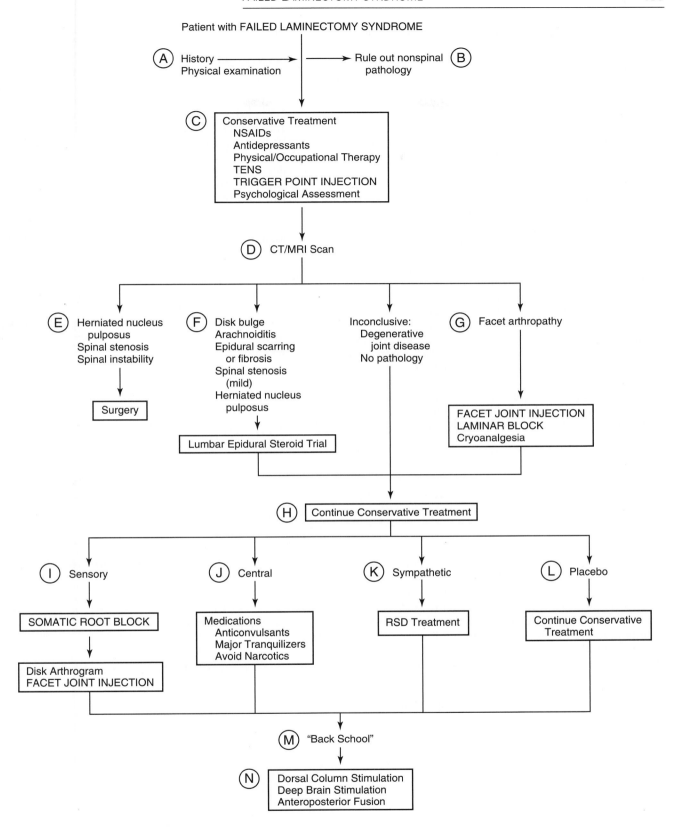

F. Lumbar epidural steroid injections (ESIs) appear to have the highest efficacy in patients with low back pain and radicular symptoms. Patients with arachnoiditis or epidural scarring may respond to lumbar ESI, but if fibrosis is present the antiinflammatory effect of the steroids will be of little benefit.

G. Facet syndrome may mimic the signs and symptoms of nerve root compression. It tends to be forgotten as an entity in the differential diagnosis of FLS. Facet joint injections with a local anesthetic and steroid can be performed, or the nerve supply to the joint can be interrupted. If these are effective but demonstrate short-lived pain relief, cryoanalgesia radiofrequency lesion, or neurolytic block can be attempted for long-term pain control.

H. Other conservative methods may be added to the regimen at this time. Biofeedback, relaxation techniques, and hypnosis may be useful. Dosages of NSAIDs and antidepressants may be increased or the medications changed as appropriate.

I. Lumbar or transsacral nerve root blocks can be effective forms of treatment in these patients. Temporary relief of pain after a series of blocks may indicate nerve root compression. Causes of this compression should be actively sought. Failure of these blocks may indicate disk pain or facet pain. A disk arthrogram that reproduces the patient's pain is justification for surgical intervention. If a facet joint injection has not been attempted recently, it should be performed at this time.

J. Patients with a central pain syndrome may benefit from a trial of anticonvulsant medications. Narcotics are unlikely to be useful.

K. Sympathetically mediated pain should be managed as reflex sympathetic dystrophy.

L. Some patients respond to placebo or show evidence of psychologically mediated pain; these individuals are best treated conservatively.

M. "Back school" should be started in patients when no further interventional therapy is planned. This should involve operant conditioning, behavior modification, PT/OT, and often drug detoxification. Success rates of greater than 70% have been achieved in these intensive programs. Opponents cite the high relapse rates as one problem with this approach.

N. Dorsal column stimulation to spinal cord stimulation has proved effective in some patients. In one study of 89 patients with arachnoiditis and FLS, an excellent response was seen in 85% after 3 months of implantation, but this decreased to only 35% after 4 to 8 years of follow-up. A 24% complication rate was also noted, electrode migration and infection being the most common. For patients not responding to spinal cord stimulation, deep brain stimulation has been attempted. Medial thalamus stimulation appears to be more effective for deep, crushing pain. Burning, sharp, and searing pain is controlled with lateral thalamus stimulation. Some studies using periventricular gray stimulation have produced 80% success rates. Complications cited include intraventricular hemorrhage, infection, and electrode movement.

Simultaneous combined anterior and posterior fusion has been recommended for patients with disabling low back pain. With this technique, 61% of patients showed good results and 14% had fair pain relief; a complication rate of 23% was experienced. Patients with combined multilevel pathology, single-level or multilevel annular tears, and herniated nucleus pulposus responded best, whereas those with multilevel degenerative disk disease fared poorly.

REFERENCES

Bogduk N: Back pain: zygapophyseal blocks and epidural steroids. In: Cousins MJ, Bridenbaugh PO (eds) *Neural Blockade in Clinical Anesthesia and Management of Pain*, 2nd ed. Philadelphia, JB Lippincott, 1988, p. 935.

Burton CV, Kirkaldy-Willis WH, Yong-Hing K, et al: Causes of failure of surgery on the lumbar spine. *Clin Orthop* 1981;157:191.

Finnegan WJ, Fenlin JM, Marvel JP, et al: Results of surgical intervention in the symptomatic multiply-operated back patient. *J Bone Joint Surg* 1979;61A:1077.

Kosak JA, O'Brien JP: Simultaneous combined anterior and posterior fusion. An independent analysis of a treatment of the disabled low-back pain patient. *Spine* 1990;15:322.

Long DM, Filtzer DL, BenDebba M, Hendler NH: Clinical features of the failed back syndrome. *J Neurosurg* 1988;69:61.

Plotkin R: Results in 60 cases of deep brain stimulation for chronic intractable pain. Proceedings of the 8th meeting World Society of Stereotactic and Functional Neurosurgery, Part 1, Zurich, 1981. *Appl Neurophysiol* 1982;45:201.

Siegfried J, Lazorthes J: Long-term follow-up of dorsal cord stimulation for chronic pain syndrome after multiple lumbar operations. Proceedings of the 8th Meeting World Society of Stereotactic and Functional Neurosurgery, Part 1, Zurich, 1981. *Appl Neurophysiol* 1982;45:201.

Facet Joint Syndrome

MAURICE G. SHOLAS

Approximately 15% to 40% of low back pain is due to dysfunction or inflammation of the facet (zygapophyseal) joints. Goldwaith, in 1911, was the first scientist credited with proposing facet joint involvement in low back pain. The term facet joint syndrome was formally coined by Ghormley et al. in 1933. The precise pathophysiology of facet joint syndrome is unclear. Two medial branches of the dorsal rami provide innervation. Any of the elements of the articulating surface or its innervation may be responsible. There are thus no pathognomonic data provided by the patient's history or physical examination. Nor is any laboratory, radiologic, or electrophysiologic test diagnostic. By convention, the diagnosis is based simply on a constellation of findings.

A. The patient's history is likely to include complaints of deep, achy, nonspecific low back pain localized over the affected facet joint. Radiation to the buttocks or proximal thigh is possible. Radiation distal to the knee is uncharacteristic. The patient may report that the symptoms are worse with lumbar extension, extensive walking, or sitting for long periods of time. There is no bowel or bladder dysfunction.

B. On physical examination, the patient demonstrates pain with deep palpation over the affected facet joint(s). There may be increased muscle tone in the paraspinal musculature overlying the affected joint(s). A loss of lordosis, a decrement in spinal extension, and pain prominent with "quadrant loading" may be present. The patient does not have focal or segmental muscle atrophy, neural tension signs, or true strength deficits.

C. Diagnostic tests may demonstrate specific facet joint pathology but are more important for ruling out other, more ominous reasons that present with a similar clinical presentation. Plain films of the spine are appropriate. Magnetic resonance imaging (MRI) is useful as well. Electrodiagnostic studies are normal and so are not indicated if one suspects facet joint syndrome.

D. Once all myelopathic processes have been ruled out, a 4- to 6-week course of conservative therapy is indicated. It should include the use of an antiinflammatory agent taken on a routine, not as-needed, basis. The use of muscle relaxants in this setting is controversial. Physical therapy is useful, as are teaching abdominal strengthening, flexibility training, educating the patient about body mechanics, and providing home exercise program instruction. There is a role for manipulation as well.

E. A surgical consultation is indicated when an acute myelopathic process is identified, there is progressive neurologic loss, or an unstable anatomic lesion is identified. There are no surgical indications for true facet joint syndrome.

F. Fluoroscopically guided joint space or medial branch block injections must reduce the pain by more than 50% to be considered successful. First, the patient is injected with lidocaine. If this is successful, a second injection at a later date is performed with bupivicaine. The second injection should not only successfully relieve the pain, the relief should be of longer duration. This procedure has been used as an important diagnostic tool.

G. The technique of mixing steroids with a local anesthetic and injecting them into the facet joint is controversial. Additionally, there are conflicting data regarding the efficacy of radiofrequency ablation of the nerve supply to the facet joint.

H. Contraindications to injection include the presence of a spinal malignancy, bleeding diathesis, or local infection or an etiology of low back pain not related to facet pathology. Injection is not contraindicated in patients with nondermatomal pain that extends below the knee.

REFERENCES

Cavanaugh JM, Ozaktay AC, Yamashita T, et al: Mechanisms of low back pain: a neurophysiologic and neuroanatomic study. *Clin Orthop* 1997;335:166–180.

Dawson E, Bernbeck J: The surgical treatment of low back pain. *Phys Med Rehabil Clin N Am* 1998;9:489–495.

Dreyer SJ, Dreyfuss PH: Low back pain and the zygapophysial (facet) joints. *Arch Phys Med Rehabil* 1996;77:290–300.

Dreyfuss PH, Dreyer SJ, Herring SA: Contemporary concepts in spine care: lumbar zygapophysial (facet) joint injection. *Spine* 1995;20:2040–2047.

Leclaire R, Fortin L, Lambert R, et al: Radiofrequency facet joint denervation in the treatment of low back pain: a placebo-controlled clinical trial to assess efficacy. *Spine* 2001;26:1411–1417.

Nelemans PJ, deBie RA, deVet HC, Sturmans F: Injection therapy for subacute and chronic benign low back pain. *Spine* 2001;26:501–515.

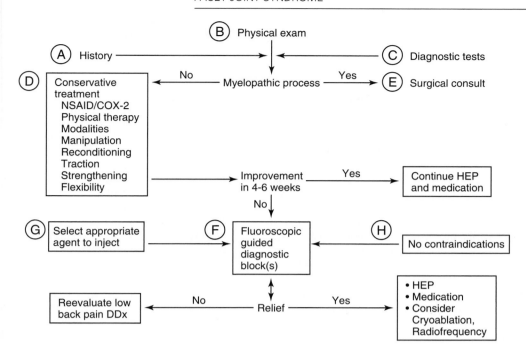

Sacroiliac Joint Pain

JAMES G. GRIFFIN

The sacroiliac joint can be a primary source of pain. Pain may be referred to the sacroiliac (SI) joint or from the SI joint to the lumbar facets, iliolumbar ligament, and gluteal, piriformis, iliopsoas, and adductor muscles. Visceral pain referral may occur from the reproductive organs in females and from the large intestine. Systemic conditions such as ankylosing spondylitis, regional ileitis, and gout can also produce pain in the SI joint. If the treatment of these sources of pain decrease but do not eliminate SI joint pain, SI joint involvement must also be considered. Conversely, SI pain unresponsive to treatment may be a symptom of another problem. The practitioner interested in an exhaustive review of the SI joint is referred to the article by Cole et al. (1996).

A. Primary SI problems are frequently the result of an accident or injury of a traumatic nature, but they also can result from an unguarded or unexpected movement, chronic strain in the workplace, or repetitive activity such as swinging a golf club. SI joint pain is not uncommon during or following pregnancy.

B. Individuals with an anatomically short leg or increased unilateral pronation can have SI joint pain as a result. Removing or correcting these stresses may easily relieve the problem. SI joint problems frequently exist in conjunction with other musculoskeletal disorders, which must be treated to ensure complete relief. Tightness and trigger points commonly exist in the musculature surrounding the SI joint and pelvis. These points respond to the methods devised by Travell (Travell and Simmons 1983), who injected a local anesthetic and subsequently stretched the muscle with use of a vapocoolant spray. A specific home exercise program may also be required.

C. Sacroiliac joint problems requiring direct attention may be treated by injection or manipulation. Such manipulation requires the practitioner to have knowledge of pelvic mechanics for evaluation and the skill to perform the appropriate manipulative technique to restore normal mechanics. Techniques used may involve high-velocity, low-amplitude thrust techniques or muscle energy techniques, which are a form of precise contract-relax stretching to mobilize the joint. By itself, manipulation may be sufficient to resolve many SI problems. An SI belt worn tightly around the pelvis just below the level of the iliac crest and above the pubic symphysis while weight-bearing can be useful in hypermobile patients, providing stability by compressing the SI joint.

D. If manual skills are unavailable, if manipulation fails, or with patients too irritable to tolerate manual treatment, injecting the joint under fluoroscopic observation is effective. An injection of 0.25% bupivacaine, distributing 1 ml to the joint and 3 ml to the posterior ligament and muscle can restore normal pelvic mechanics and relieve the pain in some patients. In some cases the combination of injecting a local anesthetic and steroid with subsequent manipulation is required to restore normal mechanics and relieve irritation in the joint. Dysfunction may exist in the lower lumbar spine and must be recognized and treated. Also, compensatory changes in the vertebral column secondary to SI dysfunction may occur even as far proximal as the cervical spine. This may be worth considering in nonresponsive patients. Patients with chronic pain suffer some degree of deconditioning and must be on a program to regain strength, flexibility, and endurance. The use of proper back hygiene is encouraged.

E. The use of a neurolytic injection may be required in persistent cases that are clearly SI joint pain and are resistant to other forms of therapy. Injection of sclerosing agents, which purportedly stabilize the joint and thus relieve pain, is supported by controlled research.

F. Surgical intervention may be required when pain is intractable or disabling, and when all other possibilities have been excluded.

REFERENCES

Aitken GS: Syndromes of lumbo-pelvic dysfunction. In: Grieve GP (ed) *Modern Manual: Therapy of the Vertebral Column*. New York, Churchill Livingstone, 1986.

Bernard TN, Kirkaldy-Willis WH: Making a specific diagnosis. In: Kirkaldy-Willis WH (ed) *Managing Low Back Pain*, 2nd ed. New York, Churchill Livingstone, 1988.

Bourdillion JF, Day EA, Bookhout MR: *Spinal Manipulation*, 5th ed. Norwalk, CT, Appleton & Lange, 1992.

Cassidy JD, Kirkaldy-Willis WH: Manipulation. In: Kirkaldy-Willis WH (ed) *Managing Low Back Pain*, 2nd ed. New York, Churchill Livingstone, 1988.

Cole AJ, Dreyfuss P, Stratton SA: The sacroiliac joint: a functional approach. *Clin Rev Phys Rehabil Med* 1996;8:125–152.

Dreyfuss P, Michaelson M, Horne M: MUJA: manipulation under joint anesthesia/analgesia: a treatment approach for recalcitrant low back pain of synovial joint origin. *J Manipul Physiol Ther* 1995; 18:537–546.

Greenman PE: *Principles of Manual Medicine*, 2nd ed. Baltimore, Williams & Wilkins, 1996.

Grieve GP: Referred pain and other clinical features. In: Grieve GP (ed) *Modern Manual: Therapy of the Vertebral Column*. New York, Churchill Livingstone, 1986.

Kirkkaldy-Willis WH: A comprehensive outline of treatment. In: Kirkaldy-Willis (ed) *Managing Low Back Pain*, 2nd ed. New York, Churchill Livingstone, 1988.

Kirkaldy-Willis WH: The site and nature of the lesion. In: Kirkaldy-Willis (ed) *Managing Low Back Pain*, 2nd ed. New York, Churchill Livingstone, 1988.

Klein RG, Eek BC, DeLong WB, Mooney V: A randomized double-blind trial of dextrose-glycerine-phenol injections for chronic low back pain. *J Spinal Disord* 1993;6:223.

Lippitt AB: Recurrent subluxation of the sacroiliac joint: diagnosis and treatment. *Bull Hosp Joint Dis* 1995;54:94–102.

Travell JG, Simmons DG: *Myofascial Pain and Dysfunction.* Baltimore, Williams & Wilkins, 1983.

Wallace LA: Limb length difference and back pain. In: Grieve GP (ed) *Modern Manual: Therapy of the Vertebral Column.* New York, Churchill Livingstone, 1986.

Wells PE: The examination of the pelvic joints. In: Grieve GP (ed) *Modern Manual: Therapy of the Vertebral Column.* New York, Churchill Livingstone, 1986.

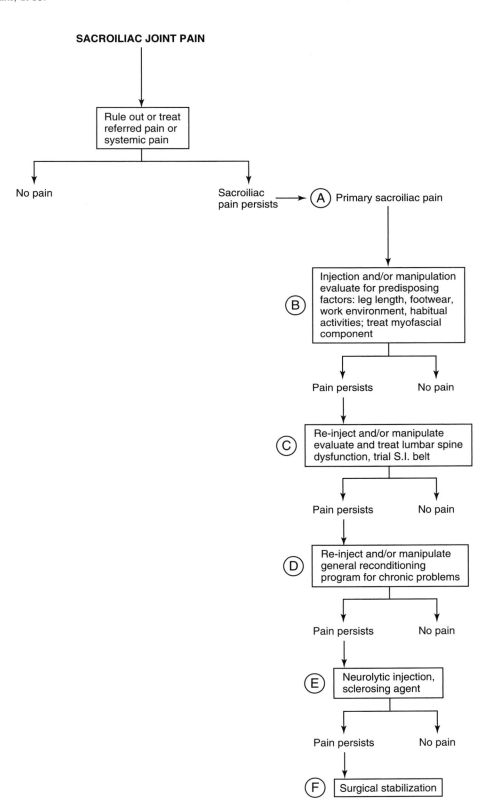

LOWER EXTREMITY PAIN

Tendonitis: Lower Extremities

Bursitis: Lower Extremities

Entrapment Syndromes: Lower Extremities

Piriformis Syndrome

Hip Pain

Knee Pain

Foot Pain

Intermittent Claudication

Tendonitis: Lower Extremities

ERIK SHAW

Tendonitis in the lower extremity is primarily due to inflammation, mainly from overuse. However, lower extremity tendonitis differs in that some or most of this overuse can be caused by abnormal biomechanics, which can be corrected from a structural basis, without surgery. It is also important to recognize whether the symptoms are from a muscle strain or tendonitis (as there can be significant overlap) or because of biomechanics that were altered to limit the pain from the original offending injury. Although the treatment is similar, it is important to recognize the clinical distinction so an appropriate treatment plan may be formulated.

A. There are specific anatomic regions that are most commonly affected, and they are discussed here proximal to distal.

1. Tensor fascia lata (TFL) involved with abduction and external rotation, is frequently referred to as a "popping hip." Ober's test can demonstrate how tight the TFL is, and this angle can be measured from the horizontal. Pain is usually noted during running, especially uphill, which requires more hip extension.

2. Adductor tendonitis can cause tremendous pain, usually near its origin at the pubis symphysis. It is noted in kicking athletes, mainly from a tensile overload. This injury is commonly associated with muscle strain. There is a loss of flexion and external rotation of the hip and weakness of the hamstrings ipsilaterally.

3. Patellar tendonitis, or jumper's knee, is noted around the insertion and is due to microtears. Commonly, there is excess stress placed on this tendon because of activity, but it can also be due to inactivity and a weak quadriceps. Pain is noted at the insertion in the tibia.

4. Shin splints are another common form of tendonitis of the leg and can be extremely painful. Although controversy surrounds their origin, they are thought to be from microtears in the insertion of the tendons of the anterior or posterior compartments of the leg. It is necessary to take care to look for a compartment syndrome, which causes pain with motion. Stress fractures, on the other hand, produce pain with weight-bearing. The muscles commonly involved are the tibialis anterior, tibialis posterior, and flexor digitorum longus. Pain is usually noted 10 to 15 cm from the insertion on the distal tibia.

5. Achilles tendonitis/tendonosis is relatively common, noted in up to 9% of long distance runners. There is some debate, but this is largely now recognized not to be an inflammatory process but, rather, mucoid degeneration of the tendon. It is considered mostly due to abnormal biomechanics, such as hindfoot varus, forefoot varus, weak gastrocnemius/soleus complex, or excessive pronation from pes planus. Pain is commonly noted 2 to 6 cm above the insertion on the calcaneus and is usually aggravated by running or walking uphill or upstairs. Rest and stretching are helpful in most cases. Some patients require immobilization for 4 to 6 weeks.

6. Plantar fasciitis, although not tendonitis, is also common in the foot and may be due to limited dorsiflexion. Pain is usually experienced just anterior to the insertion on the calcaneus. It should be noted that the commonly seen "heel spurs" are usually not the cause of pain but, rather, a result of the enthesiopathy and the body's attempt to handle it.

7. As previously noted, biomechanical imbalances, overtraining, or a change in training can cause these problems. Assessment for all the above conditions begins with a thorough history and physical examination, noting any change in training (intensity, frequency, distance, or time) or new equipment such as shoes.

B. A conservative approach includes relative rest as well as stretching and strengthening the involved muscles and their antagonists. This regimen may alleviate or eliminate the imbalance. It may be combined with other physical therapy modalities such as heat, cold, ultrasound, and massage. Nonsteroidal anti-inflammatory drugs are also indicated, and H_2-blockers or proton pump inhibitors are indicated for prevention of gastrointestinal (GI) side effects. Cyclooxygenase-2 inhibitors also limit GI side effects.

C. If biomechanical imbalance such as pes planus is still causing a problem, orthotics can be helpful for correcting abnormal pronation. In this example, the appliance helps keep the subtalar joint in neutral, maintaining neutral balance of the foot.

D. More aggressive approaches include steroid injection, with the notable exception of the Achilles tendon. If these injections do not effectively alleviate symptoms, surgical evaluation may be useful, especially in cases of patellar tendonitis and plantar fasciitis.

REFERENCES

Bracker MD: *The 5-Minute Sports Medicine Consult.* Philadelphia, Lippincott Williams & Wilkins, 2001.

Braddom RL: *Physical Medicine and Rehabilitation.* Philadelphia, Saunders, 1996.

Buschbacher RM, Braddom R: *Sports Medicine and Rehabilitation: A Sports Specific Approach.* St. Louis, Hanley & Belfus, 1994.

Choi H, Sugar R, Shatzer M, et al: *Physical Medicine and Rehabilitation Pocketpedia*. Philadelphia, Lippincott Williams & Wilkins, 2003.

Khan KM, Coo JL, Bonar F, et al: Histopathology of common overuse tendon conditions: update and implications for clinical management. *Sports Med* 1999;27:393–408.

Mellion MB: *Sport Injuries and Athletic Problems*. St. Louis, Hanley & Belfus, 1988.

Sorosky B, Press J, Plastaras C, Rittenberg J: The practical management of Achilles tendinopathy. *Clin J Sport Med* 2004;14:40–44.

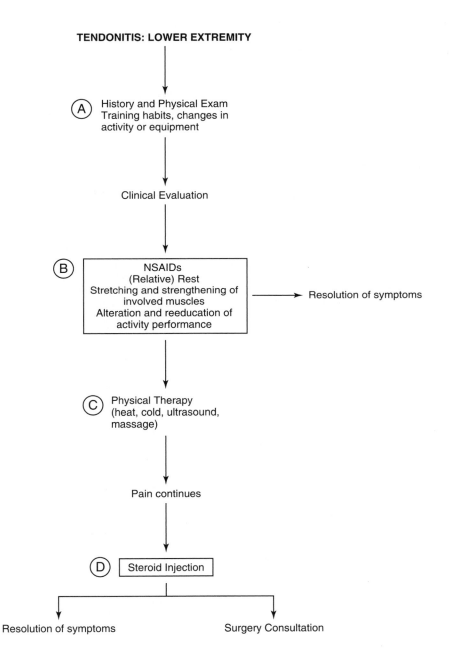

TENDONITIS: LOWER EXTREMITY

(A) History and Physical Exam
Training habits, changes in
activity or equipment

Clinical Evaluation

(B) NSAIDs
(Relative) Rest
Stretching and strengthening of
involved muscles
Alteration and reeducation of
activity performance → Resolution of symptoms

(C) Physical Therapy
(heat, cold, ultrasound,
massage)

Pain continues

(D) Steroid Injection

Resolution of symptoms   Surgery Consultation

Bursitis: Lower Extremities

MICHELE L. ARNOLD

Bursitis is a common cause of lower extremity periarticular pain, yet it is often overlooked or misdiagnosed. Bursae reduce friction between adjacent layers of bone, fascia, muscle, tendon, and skin. They are commonly injured in the setting of direct trauma or overuse.

A. A careful history includes a discussion of inciting events, exacerbating and relieving factors, similar problems in the past, and the past medical history. Typically, the pain of bursitis is localized, and radiation is not a prominent feature.

B. The physical examination reveals tenderness to palpation over the affected bursa, with varying degrees of swelling, erythema, and warmth. There may be reduced range of motion of the adjacent joint or an antalgic gait. Tenderness is localized and fairly well circumscribed. Provocative maneuvers that stretch the overlying muscle or compress the bursa may reproduce pain and help elucidate the etiology.

C. A wide range of diagnoses should be considered and typically can be differentiated with a good history and physical examination alone. Aspiration and analysis of bursal fluid should confirm the diagnosis of septic bursitis. Myofascial pain is typically regional, and radicular pain is dermatomal in nature, in contrast to the localized pain of bursitis. Radicular pain may also cross several joints, and it does not manifest with maximal tenderness upon palpation peripherally. Fibromyalgia is characterized by diffuse, widespread pain along with pain in at least 11 of 18 defined tender points. Tendinitis and ligamentous injury may be difficult to differentiate clinically from bursitis and may require further investigation with radiography or magnetic resonance imaging.

D. The more common sites encountered clinically are listed in the algorithm. Ischial bursitis, also referred to as ischiogluteal bursitis or "weaver's bottom," presents as point tenderness over the ischial tuberosity. Tenderness due to trochanteric bursitis is elicited with direct palpation over the greater trochanter. The pes anserine bursa can become tender along the anteromedial knee, inferior to the joint line where it lies underneath the tendons of insertion of the sartorius, gracilis, and semitendinosus muscles. Prepatellar bursitis, also known as "housemaid's knee," is associated with repetitive kneeling or local trauma. Subpopliteal bursitis localizes to the popliteal fossa, where it lies underneath the tendon of the popliteus. When inflamed, the semimembranosus bursa causes a popliteal Baker's cyst. Ill-fitting shoes and athletic training errors often cause inflammation of the retrocalcaneal bursa (which lies underneath the Achilles tendon) and the more superficial Achilles bursa (also referred to as Haglund's syndrome).

E. Degenerative joint disease may be a concurrent condition, and nearby osteophytes may be a potential etiologic factor. Biomechanical or structural alterations may be contributing factors to the occurrence or recurrence of bursitis; such alterations include leg length discrepancy, femoral anteversion, increased Q angle, tibia vara, ankle equinus, pes cavus, and lack of flexibility or weakness in nearby musculature. Obesity may also be a coexisting and exacerbating condition.

F. Acute management should begin with conservative measures, such as relative rest, compression, and elevation. A short course of physical therapy may be warranted, including topical cryotherapy, contrasting heat and ice, ultrasound application, phonophoresis, or iontophoresis. Patients may also obtain relief from a nonsteroidal antiinflammatory agent. If these measures prove ineffective, an injection of local anesthetic or steroid medication may provide relief. A series of injections may be necessary for resolution of symptoms. Few patients require percutaneous drainage or surgical excision.

G. Bursitis is often the result of overuse injury or uncorrected biomechanical factors, ultimately causing recurrence. Decreasing pressure over the site can reduce chronic inflammation. This typically refers to a change in body positioning or mechanics or even a change in footwear to relieve pressure over the affected bursa. It also may call for the use of appropriate protective sports equipment and padding over prominent sites to prevent acute traumatic bursitis. It may be necessary to prescribe an orthotic device to correct a biomechanical or structural alteration, such as a shoe lift for a leg length discrepancy. Maintaining a home exercise program emphasizing both strengthening and flexibility is a cornerstone for preventing recurrence.

REFERENCES

Antonelli MA, Vawter RL: Nonarticular pain syndromes: differentiating generalized, regional, and localized disorders [abstract]. *Postgrad Med* 1992;91:95.

Loeser JD: *Bonica's Management of Pain,* 3rd ed. Philadelphia, Lippincott Williams & Wilkins, 2001.

Braddom RL (ed): *Physical Medicine and Rehabilitation,* 2nd ed. London, Saunders, 2000.

Butcher JD, Salzman KL, Lillegard WA: Lower extremity bursitis. *Am Fam Physician* 1996;53:2317–2324.

Reilly JP, Nicholas JA: The chronically inflamed bursa. *Clin Sports Med* 1987;6:345–370.

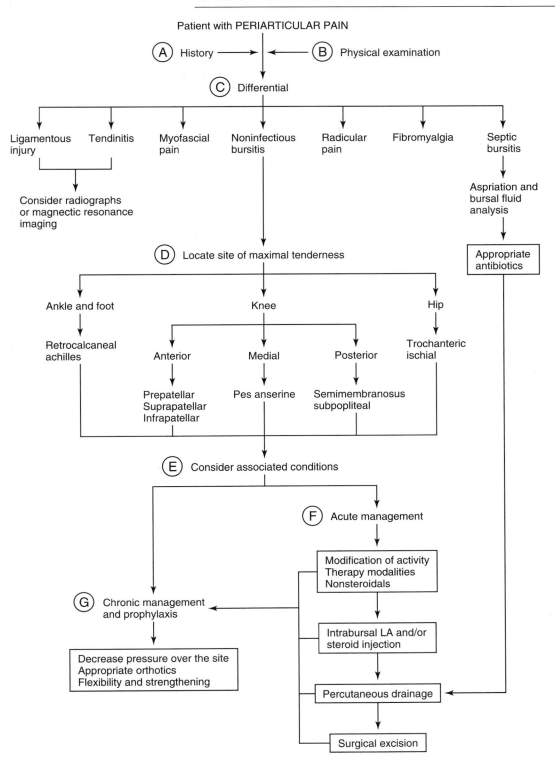

Patient with PERIARTICULAR PAIN

(A) History → ← (B) Physical examination

(C) Differential

Ligamentous injury | Tendinitis | Myofascial pain | Noninfectious bursitis | Radicular pain | Fibromyalgia | Septic bursitis

Consider radiographs or magnectic resonance imaging

Aspriation and bursal fluid analysis

Appropriate antibiotics

(D) Locate site of maximal tenderness

Ankle and foot | Knee | Hip

Retrocalcaneal achilles

Anterior | Medial | Posterior | Trochanteric ischial

Prepatellar Suprapatellar Infrapatellar | Pes anserine | Semimembranosus subpopliteal

(E) Consider associated conditions

(F) Acute management

Modification of activity Therapy modalities Nonsteroidals

(G) Chronic management and prophylaxis

Intrabursal LA and/or steroid injection

Decrease pressure over the site Appropriate orthotics Flexibility and strengthening

Percutaneous drainage

Surgical excision

Entrapment Syndromes: Lower Extremities

NIKESH BATRA

Although upper extremity entrapment syndromes are more common, those of the lower extremities carry no less importance. The commonly found lower extremity entrapment neuropathies are discussed here. For a general discussion on the entrapment syndromes, please refer to the chapter Upper Extremity Entrapment Syndromes.

A. *Lateral femoral cutaneous nerve entrapment.* The lateral femoral cutaneous nerve derives from the dorsal divisions of the ventral primary rami of the L2 and L3 spinal nerves. It emerges from the lateral border of the psoas muscle and runs down and laterally in the pelvis, lying on the iliacus muscle. It reaches the lateral end of the inguinal ligament and passes either under or through it, ending on the lateral thigh. It is vulnerable to entrapment at the anterosuperior iliac spine.

This syndrome is known as *meralgia paresthetica.* It is characterized by burning or shooting pain and paresthesias in the anterolateral aspect of the thigh. There may be sensory deficit or hyperesthesia in the affected area. It may be caused by intrinsic compression by the iliacus muscle or the inguinal ligament or by extrinsic compression, such as obesity or wearing heavy belts (policemen) or girdles. Walking or other physical maneuvers may aggravate it. This type of entrapment usually responds well to conservative management. The lateral femoral cutaneous nerve can be blocked by inserting a 25-gauge 0.5-inch needle to a point 1 inch medial to the anterosuperior iliac spine and just inferior to the inguinal ligament. The needle is inserted perpendicular to the skin until it pops through the deep fascia. Local anesthesia (5 to 7 ml) is deposited in this area in a fan-shaped manner after negative aspiration.

B. *Femoral nerve entrapment.* The femoral nerve is derived from the posterior branches of the L2, L3, and L4 nerve roots. The roots fuse together in the psoas muscle and descend laterally between the psoas and iliacus muscles to enter the iliac fossa. The femoral nerve then passes underneath the inguinal ligament to enter the thigh. It innervates the anterior portion of the thigh and medial calf.

The femoral nerve may be entrapped in the psoas muscle or the inguinal ligament, causing inguinal pain, burning pain, and paresthesias in the anterior thigh or anteromedial leg. On examination it may show quadriceps weakness with or without iliopsoas weakness, depressed patellar reflexes, and a sensory deficit. Hip adductors should have normal strength; there should be no iliopsoas weakness with inguinal compression. Femoral nerve entrapment may be caused by pelvic or inguinal compression. Being in a lithotomy position for a prolonged time may result in this neuropathy, as may hematoma or a tumor. These patients may be treated conservatively or by surgical decompression,

depending on the site and cause of entrapment. Conservative methods include rest, nonsteroidal anti-inflammatory drugs, anticonvulsant drugs, local anesthetic and steroid injections, and behavioral modification. In the thigh the femoral nerve may be blocked by inserting a needle just lateral to the pulsations of the femoral artery and just inferior to the inguinal ligament.

C. *Ilioinguinal nerve entrapment.* The ilioinguinal nerve, derived from the L1 nerve root, may be entrapped as it passes medial to the anterosuperior iliac spine through the muscles of the abdominal wall. The main symptom is burning pain over the lower abdomen that radiates down the inner thigh and into the scrotum or labia majora. There may be an area of tenderness medial to the anterosuperior iliac spine, and Tinel's sign may be elicited by tapping over the lower abdomen. A low McBurney muscle-splitting incision, inguinal herniorrhaphy, harvesting of iliac bone grant, or gynecologic and renal surgery may cause ilioinguinal neuropathy. Normal pregnancy and delivery have also been implicated, presumably by stretch or entrapment in the abdominal wall. Conservative therapy consists of avoiding activities that exacerbate pain, analgesics, anti-inflammatory medications, and local anesthetic injections. If this regimen is unsuccessful, surgery is considered. The ilioinguinal nerve is blocked by inserting a 25-gauge 1.5-inch needle at a point 2 inches superior and 2 inches inferior to the anterosuperior iliac spine at an oblique angle toward the pubic symphysis. Local anesthetic (5 to 7 ml) is injected in a fan-shaped manner as the needle pierces the fascia of the external oblique muscle.

D. *Genitofemoral nerve entrapment.* Genitofemoral neuralgia is characterized by chronic pain and paresthesia in the region of the genitofemoral nerve distribution, which may be exacerbated by hip extension. There may be significant tenderness over the inguinal canal. Genitofemoral neuropathy can be mistaken for ilioinguinal nerve entrapment because of the overlap in the sensory distribution of the two nerves. It also occurs after inguinal herniorrhaphy, appendectomy, and cesarean section.

The nerve originates from L1 and L2 nerve roots. It passes through the substance of the psoas muscle, where it divides into a genital branch and a femoral branch. The genital branch accompanies the ilioinguinal nerve in the inguinal canal for a short distance and shares the sensory supply of the scrotum or mons pubis and labium majus. It also supplies motor fibers to the cremaster muscle. The femoral branch, after passing under the inguinal ligament, supplies a small area of skin on the anterior aspect of the thigh.

CLINICAL FEATURES SUGGESTING ENTRAPMENT NEUROPATHY

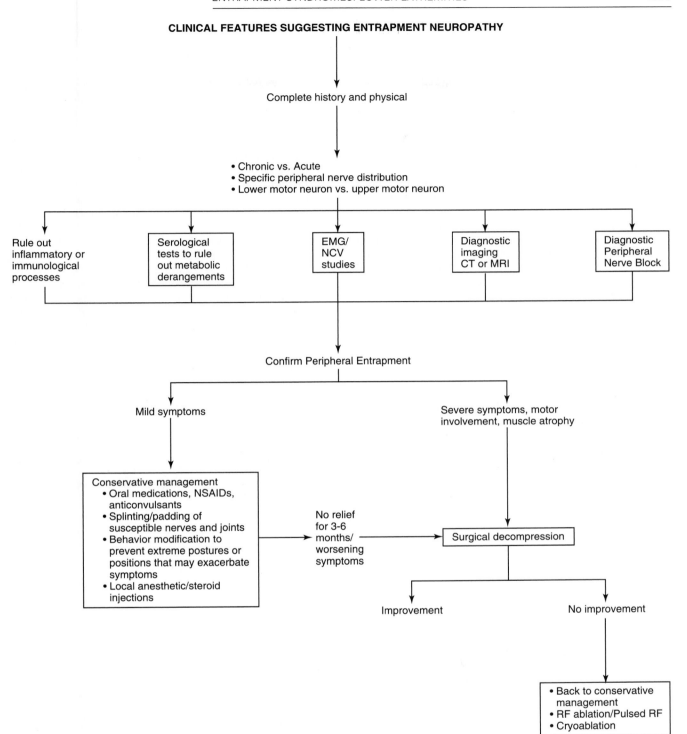

The genital branch is blocked by inserting a 25-gauge 1.5-inch needle at a point just lateral to the pubic tubercle and advancing it at an oblique angle toward the pubic symphysis. Local anesthetic (3 to 5 ml) is injected in a fan-shaped manner as the needle pierces the inguinal ligament. Care should be taken not to place the needle too deep, causing it to enter the peritoneal cavity. The femoral branch is blocked by infiltrating 3 to 5 ml of local anesthetic subcutaneously under the middle third of the inguinal ligament.

E. *Peroneal nerve entrapment.* This is the most common compressive neuropathy in the lower extremity. It is a common cause of foot drop and is usually caused by compression at the fibular head. Signs and symptoms are usually variable. There may be paresthesias in the foot, weakness, and pain in the anterior or lateral leg. On examination there may be sensory deficit in the anterolateral leg and the dorsum of the foot as well as foot drop with weak dorsiflexion and eversion. This common peroneal nerve syndrome is often seen in crossed-leg palsy.

The common peroneal nerve may be blocked by palpating the head of the fibula and inserting a 25-gauge 0.5-inch needle at a point just below the fibular head until a paresthesia is elicited or the needle contacts bone. The needle is then withdrawn 1 mm, and 5 ml of 1% preservative-free lidocaine is injected.

F. *Tibial nerve entrapment.* The tibial nerve provides sensory innervation to the posterior portion of the calf, the heel, and the medial plantar surface. The tibial nerve splits away from the sciatic nerve at the superior margin of the popliteal fossa and descends downward between the two heads of the gastrocnemius muscle, deep to the soleus muscle. The nerve courses medially between the Achilles tendon and the medial malleolus, where it divides into the medial and lateral plantar nerves, providing sensory innervation to the heel and medial plantar surface. It is subject to compression at this point, where it is entrapped in the flexor retinaculum. This is known as the tarsal tunnel syndrome. There is pain and paresthesias in the sole of the foot. On physical examination, weakness and atrophy of the abductor digiti minimi and tenderness on palpation of the flexor retinaculum are seen. The tibial nerve is blocked by placing the patient in the prone position and having the patient flex his or her leg against resistance, this maneuver identifies the margins of the semitendinosus and biceps femoris muscles. A triangle is formed by the margins of the two muscles, with the base being formed by the skin crease of the knee. A 25-gauge 1.5-inch needle is inserted at the center of this triangle until paresthesia is elicited, and 8 to 10 ml of local anesthetic can be injected.

G. *Digital nerve entrapment.* The digital nerves of the foot may be compressed by *Morton's neuroma,* which produces toe pain and numbness. On physical examination there is tenderness with hyperextension of the toe or palpation of the deep transverse metatarsal ligament.

REFERENCES

Katirji B: Entrapment and other focal neuropathies: peroneal neuropathy. *Neurol Clin* 1999;17(3).

Reid V, Didier C: Proximal sensory neuropathies of the leg. *Neurol Clin* 1999;17(3).

Waldman SD: *Atlas of Interventional Pain Management.* Philadelphia, Saunders, 1998.

Piriformis Syndrome

JONATHAN P. LESTER

Piriformis syndrome is a myofascial pain disorder that may closely mimic other causes of low back pain and disability. The piriformis muscle arises from the inner aspect of the sacrum, runs laterally through the sciatic notch, crosses over the sciatic nerve, and inserts on the greater trochanter. In some cases a portion of the sciatic nerve may pass through the piriformis. Contraction of the piriformis muscle assists external rotation of the hip.

A. Mild trauma to the buttocks or hips, postural overuse, or disturbance of the pelvic musculature may initiate formation of a painful trigger point in the piriformis muscle belly. Secondary spasm of the piriformis muscle may irritate the sciatic nerve and produce radicular symptoms. Piriformis muscle dysfunction is commonly associated with sacroiliac joint dysfunction and is frequently associated with tightness of the piriformis and adductor muscles. An accurate diagnosis is made based on appropriate historical information and the physical examination. Treatment is conservative, and complete resolution of symptoms is achieved in most cases.

B. Patients with piriformis syndrome may complain of an aching pain radiating to the hip, groin, buttock, or posterior thigh. The pain is often described as aching or cramping and is made worse with stooping, sitting, squatting, or lifting. Patients may also describe radicular symptoms in the distribution of the sciatic nerve. The onset of symptoms is often related to pelvic trauma or overuse. Women may complain of dyspareunia. Physical examination is remarkable for the tenderness over the piriformis muscle belly, which is exacerbated by passive internal rotation of the hip (Freiberg's sign) and resisted external rotation of the hip (Pace's sign). Rectal examination is extremely helpful for confirming the diagnosis. Other causes of low back pain and posterior thigh pain are excluded by additional physical examination techniques.

C. Conservative care consists of mobilizing the sacroiliac joint, aggressive stretching protocols for the hip girdle muscles, and nonsteroidal anti-inflammatory drugs. Opioids and muscle relaxants are not indicated. Trigger points may be present at the insertion onto the trochanter, at the point where the muscle emerges from the sciatic notch, or most commonly in the middle of the belly of the muscle. The trigger point that most accurately reproduces the patient's pain is injected with an intermediate-acting local anesthetic, such as lidocaine 0.5%. Some clinicians add steroids to the mixture. The injected local anesthetic can spread to the sciatic nerve, producing nerve block and leg weakness, thereby requiring observation in the clinic for the duration of the block. For this reason we avoid the use of long-acting local anesthetics such as bupivacaine. After the injection, patients are taught an aggressive stretching program for the piriformis and gluteal muscles. Most cases are resolved with a few visits to the clinic. Recurrences are prevented by a maintenance stretching program. Severe cases unresponsive to conservative therapy may benefit from surgical resection of the piriformis muscle especially if magnetic resonance imaging confirms entrapment of the sciatic nerve.

REFERENCES

Bernard T, Kirkaldy-Willis W: Recognizing specific causes of nonspecific low back pain. *Clin Orthop* 1987;217:266.

Durrani Z, Winnie AP: Piriformis muscle syndrome: an underdiagnosed cause of sciatica. *J Pain Symptom Manage* 1991;6:374.

Ludvig F, Siewer P, Bernhard P: The piriformis muscle syndrome: sciatic nerve entrapment treated with section of the piriformis muscle. *Acta Orthop Scand* 1981;52:73.

Pace J, Nagle D: Piriform syndrome. *West J Med* 1976;124:435.

Steiner C, Staubs C, Buhlinger C: Piriformis syndrome: pathogenesis, diagnosis, and treatment. *J Am Osteopath Assoc* 1987;87:318.

PATIENT WITH LOW BACK, BUTTOCK, OR POSTERIOR THIGH PAIN

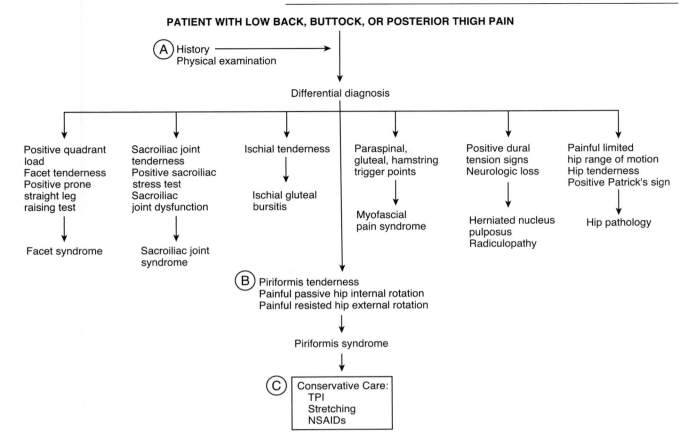

Hip Pain

BERT BLACKWELL

Hip pain is a common pain complaint, the diagnosis and treatment of which can be vexing for patient and practitioner alike. The biomechanical features of weight bearing during ambulation and multiplanar range of motion make the hip especially susceptible to injury and mechanical stress. In addition, the reinforcing structures surrounding the hip, which both simultaneously and sequentially provide support and freedom of movement, are vulnerable to routine perturbations.

A. Perhaps the most straightforward pathology affecting the hip is muscle strain. There is frequently an inciting event or trauma related to onset of acute pain in a well defined area. Commonly affected muscles in the hip region include the adductor, quadriceps, hamstring, and iliopsoas. Strains can range in severity from soreness with no myotendinous disruption to complete muscle rupture. Short of complete rupture, treatment is essentially the same and follows the RICE (rest, ice, compression, and elevation) algorithm with or without nonsteroidal antiinflammatory drug (NSAID) use. After the acute period of rest (which varies depending on severity), active range of motion can begin that is directed at restoring functional range. Passive ranging should not begin for a minimum of 4 to 6 weeks. Complete ruptures require expedient surgical consultation.

B. In contrast to strains, bursitis around the hip joint rarely presents acutely unless there is a septic etiology. The most commonly affected bursae about the hip are the iliopectineal, ischial, and trochanteric. Treatment is essentially the same as for any other bursitis of the lower extremity.

C. Hip fractures occurring either in the pelvis or proximal femur almost always present acutely following some degree of trauma. Imaging studies are essential in working up hip pain in order to ascertain fracture. An evaluation for neoplasm (primary or metastatic) should be undertaken when inciting events are slight. Surgical evaluation is mandatory.

D. Although plain radiographs can easily lead to a diagnosis of hip fracture, the diagnosis of avascular necrosis (AVN) can be somewhat more elusive. If radiographs are negative in the setting of persistent hip or groin pain that is exacerbated by weight bearing and no other source of pain is readily identifiable, the possibility of AVN should be considered. Magnetic resonance imaging (MRI) is essential in making the diagnosis of AVN. If bone necrosis is evident, a non-weight-bearing status should be maintained and surgical consultation requested.

E. Hip pain in the setting of a "snapping" sensation about the hip with ambulation is not uncommon. The sensation usually results from the iliotibial band "snapping" across the greater trochanter. Trochanteric bursitis is a common sequela. Similarly, the iliopsoas can "snap" across the iliopectineal eminence and result in iliopectineal bursitis. Treatment is directed at restoring normal muscle balance between agonist and antagonist muscles. Other less common causes of this sensation include labral tears and intraarticular loose bodies. If reconditioning and treatment of potential underlying bursitis does not result in swift improvement of symptoms, more advanced imaging studies and possible surgical intervention may be required.

F. Pain that is present primarily over the pubis and exacerbated during midstance when the hemipelvis drops, may result from an inflammation of the symphysis pubis. The resulting osteitis pubis can be demonstrated on radiographs by periosteal reaction, demineralization, and sclerosis. This condition usually occurs in active individuals who rapidly increase their exercise program. Treatment consists of relative rest for up to 2 months with or without NSAIDs. Lower extremity reconditioning should be undertaken only when the area is pain free. Graduated activity is essential to prevent recurrence. Surgical intervention is rarely required but arthrodesis of the symphysis has been performed.

G. Piriformis syndrome can contribute to hip pain. Restriction of internal hip rotation with the patient prone can demonstrate piriformis tightness on the affected side. Although there may be electromyography (EMG) and MRI findings, they are very late findings and, hence, are of little value in treating the vast majority of patients. Both of these studies can be helpful in excluding the diagnosis of concomitant radiculopathy. The sacroiliac joint should also be scrutinized for any contributing role. Treatment consists of reducing acute pain and stretching of the piriformis. Strengthening of internal hip rotators is mandatory to prevent recurrence.

REFERENCES

Braddom RL: *Physical Medicine and Rehabilitation.* Philadelphia, WB Saunders, 1996.

Delee JC, Drez D: *Orthopaedic Sports Medicine.* Philadelphia, WB Saunders, 1994.

Kuland DN: *The Injured Athlete,* 2nd ed. Philadelphia, JB Lippincott, 1988.

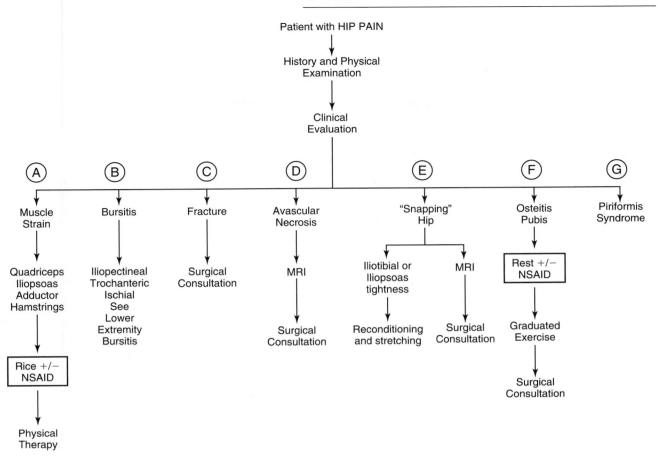

Patient with HIP PAIN

History and Physical Examination

Clinical Evaluation

Ⓐ Muscle Strain

Quadriceps
Iliopsoas
Adductor
Hamstrings

Rice +/−
NSAID

Physical Therapy

Ⓑ Bursitis

Iliopectineal
Trochanteric
Ischial
See
Lower
Extremity
Bursitis

Ⓒ Fracture

Surgical Consultation

Ⓓ Avascular Necrosis

MRI

Surgical Consultation

Ⓔ "Snapping" Hip

Iliotibial or Iliopsoas tightness

Reconditioning and stretching

MRI

Surgical Consultation

Ⓕ Osteitis Pubis

Rest +/−
NSAID

Graduated Exercise

Surgical Consultation

Ⓖ Piriformis Syndrome

Knee Pain

STEPHEN W. DINGER

Knee pain is a common presenting complaint in patients of all ages. It is present in approximately 20% to 25% of the general population, and commonly occurs secondary to trauma, sport related activities, overuse syndromes, and degenerative changes. The most common etiology of knee pain are strains and sprains (42%), osteoarthritis (OA) (34%), meniscus (9%), collateral ligament (7%), cruciate ligament (4%), gout (2%), fracture (1.2%), rheumatoid arthritis (0.5%), infectious arthritis (0.3%), and pseudogout (0.2%). In people older than 55 years of age, the most common cause of disability related to knee is pain secondary to osteoarthritis.

A. When formulating a differential diagnosis, the history and mechanism of injury are key components that further direct the physical exam, laboratory testing, and imaging. Important information to obtain includes the following: how the injury occurred, any trauma, previous injury, "pop" or "tearing" sound or sensation (common with ligament or meniscus injury), swelling, hyperthermia, ecchymosis, visual deformity, or atrophy. Valgus and varus stress to the knee usually leads to medial collateral ligament injury (MCL) and lateral collateral ligament (LCL) injury, respectively. Hyperextension and twisting injuries can lead to anterior cruciate ligament (ACL) and meniscus injury. Posterior translation of the tibia and dashboard impact can lead to posterior cruciate ligament (PCL).

B. Physical examination involves inspection of the knee and leg, general alignment, evaluation of gait, ability to bear weight, palpable bony or soft tissue deformities, scars, position of the patella, and systemic involvement. Range of motion of the knee, audible or palpable crepitus, and point tenderness over anatomic structures should be documented, and help narrow the differential diagnosis.

C. Most injuries can be separated into spontaneous occurring pain and posttraumatic pain. Traumatic injuries commonly lead to ligament, meniscus, and/or bone injuries. Ligament and meniscus injuries are best diagnosed with a good musculoskeletal examination and special provocative tests, and the severity can range from mild sprain to complete tear. The Lachman test, pivot shift test, and anterior draw assess ACL injuries. Joint line pinpoint tenderness and reproduction of pain with the McMurray test suggest meniscus injury. Posterior draw assesses PCL integrity. Pain to palpation of the patella facets and patella instability/apprehension support the diagnosis of patella subluxation/dislocation.

D. The location of pain is important in formulating a diagnosis. For example, anterior knee pain is usually secondary to patella femoral pain syndrome (PFPS); medial knee pain from medial plica syndrome, pes anserine bursitis, medial compartment OA, MCL, or medial meniscus injury; lateral knee pain may be iliotibial band, lateral compartment OA, LCL, or lateral meniscal injury; posterior knee pain may include popliteal (Baker's) cyst and PCL injury.

E. The presence and location of swelling may suggest particular diagnoses. Extracapsular swelling may indicate prepatellar bursitis when anterior, or popliteal cyst when posterior. Intracapsular effusion can occur with multiple injuries and is nonspecific. They can range from small to large, and moderate to large intracapsular effusion should be considered for an arthrocentesis. Immediate swelling following an injury suggests a hemarthrosis, and is associated with fracture, patella dislocation, and ligament and/or peripheral meniscus tear. A warm, erythematous, and swollen knee with no history of trauma suggests septic or crystal-induced arthritis. Arthrocentesis will provide a sample for cell count, Gram stain, culture, and crystal. A cell count greater than 50,000 per mm^3, with more than 75% neutrophils is consistent with an infectious source. Urate (gout) and calcium pyrophosphate dihydrate crystals (pseudogout) can be identified by microscopy.

F. The American College of Rheumatology's clinical criteria for OA includes at least three of the following: age greater than 50 years, stiffness for less than 30 minutes, crepitus, bony tenderness, bony enlargement, and no palpable warmth.

G. Radiographs should be obtained if the pain occurs secondary to a fall or blow to the knee, and has at least one of four characteristics: age greater than 55 years, tenderness at the fibular head or patella, inability to bear weight, and lack of 90 degrees of flexion (Quebec rules). Radiography is helpful in assessing OA and osteochondral lesions. The Kellgren Lawrence radiographic criteria for OA included the presence of osteophytes, sclerosis, joint space narrowing, and cystic subchondral bone. If ligament or meniscus injury is suspected, magnetic resonance imaging (MRI) can help with diagnosis.

H. Other causes of knee pain include quadriceps tendon rupture, rheumatologic diseases (rheumatoid arthritis and Reiter's syndrome), avascular necrosis, neoplasm, and referred hip pain.

Treatment is directed to the underlying diagnosis. In general, conservative therapy consisting of nonsteroidal antiinflammatory drugs (NSAIDs), physical therapy, modalities, bracing/casting, and injections (steroid, anesthetic and/or hyaluronic acid) is indicated. Some injuries may require referral for further evaluation and treatment, or surgical intervention.

REFERENCES

Calmbach WL, Hutchens M: Evaluation of patient presenting with knee pain, Parts I and II. *Am Fam Physician* 2003;68:907–912, 917–922.

Hamer AJ: Pain in the hip and knee. *Br Med J* 2004;328:1067–1069.

Jackson JL, O'Malley PG, Kroenke K: Evaluation of acute knee pain in primary care. *Ann Intern Med* 2003;139:575–588.

Kozol RA, Nasser S, et al: When to call the surgeon: decision making for the primary care provider. Philadelphia, FA Davis 1999, 204–220.

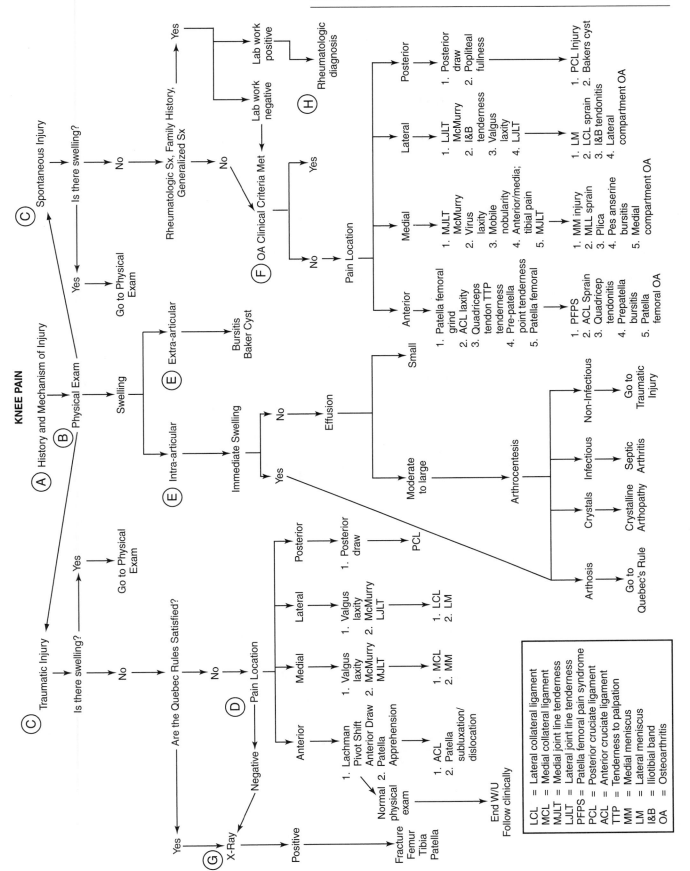

Foot Pain

JAMES G. GRIFFIN

In the presence of foot pain, obtain a careful history to determine the location of the pain, type of onset, intensity and quality of the pain, pain profile over time, and factors that aggravate or relieve the patient's pain. The physical examination should include inspection, palpation, evaluation of neurologic status, and active and passive range of motion. A biomechanical assessment should be made with the patient sitting, standing, and walking.

A. An evaluation of footwear must be a part of any treatment of foot pain. Poorly fitting or worn footwear can cause or contribute to pain in the lower extremity. The margin of error for wear may be less for athletic individuals than for sedentary people. A change of shoe brand or model may cause problems in previously nonsymptomatic persons. Individuals must find the shoe that fits their needs, not a popular style or brand. Changing to well fitting shoes or repairing or replacing worn shoes is sometimes a simple solution for foot pain.

B. The radiographic examination should include anteroposterior, lateral, and oblique radiographic views obtained while weight-bearing if possible. Special views are required to visualize the sesamoids, talocalcaneal, and talonavicular coalitions. Stress views that compare the normal and affected side may reveal instability. Bone scans reveal areas of increased uptake and are diagnostic for stress reactions. Soft tissue tumors may be evaluated with computed tomography or magnetic resonance imaging to determine size and composition.

C. Nerve conduction velocity and electromyography may be indicated for evaluation of peripheral neuropathies and tarsal tunnel entrapment. Doppler studies indicate the status of the peripheral circulation. Laboratory studies of blood, joint fluid, or tissue samples can help in suspected cases of rheumatoid arthritis, gout, or osteomyelitis.

D. Complex regional pain syndrome (CRPS) can occur as a result of even a trivial injury to the foot. Early CRPS is commonly overlooked and must be suspected when pain is greatly out of proportion to expectation. Prompt recognition and treatment can prevent progression to an irreversible, debilitating condition.

E. Soft tissue pain due to corns and calluses without foot deformity are often the result of pressure from ill-fitting footwear. Verruca pedis (plantar warts) are differentiated from calluses by their extreme sensitivity to lateral compression. Dorsal ganglia are troublesome because of constant irritation from shoes. Excision at the origin is the definitive treatment. Myofascial pain can produce discomfort following injury or immobilization of the foot or lower extremity. Pain may also be due to the loss of passive joint play in the foot as a result of injury or immobilization. These problems are common but not often considered primary causes of pain.

Techniques to treat these problems are simple and safe.

F. Bony exostoses occur in several locations in the foot and can be painful impediments to joint motion or irritating pressure points for callus formation. Surgical excision may be required if conservative efforts fail to relieve the pain.

G. The great toe is the most common site of ingrown toenails. It is subject to disorders of hypermobility, hypomobility, and deformation. The hypermobile first ray can shift weight to other areas, causing pain. It is treated with padding or orthotics to normalize weight distribution. Hallux rigidus produces pain and dorsal exostoses in the first metaphalangeal joint; it may respond to nonsteroidal anti-inflammatory drugs (NSAIDs) and a stiff rocker sole shoe. Surgery to increase motion or to fuse a degenerated joint may be indicated. Hallux valgus may be treated conservatively with accommodative footwear and orthotic control of excess pronation. Surgery may be necessary to repair a deformity and restore normal biomechanics. The sesamoids can become irritated and locally swollen. They respond to NSAIDs and decreased weight-bearing until the inflammation resolves. Gout can be well localized to the first metaphalangeal joint, but it may affect the entire medial column of the foot. Medication can control the condition, but surgery may be needed for advanced degeneration.

H. Deformation of the small toes can result in corns and calluses. Severe deformities and painful keratoses may require surgical intervention to restore normal weight-bearing. A long second ray with a hypermobile first ray can produce a painful maldistribution of weight across the metatarsal heads. Padding or orthotic support may be required.

I. Forefoot pain under the metatarsal heads may occur with a splayed or pronated foot, resulting in disproportionate weight-bearing. A metatarsal bar or selective padding may be sufficient treatment. Surgical intervention may be required to restore normal weight distribution. Morton's neuroma is common, but not exclusive, to the space between the third and fourth toe. These neuromas may respond to steroid injection with adequate footwear, padding, or both. Surgical excision requires care to remove all branches of the neuroma. Stress reactions should be suspected with forefoot pain following initiation of, or an increase in, weight-bearing activity. Radiographs and bone scans are negative acutely. Pain with activity and relieved with rest may be the only finding. Although common in the metatarsals, stress reactions may occur in any bone in the foot.

J. Midfoot discomfort from arch strain may occur as an interaction of foot mechanics, usually excessive pronation, activity, poor footwear, and insufficiency

FOOT PAIN

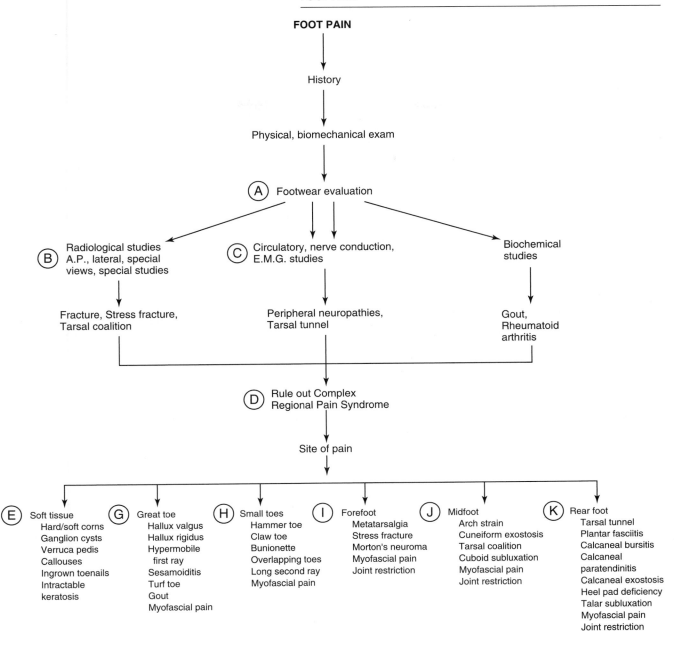

History

↓

Physical, biomechanical exam

↓

Ⓐ Footwear evaluation

Ⓑ Radiological studies
A.P., lateral, special
views, special studies

↓

Fracture, Stress fracture,
Tarsal coalition

Ⓒ Circulatory, nerve conduction,
E.M.G. studies

↓

Peripheral neuropathies,
Tarsal tunnel

Biochemical
studies

↓

Gout,
Rheumatoid
arthritis

Ⓓ Rule out Complex
Regional Pain Syndrome

↓

Site of pain

Ⓔ Soft tissue
Hard/soft corns
Ganglion cysts
Verruca pedis
Callouses
Ingrown toenails
Intractable
keratosis

Ⓖ Great toe
Hallux valgus
Hallux rigidus
Hypermobile
 first ray
Sesamoiditis
Turf toe
Gout
Myofascial pain

Ⓗ Small toes
Hammer toe
Claw toe
Bunionette
Overlapping toes
Long second ray
Myofascial pain

Ⓘ Forefoot
Metatarsalgia
Stress fracture
Morton's neuroma
Myofascial pain
Joint restriction

Ⓙ Midfoot
Arch strain
Cuneiform exostosis
Tarsal coalition
Cuboid subluxation
Myofascial pain
Joint restriction

Ⓚ Rear foot
Tarsal tunnel
Plantar fasciitis
Calcaneal bursitis
Calcaneal
paratendinitis
Calcaneal exostosis
Heel pad deficiency
Talar subluxation
Myofascial pain
Joint restriction

of the musculature supporting the medial arch. The closed-chain mechanics of the lower extremity make it possible for pain also to occur in the knee or hip stemming from distal stresses produced by excessive pronation. Treatment may include supportive footwear, activity modification, and orthotic devices to control pronation of the foot. Severe injury may result in instability of the metatarsocuneiform joints, requiring casting or surgical stabilization. The cuboid may sublux with an inversion injury and be mistaken for a "chronic ankle sprain." This injury responds to manipulation and supportive padding or orthotics. Tarsal coalition produces pain with activity and may result in arthritis of the subtalar or other joints. Pain, lack of subtalar motion, and radiographic studies confirm the diagnosis. Conservative treatment with supportive shoes and biomechanical support precede surgical intervention.

K. Rear foot pain may be produced by a talar subluxation secondary to inversion stress. Like the cuboid subluxation, it is often treated as a "chronic sprain." This entity may require injection of the sinus tarsi followed by manipulation of the talus plus ankle rehabilitation. Orthotic support may be required (Beirne et al. 1984). Tarsal tunnel syndrome produces burning pain or numbness in the distribution of the posterior tibial nerve as it is trapped by the flexor retinaculum in the tarsal tunnel. The nerve is tender, and Tinel's sign may be present. It is treated conservatively with correction of hyperpronation, NSAIDs, transcutaneous electrical nerve stimulation, or injection of local anesthetic and steroids. Persistent symptoms require surgical decompression. Plantar fasciitis is irritation of the proximal insertion of the plantar fascia in which tenderness is found on the anteromedial aspect of the heel. Treatment consists of NSAIDs and well made shoes with medial arch support. Injection, a walking cast, or rarely surgical release is required in resistant cases (Bonica and Lippert 1990). Posterior heel pain can originate with irritation of the insertion of the Achilles tendon, the bursa, or the loose tissue immediately around the Achilles insertion. Generally, it is treated conservatively with NSAIDs, use of a heel lift, moderation of activity, ice massage, and stretching the Achilles tendon. If simple measures fail, a short leg cast and immobilization may be required. Surgical removal of inflamed tissues is rarely required. Orthotic control of foot mechanics may be required, ranging from off-the-shelf products to custom-made devices. The goal is to maintain the foot in a biomechanically sound position and equally distribute stress. A suitable orthotic may have to compensate for biomechanical disparities in the foot, ankle, and lower extremity to achieve optimal results.

REFERENCES

Beirne DR, Burckhardt JG, Peters VJ: Subtalar joint subluxation. *J Am Podiatry Assoc* 1984;74:529–523.

Bonica JJ, Lippert FG: Pain in the leg, ankle, and foot. In: Bonica JJ (ed) *The Management of Pain*, 2nd ed, vol 2. Philadelphia, Lea & Febiger, 1990.

McRae R: *Clinical Orthopedic Examination*, 3rd ed. New York, Churchill Livingstone, 1990.

Mennell JM: *Joint Pain*. Boston, Little, Brown, 1964.

Newell SG, Woodle A: Cuboid syndrome. *Physician Sports Med* 1981; 1:71–76.

Travell JG, Simmons DG: *Myofascial Pain and Dysfunction*. Baltimore, Williams & Wilkins, 1983.

Wooden MJ: Biomechanical evaluation for functional orthotics. In: Donatelli R (ed) *The Biomechanics of the Foot and Ankle*. Philadelphia, Davis, 1990.

Intermittent Claudication

SOMAYAJI RAMAMURTHY

Intermittent claudication is the most common presenting symptom of chronic obstructive peripheral arterial disease. Patients complain of buttock and leg pain with ambulation, which is quickly relieved with rest. Pain in the buttocks and legs, extreme fatigue, and muscle cramping all occur more quickly if the speed of ambulation increases or the patient walks uphill. Atherosclerotic occlusive disease has a slow, insidious onset. The prevalence of claudication ranges from 1.3% to 5.8% of persons older than 60 years of age. The site of pain correlates well with the site of obstruction, occupation, and lifestyle.

A. Characteristic history and physical signs of decreased lower extremity perfusion diagnose intermittent claudication.

B. Pain while walking that is relieved promptly with the rest is characteristic. Unlike neurogenic claudication, the patient need not sit, squat, or recline to achieve relief. Dependent rubor is common, as is pallor with elevation. In severe cases, the pain diminishes with placement of the limb in a dependent position.

C. A differential diagnosis includes spinal stenosis, arthritis, degenerative disk disease, myofascial pain, thromboangiitis obliterans, acute arterial occlusion, compartment syndrome, muscle cramps, and McArdle's disease.

D. A comparison of systolic pressures between the arm and thigh, calf and ankle provides noninvasive confirmation of the area of occlusion. Normal ankle–arm indices are >1. Sphygmomanometer determinations in diabetes are often not obtainable because of noncompressible calcified vessels. Other flow studies such as directional Doppler flow velocity detection and pulse volume recording provide noninvasive means to study the blood flow to an extremity both before and after exercise. Postexercise values will relate better with the extent of the disease.

E. In mild to moderate disease, pain occurs with activity and does not interfere with vocation or lifestyle.

F. Cessation of smoking is imperative. Exercise (e.g., walking, bicycling) is beneficial when done daily for 30 to 60 minutes at a nonpainful level. The blood pressure should be controlled, maintaining diastolic pressure near 90 mm Hg to ensure collateral perfusion. Foot care is essential, including trimming of the nails; avoiding cold exposure; keeping the skin warm, dry, supple; and inspecting the feet daily. Underlying systemic disease such as congestive heart failure, chronic obstructive pulmonary disease, and diabetes must be rigorously controlled. Treat polycythemia to keep the hematocrit less than 55%. Weight loss and control of hyperlipidemia are also recommended.

Give nonsteroidal antiinflammatory drugs (NSAIDs) for pain; more severe pain may require aspirin or acetaminophen with codeine. Vasodilators and anticoagulants are no longer considered an effective treatment. Pentoxifylline efficacy is undetermined and fibrinolytic therapy has negligible benefit in chronic occlusion.

G. Severe chronic obstructive peripheral arterial disease is characterized by pain at rest, ulcers, ischemic neuropathy causing numbness, dysaesthesias, or an ankle arm index <0.6 in addition to intermittent claudication.

H. Incapacitating symptoms that interfere with lifestyle or livelihood require surgical evaluation. Gangrene, nonhealing ulcers, ankle systolic pressure less than 45 mm Hg, and ischemic pain at rest are other surgical indications.

I. Patients with substantial surgical risk or nongraftable lesions are not candidates for surgery.

J. Surgical revascularization procedures include femoral popliteal bypass graft, or aortoiliac endarterectomy or graft, femorotibial graft, femoroperoneal vein graft, infrapopliteal bypass graft, and percutaneous transluminal angioplasty for aortoiliac disease. Use of an adequate caliber vein (4 mm) is preferable to an artificial graft. When possible, use regional anesthesia for these procedures. Amputation is the alternative for life-threatening, intractable disease.

K. A successful trial of spinal cord stimulation using an epidural lead can be followed by implantation of a spinal cord stimulation system to provide pain relief.

L. Chemical sympathectomy can provide significant relief to most nonsurgical candidates, relief being obtained from rest pain rather than from claudication pain and percutaneous sympathetic blockade can be done as an outpatient procedure.

REFERENCES

Bonica JJ: Pain due to vascular disease. In: Bonica JJ (ed) *The Management of Pain*, 2nd ed. Philadelphia, Lea & Febiger, 1990, p. 506.

Jivergard LE, Augutinsson LE, Holm J, et al: The effectiveness of spinal cord stimulation (SCS) in patients with inoperable severe lower limb ischemia: a prospective randomized to study. *Eur J Vasc Endovasc Surg* 1995;9:421.

Radack K, Wyderski R: Conservative management of intermittent claudication. *Ann Intern Med* 1990;113:135.

Whittemore AD, Mannick JA: Intermittent claudication. In: Branch WT Jr (ed) *Office Practice of Medicine*, 2nd ed. Philadelphia, WB Saunders, 1987, p. 182.

Patient with LEG PAIN WITH AMBULATION

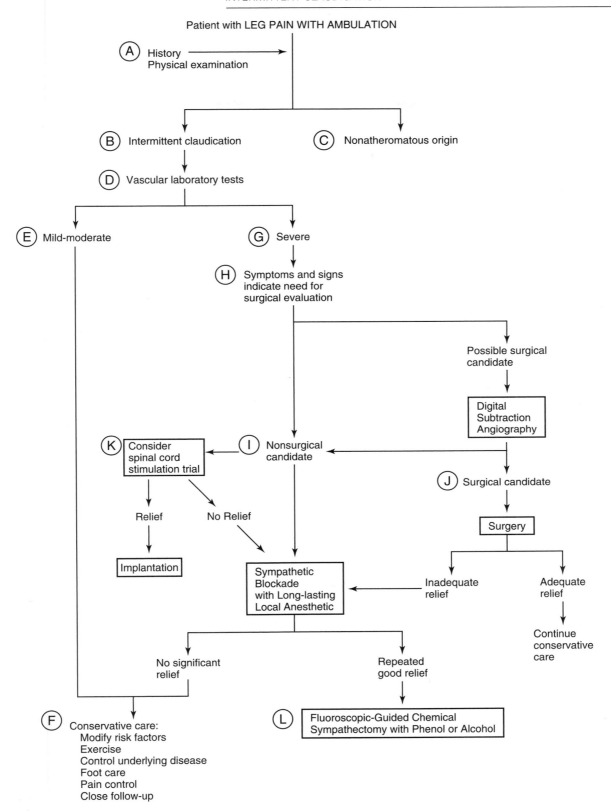

(A) History
Physical examination

(B) Intermittent claudication

(C) Nonatheromatous origin

(D) Vascular laboratory tests

(E) Mild-moderate

(G) Severe

(H) Symptoms and signs
indicate need for
surgical evaluation

Possible surgical
candidate

Digital
Subtraction
Angiography

(K) Consider
spinal cord
stimulation trial

(I) Nonsurgical
candidate

(J) Surgical candidate

Relief

No Relief

Surgery

Implantation

Sympathetic
Blockade
with Long-lasting
Local Anesthetic

Inadequate
relief

Adequate
relief

Continue
conservative
care

No significant
relief

Repeated
good relief

(F) Conservative care:
Modify risk factors
Exercise
Control underlying disease
Foot care
Pain control
Close follow-up

(L) Fluoroscopic-Guided Chemical
Sympathectomy with Phenol or Alcohol

PEDIATRIC PAIN

Management of Painful Procedures in
Pediatric Patients

Chronic Benign Pain in Children

Cancer-Related Pain in Children

Management of Painful Procedures in Pediatric Patients

LYNDA WELLS

The physical and psychological components of pain are inseparable. The key to the successful management of painful procedures in pediatric patients relies on both the prevention of pain and the alleviation of anxiety. This can be achieved by pharmacologic and nonpharmacologic interventions.

A. The first step is to establish a rapport with the patient and the caregiver. Individual coping styles should be recognized and respected. Patients who are "information gatherers" should be included in the consent process and their questions answered as fully as is appropriate for their development age. Patients who are "information avoiders" should be included only in as much as is necessary to enable their cooperation.

B. Preemptive analgesia is preferable. This includes the use of topical local anesthetic preparations, for EMLA cream, prior to all needlesticks. EMLA cream should be applied for 60 to 90 minutes to ensure effective analgesia. Pharmacologic premedication with a sedative or sedative–analgesic combination of drugs is often most appropriate. Oral medications should be preferred whenever possible and time allowed for them to become effective before embarking on any painful procedures. Sedative and/or anxiolytic drugs (e.g., benzodiazepines) should not be used in place of analgesics. The choice of medication should be guided by anticipated duration of the procedure and the severity of the pain expected during and after the procedure.

Ketamine, a phencyclidine derivative, has both sedative and analgesic properties at lower doses. At higher doses it will induce general anesthesia. Ketamine can be given orally or parenterally and produces a dissociative state. Its use is associated with increased salivation and pulmonary secretions, so an antisialogogue should also be used. Ketamine administration has been associated with emergence delirium, particularly when used for general anesthesia, and the concomitant use of a benzodiazepine, barbiturate, or opioid is recommended to minimize this risk.

Nitrous oxide is an inhaled analgesic, amnesiac, and sedative drug. It is given mixed with oxygen in a 50:50 mixture. In Europe, premixed nitrous oxide:oxygen tanks (Entonox) are available for this purpose. Although a 70:30 nitrous oxide to oxygen mixture is also effective there is a 30% risk of loss of consciousness while inhaling the drug at this concentration.

Nitrous oxide provides profound analgesia from 45 seconds after inhalation commences to approximately 60 seconds after cessation. Thus it is ideal for providing analgesia and sedation to cover needle sticks; procedures in which standard analgesics are inadequate, for example, bone marrow aspiration; and short procedures in which postprocedural pain is not expected. A mechanism for scavenging the exhaled gas and a closed, facemask delivery system is required. Monitoring is the same as when using other sedative/analgesic drugs.

C. Nonpharmacologic interventions can be used alone or in combination with pharmacologic therapies. These include distraction, guided imagery, hypnosis, meditation, and so forth. Parental presence may or may not be helpful. Each situation should be assessed on its merits. Parents should never be coerced to remain with their child. However, a designated adult must be present to comfort, distract, and reassure the child.

Local or general anesthesia should be considered based on the requirements and characteristics of the procedure and of the patient. Local anesthesia can take the form of skin infiltration, peripheral nerve blocks, or plexus blocks. If the procedure is long, or requires the patient to remain immobile, general anesthesia may be preferable. If significant pain is anticipated after the procedure local anesthesia for postprocedural analgesia can be combined with general anesthesia.

The American Academy of Pediatrics guidelines on monitoring and managing sedated pediatric patients should always be followed whenever sedation/analgesia is provided to a child.

REFERENCES

American Academy of Pediatrics Committee on Drugs: Guidelines for monitoring and management of pediatric patients during and after sedation for diagnostic and therapeutic procedures. *Pediatrics* 1992;89:1110–1115.

Anderson C, Zeltzer L, Fanurik D: Procedureal pain. In: Schechter N, Berde C, Yaster M (eds) *Pain in Infants, Children and Adolescents.* Baltimore, Williams & Wilkins, 1993.

Bjerring P, Arendt-Nielsen L: Depth and duration of skin analgesia to needle insertion after topical application of EMLA cream. *Br J Anaesth* 1990;64:173–177.

MANAGEMENT OF PAINFUL PROCEDURES IN CHILDREN

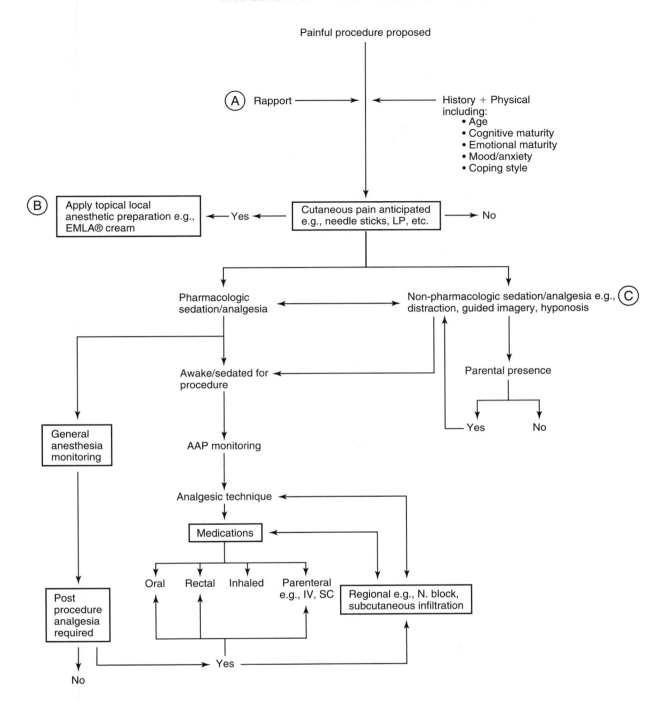

Chronic Benign Pain in Children

KENNETH R. GOLDSCHNEIDER, ANNA M. VARUGHESE,
AND NORBERT J. WEIDNER

Chronic pain during childhood is far more common than might be thought. Common pain sites include the head, abdomen, back, extremities, and chest. Although the distribution of pain is similar to that in adults, the disease entities differ. Clinicians must be alert to the multiple facets of pediatric pain, at least as much as they do for adults. Pediatric pain commonly presents as a family issue as well as an individual's symptom. Attention to pain's effect on the family is an important and unique function of the pediatric pain clinician. Parents do not expect children to have pain, and so a fair amount of anxiety over the etiology of the pain may be seen. Patients usually arrive at the pain clinic after being evaluated by their pediatrician or site-specific specialists (e.g., an orthopedic surgeon for foot pain).

A. The initial visit to the pain clinic optimally includes evaluation by a pain physician, a psychologist, and a physical therapist. Rarely does a child have pain that would not benefit from the expertise of at least two of these three disciplines. Follow-up visits depend on the specific diagnosis and needs of the child and family.

B. The pain physician reviews the general and specific histories obtained from the patient and adult caretaker ("parent" for our purposes, although this is not always the case). A full physical and comprehensive history help set the groundwork for proper diagnostic and therapeutic decisions as well as accurate and informative follow-up. Attention is paid to the social history because school avoidance can be significant and resemble adult disability behaviors. "Red flags" must be sought to reassure the family as well as ensure the safety of the patient. Some of the items requiring further investigation include fever, weight loss, change in bowel or bladder function, spinal point tenderness, peritoneal signs in the abdomen, change in level of consciousness or neural function, history of malignancy.

C. Diagnosis is optimally based on input from all practitioners. Although a specific pain site or condition may be evident from the physical examination, the effect on physical function and exacerbating issues, stresses, and impediments to therapy can be identified by physical therapy and psychology evaluations and should be included in the diagnostic and therapy-planning process. Input from all disciplines should be provided to the patient and family when the diagnosis and proposed therapy are discussed with them.

D. Treatment is tailored to the needs of the individual. Education plays a key role in reducing fear and anxiety, making expectations realistic and aiding compliance with the overall therapeutic plan. Patients should be helped to understand that their pain condition is not their fault, but care of their body is their responsibility.

A general approach that focuses on optimal physical and psychological function with the aid of appropriate medications is desirable. Many of the anticonvulsants, muscle relaxants, and antidepressants that are useful in adults are also appropriate in children, taking care to adjust for weight and medical conditions. Children generally do not tolerate needle procedures, and the disease entities from which they suffer are often not amenable to injection therapy. Therefore a noninvasive, holistic approach is usually best tolerated.

Opioid use for benign pain has been a point of contention among pain physicians. The use of opioids in children should be limited to a few scenarios. First, they may be used for cancer-related pain (see Chapter 86, p. 234). Second, opioids may be used for short periods of time while therapy is just beginning and after a surgical intervention. Long-term use may be appropriate for patients such as those with sickle cell disease or severe juvenile rheumatoid arthritis. These patients have pain that is expected to last their lifetimes, for which other interventions may be of limited benefit. An opioid contract delineating the terms of opioid use is appropriate and should be signed by the patient and the parents of minors.

E. Psychology is a key component in the treatment of chronic pain in children. Interventions such as biofeedback, relaxation training, coping skills training, and parent skills training are effective. Often families resist the involvement of psychology, fearing that the clinician believes the pain is feigned or imagined. The clinician should have a matter-of-fact approach that psychology is useful to the child, and that the main issue is helping to relieve the pain, not judging the mental health of the child. Physical therapy, too, is critical to the recovery of most pediatric pain patients. Stretching using the proper technique cannot be overemphasized. General or focused strengthening and range-of-motion exercises can be useful. Desensitizaton for complex regional pain syndromes and myofascial release techniques for myofascial pain are other examples of physical therapy interventions. Transcutaneous electrical nerve stimulation usually falls under the purview of a physical therapist. This modality can help with a variety of localized pain conditions and is well accepted by pediatric patients.

F. Rarely, a combination of physical, psychological, and logistical issues prevents resolution of the painful condition. At times, an intensive inpatient program can be constructed to achieve maximal benefit within a relatively short time. For regional pain, indwelling neuraxial or sympathetic catheters may help. The patient's day should be structured, with time included for completion of schoolwork and a limitation on passive activities and nonessential bed rest.

REFERENCES

Borge AI, Nordhagen R, Moe B, et al: Prevalence and persistence of stomachache and headache among children: follow-up of a cohort of Norwegian children from 4 to 10 years of age. *Acta Paediatr* 1994;83:433–437.

Leboeuf-Yde C, Kyvik KO: At what age does low back pain become a common problem? A study of 29,424 individuals aged 12-41 years. *Spine* 1998;23:228–234.

Scharff L: Recurrent abdominal pain in children: a review of psychological factors and treatment. *Clin Psychol Rev* 1997;17:145–166.

Schecter NL, Berde CB, Yaster M: *Pain in Infants, Children, and Adolescents.* Baltimore, Williams & Wilkins, 1993, p 691.

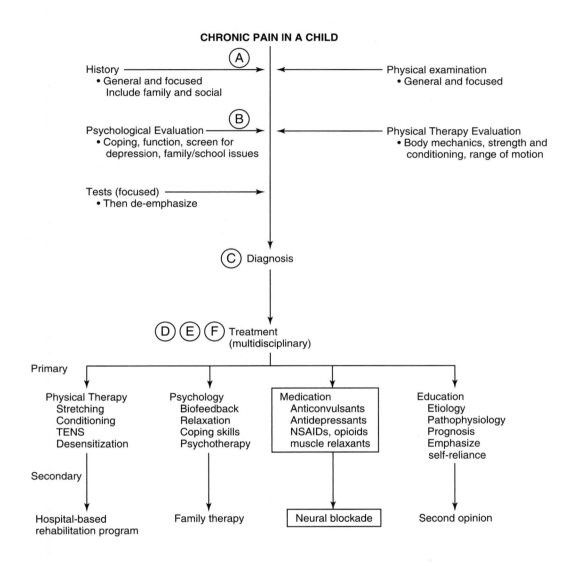

Cancer-Related Pain in Children

NORBERT J. WEIDNER, KENNETH R. GOLDSCHNEIDER, AND
ANNA M. VARUGHESE

The difficulty of caring for a child with a life-threatening illness such as cancer is that pain management is only one facet of the care of the child and the parents. Ideally, the management team constructs a care program centered on cure, simultaneously focusing on symptom management, and ultimately dealing with end-of-life issues. Pain can befall a child during the course of cancer in a number of situations. The pain can be caused by the cancer itself, which may involve visceral or abdominal pain; there may also be somatic pain, caused by direct invasion of anatomic structures, and bone and joint pain due to primary hematologic or metastatic disease. Moreover, when a tumor invades the peripheral or central nervous system, pain is a significant component. Pain caused by the invasive diagnostic and therapeutic procedures used in cancer patients is seen more often in pediatric cancer patients. It is this diagnostic/treatment-related pain that is most feared by children suffering from cancer.

A. As for most types of pain, a thorough history is important; one should obtain both a medical and an oncologic history. An age and developmentally appropriate pain scale must be used. It is important not only to measure the pain using an appropriate tool but also to involve the parents and other caregivers when formulating the assessment by relying on their observations. The medical examination should include a neurologic evaluation, looking for clues as to the nature of the process. Cancer and its therapy are dynamic processes that require regular, sometimes frequent reassessment of the pain.

B. Procedure-related pain is amenable to appropriate sedation or anesthetic protocols (or both). Cognitive and behavioral adjuncts are often included in these protocols. However, if pain is either disease- or treatment-related, a more traditional opioid pharmacologic approach is recommended. It is important to recognize that the three-step analgesic ladder of the World Health Organization remains the mainstay of pharmacologic management. For advanced cancer, nonopioid analgesics are of limited value. Opioid dosing should be titrated to the point of providing pain relief or the development of recognized side effects. Remember to include palliative and potential curative anticancer therapy when considering a treatment plan.

C. The appropriate route of administration depends on the interplay of the intensity of the pain and the availability of the various routes. The oral route should be used as a first-line approach for most patients when initiating opioid therapy. When oral opioids are not appropriate, alternate techniques include subcutaneous, intermittent intravenous, patient-controlled analgesia (PCA), nurse/parent-controlled analgesia (NCA), continuous infusions, and transdermal routes of administration. As for adults, opioids should be administered on a regular schedule with the provision of breakthrough or rescue medications on an as-needed basis.

D. During opioid therapy one must anticipate, recognize, and treat opioid-related side effects. Adjunct medications can be beneficial in limiting the amount of opioid required and for diminishing opioid-related side effects. Corticosteroids can help with pain resulting from acute nerve compression, visceral distension, soft tissue infiltration, or increased intracranial pressure. Anticonvulsants may be beneficial when neuropathic pain is present. Tricyclic antidepressants also are beneficial for neuropathic pain, as well as to treat depression and help with insomnia. Psychostimulants, such as methylphenidate or dexamphetamine, are beneficial for combatting the somnolence of opioid therapy and for adding analgesia to the regimen. Neuroleptics may be beneficial when dealing with hallucinations during opioid therapy.

E. When titrating opioids to effect, it is important to reassess the adequacy of the pain relief or the development of side effects at regular intervals. If adequate relief is obtained, simply continuing opioid therapy with periods of reassessment is indicated. If side effects develop, appropriate adjunctive treatment is warranted. However, if pain relief is inadequate, dose escalation of at least 25% to 50% is indicated to achieve an adequate effect. If at this point relief is still inadequate despite dose escalation, or if it is difficult to manage unpleasant side effects despite appropriate therapy, it is important to switch or rotate opioids. When switching opioids, it is important to bear in mind the relative differences in opioid potency. Initial doses of new opioids should be 25% to 50% less than the estimated equivalent dose of the prior opioid to allow incomplete cross-tolerance. Importantly, if rotation to methadone is planned, one must reduce the equianalgesic dose by 75% to avoid significant sedation. If the new regimen provides adequate relief and management of side effects, there should be continued reassessment of the process and continuation of the opioid therapy.

F. If opioid rotation and dose escalation thereof are not providing analgesia or relieving the side effects, one must consider invasive approaches. This might include spinal or epidural drug delivery or surgical or neuroablative procedures, depending on the nature of the tumor process. Unfortunately, a small percentage of patients still finds no relief despite aggressive, invasive therapy. At this point, one should meet with the family to consider terminal sedation. This is an infrequently used treatment arm in pediatric cancer management because 90% of patients who experience pain find relief with opioids alone.

REFERENCES

Cancer: Pain Relief and Palliative Care in Children. Geneva, World Health Organization, 1998.

Cherny NI, Portenoy RTK: Sedation and the management of refractory symptoms: guidelines for evaluation and treatment. *J Palliat Care* 1994;10:31–38.

Collins JJ, Grier HE, Sethna NF, et al: Regional anesthesia for pain associated with terminal malignancy. *Pain* 1996; 65:63–69.

Haine R: Pain scales in children: a review. *Palliat Med* 1997; 11:341–350.

Practice guidelines for cancer pain management. *Anesthesiology* 1996; 84:1243–1257.

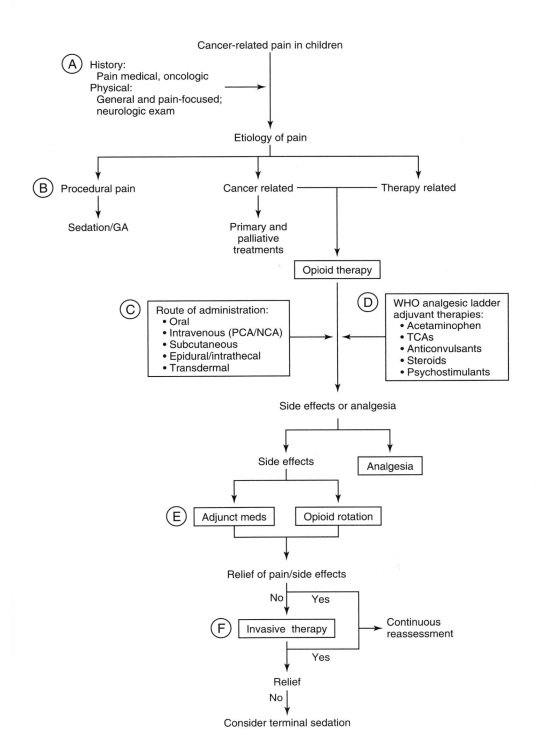

PHARMACOLOGY

Local Anesthetic Choice

DOUGLAS M. ANDERSON AND JERRY A. BEYER

Regional anesthesia techniques can be divided into five categories: infiltrative anesthesia, intravenous regional anesthesia, topical anesthesia, peripheral nerve blocks, and neuraxial blocks. Consider several factors when choosing a local anesthetic for a given technique (Table 1). Review the onset, duration, allergic potential, toxicity, and metabolism of the various local anesthetics. Become familiar with the local anesthetics used to perform short-, intermediate-, and long-duration regional techniques.

Local anesthetics temporarily impair the transmission of neural impulses by inhibiting the opening of sodium channels and the subsequent influx of sodium ions associated with depolarization. The ability of local anesthetics to slow the rate of depolarization and inhibit the propagation of an action potential depends on the ability of the local anesthetic to traverse a hydrophobic environment and bind to intracellular sodium channels. The ultimate effect achieved with a given regional anesthetic technique depends on many factors (Figure 1), including the local anesthetic used, the concentration and volume of the local anesthetic injected, the injection site, and the pH of the environment into which the medication is injected.

Local anesthetics are weak bases consisting of a lipophilic unsaturated benzene ring and a hydrophilic amine connected by an ester or amide linkage. Local anesthetics are classified as esters or amides based on the type of linkage connecting the two ends of the molecule. The clinical differences between amides and esters relates to metabolism (i.e., liver versus pseudocholinesterase) and allergic potential (esters > amides). At physiologic pH, local anesthetic molecules carry a positive charge (NH_3^+) on the amine group. Local anesthetics are distributed in acidic solutions (pH 6 to 7) to enhance the solubility. Interestingly, the positively charged (NH_3^+) species is the physiologically active form of the molecule at the intracellular receptor site in the sodium channel. However, for the local anesthetic to reach the receptor site, it must transverse a hydrophobic environment. This is best accomplished when the amine group is in an uncharged (NH_2) state. This is the principle behind the alkalization of local anesthetics and the difficulty encountered when anesthetizing inflamed (acidic) tissues. Because epinephrine is unstable in alkaline solutions, commercially prepared local anesthetic solutions containing epinephrine have a pH of 4 to 5. Thus it is best to add the epinephrine immediately before using it to maintain as much unprotonated (uncharged) local anesthetic as possible.

The pH at which a drug in solution has an equal number of ionized and nonionized species is referred to as the pKa of the drug. Local anesthetic medications have pKa values in the range of 7.6 to 9.0. Local anesthetics with a pKa closer to physiologic pH have a higher percentage of unprotonated (uncharged) species, which speeds the onset of action. Warming local anesthetic solutions serves to lower the pKa and thus speeds the onset of action.

The use of alkalinized or carbonated local anesthetic solutions is somewhat controversial. Based on our understanding of how local anesthetics work, alkalinization should speed the onset of action, improve the quality of the block, and prolong the duration of the blockade. However, several clinical studies have had conflicting results. For lidocaine and mepivacaine, 1 mL of 8.4% sodium bicarbonate is added for every 10 mL of local anesthetic. For bupivacaine, 0.1 mL of 8.4% sodium bicarbonate is added for every 10 mL of bupivacaine. The use of alkalinized local anesthetic solutions is highly effective for decreasing pain during subcutaneous infiltration.

The addition of epinephrine or, less frequently, phenylephrine to local anesthetic solutions causes vasoconstriction at the site of administration. This slows the distribution of local anesthetic to the central circulation, resulting in a prolonged block (greatest with intermediate-duration local anesthetics), decreased local anesthetic serum concentrations, and increased intensity of the block. Some of the suggested beneficial effects of vasoconstrictors may be mediated by mechanisms other than vasoconstriction.

The concept of a differential conduction blockade relates to the difficulty with which certain nerve fibers are blocked with a local anesthetic. Typically, preganglionic sympathetic B fibers are the first nerve fibers to be blocked. They require only a minimal local anesthetic concentration. Loss of sensation for pain and temperature requires a slightly higher concentration of local anesthetic. Successful motor blockade followed by loss of touch and proprioception requires the highest concentration of local anesthetic and is often difficult to achieve with certain regional techniques.

Local anesthetics have varying degrees of cardiac and central nervous system (CNS) toxicity, with long-acting drugs (e.g., bupivacaine, etidocaine) being the most toxic. In an effort to produce long-acting local anesthetics with less toxicity, much research and development has gone into the study of stereoisomers. Bupivacaine is a racemic mixture of two stereoisomers: S-(−)-enantiomer and R-(−)-enantiomer. Recently, levobupivacaine, the pure S-(−)-enantiomer of bupivacaine, has been marketed. This drug is similar to ropivacaine, which is a pure S-(−)-enantiomer of a propyl homologue of bupivacaine. These drugs appear to be less toxic to cardiac and CNS structures than bupivacaine on a milligram per milligram basis. However, much controversy surrounds the potency of ropivacaine. Several studies have shown that ropivacaine may be 40% to 50% less potent than bupivacaine. Many practitioners believe the decreased potency accounts for its "improved" safety profile and enhanced differential blockade. Research on levo-bupivacaine suggests that this drug is at least as potent as bupivacaine but has a safety profile intermediate between those of bupivacaine and ropivacaine. The major disadvantage of these new stereo-specific long-acting local anesthetics is the expense.

REFERENCES

D'Angelo R: Are the new local anesthetics worth their cost? *Acta Anaesthesiol Scand* 2000;44:639–641.

McLeod GA, Burke D: Levobupivacaine. *Anaesthesia* 2001;56:331–341.

Stoelting RK: *Local Anesthetics. Pharmacology and Physiology in Anesthetic Practice,* 3rd ed. Philadelphia, Lippincott-Raven, 1999, pp 158–181.

Tucker GT, Mather LE: Properties, absorption, and disposition of local anesthetic agents. In: Bridenbaugh PO (ed) *Neural Blockade in Clinical Anesthesia and Management of Pain,* 3rd ed. Philadelphia, Lippincott-Raven, 1998, pp 55–95.

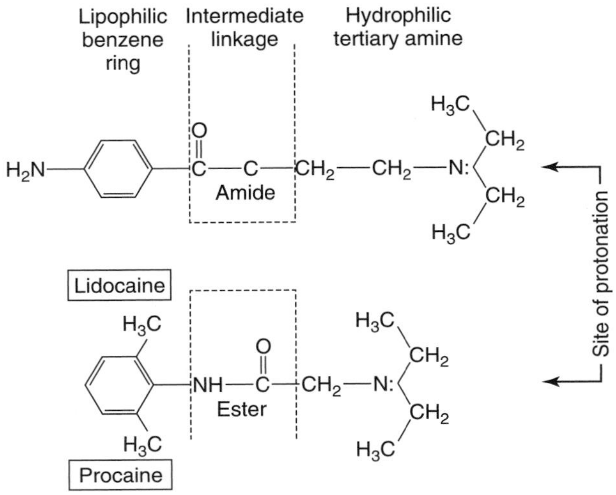

FIGURE 1 Local anesthetic: ester or amide.

TABLE 1
Local Anesthetics Used for Blocks

Local Anesthetic	Infiltrative Anesthesia	IV Regional Anesthesia	Topical Anesthesia	Peripheral Nerve Blocks	Neuraxial Blocks	Max. Dose* (mg/kg)
Amides						
Long duration						
Bupivacaine	0.25–0.5% Common	Not recommended		0.25–0.5% Common	Commonly used	2.5–3.5
Ropivacaine	0.25–0.5% Common	Not recommended		0.25–0.5% Common	Commonly used	2.5–3.5
Levobupivacaine	0.25–0.5% Common	Not recommended		0.25–0.5% Common	Commonly used	2.5–3.5
Etidocaine	Can be used	Has been successfully used No epinephrine		Motor block may outlast sensor block Fast onset	Can be used Dense motor block Motor block may outlast sensory block Fast onset	4.0–5.5
Intermediate duration						
Lidocaine	0.5–2.0% Common	3 mg/kg (40 cc of 0.5%) Preservative-free No epinephrine Only LA FDA approved for IV regional anesthesia	2–4% Topical or nebulized Part of EMLA 5% Ointment Lidoderm patch	1–2% Common	Can be used SAB associated with syndrome of transient neurologic symptoms	7
Mepivacaine	0.5–2.0% Common	Has been used successfully		1–2% Common	Can be used SAB associated with syndrome of transient neurologic symptoms	7
Short duration						
Prilocaine	Can be used	3 mg/kg (40 cc of 0.5%) Preservative free No epinephrine Methemoglobinemia[†]	Part of EMLA Methemoglobinemia[†]	Can be used Methemoglobinemia[†]		8
Esters						
Intermediate duration						
Tetracaine	Can be used		1–2% Common	Can be used	Can be used	2
Short duration						
Chloroprocaine	Can be used	Not recommended because of thrombophlebitis	Poor choice	Can be used	Can be used epidurally and intrathecally Associated with syndrome of transient neurologic symptoms Preservatives, large doses, pH-related problems	12–15
Procaine	Can be used	Has been used successfully No epinephrine	Poor choice	Can be used	SAB associated with syndrome of transient neurologic symptoms SAB associated with N/V	10–14
Benzocaine			Mucosal application Subcutaneous application Methemoglobinemia			200 mg total

EMLA, eutectic (easily melted) 1:1 mixture of 5% lidocaine and 5% prilocaine in an oil-in-water emulsion; N/V, nausea and vomiting; SAB, subarachnoid block.
*Higher doses with the use of 1:200,000 epinephrine.
Clinically significant methemoglobinemia associated with prilocaine doses higher than 600 mg.

LOCAL ANESTHETIC CHOICE

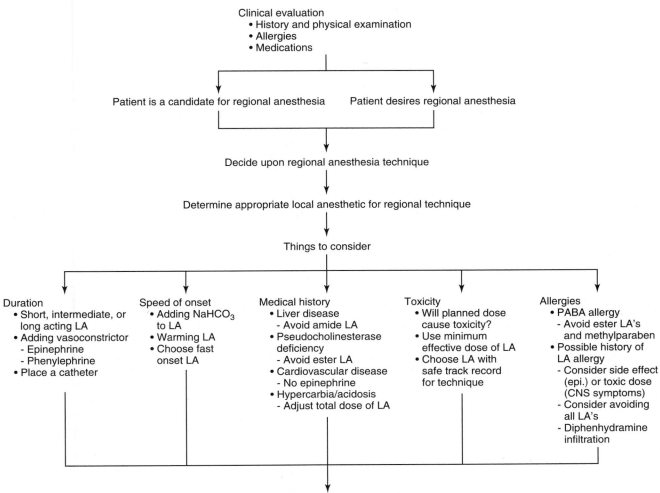

Clinical evaluation
- History and physical examination
- Allergies
- Medications

Patient is a candidate for regional anesthesia   Patient desires regional anesthesia

Decide upon regional anesthesia technique

Determine appropriate local anesthetic for regional technique

Things to consider

Duration
- Short, intermediate, or long acting LA
- Adding vasoconstrictor
  - Epinephrine
  - Phenylephrine
- Place a catheter

Speed of onset
- Adding NaHCO$_3$ to LA
- Warming LA
- Choose fast onset LA

Medical history
- Liver disease
  - Avoid amide LA
- Pseudocholinesterase deficiency
  - Avoid ester LA
- Cardiovascular disease
  - No epinephrine
- Hypercarbia/acidosis
  - Adjust total dose of LA

Toxicity
- Will planned dose cause toxicity?
- Use minimum effective dose of LA
- Choose LA with safe track record for technique

Allergies
- PABA allergy
  - Avoid ester LA's and methylparaben
- Possible history of LA allergy
  - Consider side effect (epi.) or toxic dose (CNS symptoms)
  - Consider avoiding all LA's
  - Diphenhydramine infiltration

See table for guidance in choosing appropriate local anesthetic

Local Anesthetic Toxicity

DOUGLAS M. ANDERSON AND JERRY A. BEYER

Local anesthetic toxicity can be classified as *systemic* (cardiovascular and central nervous system), *localized* (neural and skeletal muscle damage), and *special* side effects including methemoglobinemia, allergy, and addiction.

A. The development of toxicity to a local anesthetic is the result of a critical number of local anesthetic molecules reaching and binding to a potentially hazardous effector site, that is, brain and heart, at a given point in time. Since the consequences of such a reaction can be grave, the best defense against such a scenario is prevention and preparedness to treat any complications. Relying on total doses quoted in the literature to be safe is simplistic. The literature provides us with some "recommendations" of safe doses for a given local anesthetic. However, these "recommendations" fail to take into account the site and speed of injection, the amount of protein binding, the age of the patient, elimination, concomitant disease processes, and confounding medications. Studies have determined that the resultant serum concentrations of local anesthetic injections in various regions of the body are as follows:

> intravenous > airway > intercostal > caudal
> > epidural > brachial plexus > sciatic/femoral

The addition of epinephrine (1:200,000) to local anesthetics acts as a "chemical tourniquet" with resultant decreased peak serum concentrations. The total dose of epinephrine administered should not exceed 250 mcg in any patient. The use of epinephrine in a patient with moderate to severe coronary artery disease, uncontrolled hypertension, and an immediate history of cocaine use is contraindicated. Also, epinephrine should not be used on appendages with limited or single pathways of blood supply such as fingers, toes, ears, and the penis. Important issues in preventing systemic reactions to local anesthetics include using the smallest effective dose of local anesthetic, utilizing a *test dose*, premedication with a benzodiazepine to raise the seizure threshold, and fractionated injection of local anesthetic with confirmation of negative aspiration of blood after *every* 5 to 10 ml is injected.

B. Toxic levels of local anesthetics in the CNS generally manifest first with light-headedness and numbness of the tongue. If the serum concentration continues to rise, the patient may experience visual and auditory disturbances followed by muscle twitching, unconsciousness, convulsions, coma, and finally respiratory arrest. The early excitatory symptoms of local anesthetic toxicity are thought to result from inhibition of inhibitory pathways in the cerebral cortex. Interestingly, high-dose lidocaine is a treatment for resistant status epilepticus. All local anesthetics are potentially toxic to the central nervous system (CNS) and the dose required to produce symptoms is proportional to serum Pco_2, and pH. The dose of local anesthetic required to produce CNS toxicity correlates with the potency of the local anesthetic. Procaine is least toxic with lidocaine/mepivacaine/prilocaine having intermediate toxicity followed by etidocaine and bupivacaine being the most toxic. Bupivacaine is approximately four times more toxic to the CNS than lidocaine.

C. The most feared systemic complication of local anesthetics is cardiovascular toxicity. High systemic serum concentration of local anesthetics can produce a diffuse sympathectomy resulting in profound vasodilatation and subsequent cardiovascular collapse. Direct cardiac effects and brain stem–mediated effects of local anesthetic toxicity include electrophysiologic and myocardial depression. The character of the arrhythmias caused by a toxic dose of bupivacaine is unique from all other local anesthetics. Lidocaine and other local anesthetics tend to produce only bradycardia with associated hypotension and cardiovascular collapse. However, bupivacaine toxicity usually results in progressive QRS widening, ventricular dysrhythmias, electromechanical dissociation, and finally refractory asystole. Although all local anesthetics bind Na^+ channels in the open configuration with similar ease, the kinetics of dissociation vary. The unique arrhythmias caused by bupivacaine are related to its kinetics in relation to its dissociating from Na^+ channels. Bupivacaine and lidocaine dissociate from inactivated Na^+ channels with a time constant of 1.50 seconds and 0.15 seconds, respectively. Thus, bupivacaine incompletely dissociates from the Na^+ channel during diastole, leading to accumulation of blockade. This phenomenon has led to the terms fast-in, slow-out for bupivacaine and fast-in, fast-out for lidocaine. Although blockade of Na^+ channels is believed to play the major role in the cardiac toxicity of local anesthetic, new studies suggest that blockade of K^+ and Ca^{2+} channels may be contributory.

D. Toxic doses of bupivacaine and, to a lesser extent, etidocaine can result in severe cardiac conduction abnormalities including ventricular fibrillation and reentrant type arrhythmias such as torsades de pointes. Ventricular arrhythmias are rarely seen with other local anesthetics. Amiodarone (Haasto et al. 1990) and bretylium (Kasten and Martin 1985) are reported in the literature as possible effective agents in the treatment of local anesthetic–induced arrhythmias. In a study of 30 anesthetized pigs with bupivacaine-induced cardiac toxicity, 90% of the pigs treated with amiodarone survived. This compares with 40% survival with bretylium and 60% survival in the control group. It should be noted, however, that because of the size of the study ($n = 30$) the difference in survival was not statistically significant (Haasto et al. 1990).

Despite the scarcity of good scientific data and conflicting views (de La Cousssaye et al. 1991) amiodarone is probably the antiarrhythmic agent of choice to treat bupivacaine-induced cardiac arrhythmias, given the difficulty encountered in acquiring bretylium, since it has been largely eliminated from the current advanced cardiac life support (ACLS) protocols. The use of beta-blockers to prevent or treat local anesthetic–induced arrhythmias is controversial. Beta-blockers have been reported to both protect and to predispose patients to bupivacaine-induced cardiac toxicity.

E. Local anesthetics produce a direct dose-dependent reduction of myocardial contractility. Bupivacaine appears to be a mitochondrial toxin. Bupivacaine inhibits metabolism of fatty acids, the heart's preferred fuel, at concentrations that do not adversely affect pyruvate metabolism (Weinber and VandeBoncouer 2001). Infusions of glucose–insulin–potassium have been shown to reduce bupivacaine cardiac toxicity, perhaps by promoting pyruvate availability for mitochondrial metabolism. Amrinone, milrinone, dopamine, norepinephrine, epinephrine, and isoproterenol have been investigated as possible methods of treating bupivacaine-induced asystole. However, there is no consensus regarding which drug is the most efficacious and often the study results are conflicting. Finally, it has been reported that bupivacaine has increased cardiac toxicity in animals under light halothane anesthesia with hypoxia and hypercarbia (Heavner et al. 1995). This suggests the possibility of increased risk when combined regional–general anesthesia is utilized without careful attention to PaO_2 and $PaCO_2$.

F. Lidocaine has been associated with both a permanent and a temporary form of nerve damage when used for spinal anesthesia. Some patients have surgical procedures for which an ultra-low dose of lidocaine (20 mg combined with 25 mcg of fentanyl) is appropriate. When used in this way, lidocaine appears to produce transient neurologic symptoms (TNS) with an incidence of approximately 3%. More conventional doses of intrathecal lidocaine are associated with a 30% incidence of TNS. The incidence of TNS appears to be increased with the addition of a vasoconstrictor such as epinephrine. Most severe neurologic injuries (cauda equina syndrome) associated with local anesthetics such as lidocaine, tetracaine, and chloroprocaine are related to large subarachnoid doses and the use of microcatheters.

G. The injection of chloroprocaine into the subarachnoid space or epidural space has been associated with prolonged motor and sensory deficits in several patients. Although chloroprocaine itself does not appear to be a neurotoxin, certain commercial preparations of this local anesthetic can be neurotoxic. The deficits occurred with large injections of chloroprocaine combined with 0.2% sodium bisulfite *and* a low pH. Newer preparations of chloroprocaine utilize EDTA as a preservative or are completely preservative free and appear to have a lower incidence on complications. However, there are reports of transient, severe back pain after epidural administration of chloroprocaine containing EDTA. Large doses of chloroprocaine (>40 cc), EDTA preservative, and low pH have all been implicated as possible causes of these problems (Hodgson et al. 1999).

H. The injection of various local anesthetics into skeletal muscle is associated with reversible histologic changes. Muscle regeneration occurs very rapidly with complete recovery within 2 weeks. The degree of muscle damage seems to be related to the potency or duration of the local anesthetic, with bupivacaine and etidocaine being the most damaging.

I. Allergic reactions to local anesthetics are very rare, with fewer than 1% of all reported cases of local anesthetic allergies being "true" allergies. There are few published reports of allergic reactions with a confirmed immunological component. Most claims of allergy are related to the addition of epinephrine, systemic toxicity, or side effects of other drugs given concomitantly. Allergic reactions to ester compounds are more common than to amide compounds, with no cross-reactivity between groups. The immunologic trigger is usually paraaminobenzoic acid (PABA), the product of ester compound metabolism by plasma esterases. Methylparaben is structurally related to PABA and is a common preservative in amide and ester compounds packaged in multiple-dose vials. People allergic to ester compounds may react to amide compounds preserved with methylparaben. In patients with a known allergy or an unreliable history of local anesthetic allergy, skin infiltration with diphenhydramine is an acceptable method of producing analgesia.

J. Clinically significant methemoglobinemia has been associated with both prilocaine (>600 mg) and benzocaine local anesthetic use. This complication can be treated with IV methylene blue 1-2 mg/kg over 5 minutes. However, most cases of methemoglobinemia are mild and clinically insignificant. Most serious complications associated with methemoglobinemia are the result of failure to diagnose this easily treatable problem.

K. The treatment of systemic local anesthetic toxicity is largely encompassed in the principles of basic life support. If a patient starts to experience signs and symptoms consistent with CNS toxicity, the patient's airway, breathing, and circulation should be assessed and supported as necessary. The primary cause of death related to local anesthetic toxicity is status epilepticus and unrecognized or unsuccessfully treated apnea. Researchers report that most toxic reactions to local anesthetics are transient and respond very well to simple hyperventilation and supplemental oxygen. However, if convulsions persist, a small dose of intravenous benzodiazepine or thiopental (50 to 100 mg) can be given to terminate the seizure. Fortunately, cardiovascular toxicity is not a common problem but can be very serious in situations where large doses of bupivacaine are used or an intravascular injection has occurred. The treatment for cardiovascular toxicity resulting in hypotension is largely fluids, elevation of the legs, and pressor support. Should severe cardiac arrhythmias occur, the drug of choice is probably amiodarone. In severe cases of resistant ventricular fibrillation cardiopulmonary bypass has been successfully used to treat bupivacaine toxicity.

REFERENCES

de La Coussaye JE, Bassoul BR, Gagnol JP, et al: Experimental treatment of bupivacaine cardiotoxicity: what is the best choice? *Reg Anesth* 1991;16:120–122.

Haasto J, Pitkanen MT, Kytta J, Rosenberg PH: Treatment of bupivacaine-induced cardiac arrhythmias in hypoxic and hypercarbic pigs with amiodarone or bretylium. *Reg Anesth* 1990;15:174–179.

Heavner JE, Badgwell JM, Drvden CF Jr, Flinders C: Bupivacaine toxicity in lightly anesthetized pigs with respiratory imbalances plus or minus halothane. *Reg Anesth* 1995;20:20–26.

Hodgson PS, Neal JM, Pollock JE, Liu SS: The neurotoxicity of drugs given intrathecally (spinal). *Anesth Analg* 1999;88:797–809.

Kasten GW, Martin ST: Bupivacaine cardiovascular toxicity: comparison of treatment with bretylium and lidocaine. *Anesth Analg* 1985;64:911–916.

Weinber G, VandeBoncouer T: Improved energetics may explain the favorable effect of insulin infusion on bupivacaine cardiotoxicity. *Anesth Analg* 2001;92:1075–1076.

LOCAL ANESTHETIC TOXICITY

(A) **PREVENTION**

- Hx and PE for contraindications
- Prepare for toxic reactions before block
- Use lowest effective dose
- Monitor vitals during and after injection
- Pre-medicate to raise seizure threshold
- Avoid intravascular injection
  - Use test dose
  - Fractionated injection

Types of Reactions

Systemic

Immediate
- Intravascular injection LA
- Intravascular injection Epi
Delayed
- 20 min after injection

(F) (G) **TNS**

SAB lidocaine, tetracaine and chloroprocaine
- Avoid preservatives if possible
- Use lowest effective dose
- Avoid vasoconstrictors if possible

(H) **Local Tissue**

(I) **Allergic**

(J) **Methemoglobinemia**

Prilocaine
Benzocaine
- Usually transient
- Can tx with methylene blue

Esters

By-product of metabolism
- PABA
Multiple dose vials
- Methylparaben

Amides

Mult dose vials
- Methylparaben

(B) **CNS**

Initial excitation followed by
- Convulsions, and finally
- CNS depression
  - Respiratory arrest
  - Coma

(C) (D) (E) **Cardiovascular**

CV stimulation secondary to convulsions
CV depression
- Usually occurs after CNS depression
- Negative inotropic
- Impaired conduction
- Peripheral vasodilation
Ventricular arrhythmias
- Most common with bupivacaine

(K) **Treatment**

Stop Convulsions

Benzodiazepine
Pentothal 50-100 mg

Basic/Advanced Cardiac Life Support

Maintain or provide an airway
- Succinylcholine may be necessary
- Suction if needed
Evaluate and assist ventilations
- Provide 100% oxygen
Evaluate and support CV system
- Increase IVF and elevate legs if BP low
- Consider pressor support for severe or persistent hypotension
- Consider glucose/insulin/potassium infusion
- Treat severe arrhythmias with amiodarone or bretylium

Nonsteroidal Antiinflammatory Drugs

EULECHE ALANMANOU

Nonsteroidal antiinflammatory drugs (NSAIDs) include aspirin, several other classes of organic acids (acetic acid derivative, propionic acid derivative, enolic acid derivative), and selective cyclooxygenase-2 (COX-2) inhibitors. When activation occurs, arachidonic acid is liberated from membrane-bound phospholipids by phospholipase A_2. The enzyme COX catalyzes the formation of prostanoids from arachidonic acids. Those prostanoids include thromboxane A_2 and prostaglandins such as PGD_2, PGE_2, PGF_2, and PGI_2 (prostacyclin). Under normal physiologic condition, prostaglandins are essential for cytoprotection of the gastric mucosa, hemostasis, renal physiology, pregnancy, and labor. Prostaglandins also sensitize nociceptive nerve endings to other mediators (bradykinin and histamine). They enhance nociception in the dorsal horn of the spinal cord. Prostaglandin may also inhibit the descending noradrenergic pathway involved in pain inhibition. COX-1 is constitutively expressed and present in most cells. COX-2 expression is almost undetectable in most tissues under normal physiologic condition. COX-2 expression is induced in the setting of inflammation and cellular transformation. It is, however, present under basal conditions in the brain and the renal cortex.

Aspirin causes irreversible inhibition of both COX-1 and COX-2. The other traditional NSAIDs cause reversible inhibition of COX-1 and COX-2. The antipyretic, analgesic, and antiinflammatory actions of NSAIDs are related to their ability to inhibit COX-2. Selective COX-2 inhibitors were developed to spare COX-1 and its cytoprotective function. Complications such as gastrointestinal bleeding and renal toxicity result from inhibition of COX-1.

NSAID-induced gastrointestinal toxicity (dyspepsia, abdominal pain, gastric or duodenal ulcer, perforation, bleeding) is caused by COX-1–related suppression of thromboxane A_2 (TXA_2) in platelets, concomitantly with loss of PGE_2-mediated gastrointestinal (GI) cytoprotective effect. The following risk factors for GI bleeding have been identified: (1) concomitant use of medications such as anticoagulants and corticosteroids, (2) concomitant use of low-dose aspirin or other NSAIDs, (3) increasing age ($\geq$60 years), (4) increasing dose, (5) previous history of GI bleeding, and (6) concomitant use of alcohol. The prevention of GI toxicity includes the use of synthetic analog of PG (misoprostol), sucralfate, proton pump inhibitor (omeprazole).

Impaired regulation of renal blood flow by suppression of prostaglandin may explain NSAIDs-induced renal toxicity. Risk factors include underlying kidney disease, age 65 years or older, renal prostaglandin–dependent states (volume depletion, congestive heart failure, hypertension, diabetes).

Cardiovascular effects of NSAIDs use are currently the subject of heated debate. Data from controlled trials show that COX-2 selective agents (rofecoxib, celecoxib, valdecoxib) may be associated with an increased risk of serious cardiovascular events (myocardial infarction and stroke), especially when used for long periods of time or immediately after cardiac surgery. A clinical trial also suggests that long-term use of naproxen may be associated with an increased cardiovascular risk compared with placebo. In the vasculature, COX-2 is the main enzyme responsible for the production of the vasodilatory and antithrombotic prostacyclin. In platelets, production of the prothrombotic prostanoid TXA_2 is due to COX-1. Aspirin irreversibly blocks COX, which means, in the platelet, inability to synthesize COX-1 and consequently TXA_2. It takes 7 to 10 days for the formation of platelets but bleeding time normalizes sooner after the suspension of aspirin use. Aspirin also suppress COX-2, thus prostacyclin; but the suppression of thromboxane predominates. This explains the cardioprotection offered by aspirin. Other nonselective NSAIDs induce reversible inhibition of COX-1–derived thromboxane and COX-2–derived prostacyclin to a similar degree that does not offer cardiovascular protection.

Inhibition of COX-2–derived prostacyclin and lack of suppression of COX-1–derived TXA_2 may be to blame in the increased risk of cardiovascular events with the use of selective COX-2 inhibitors.

Aspirin given during fever or viral illness in children has been associated with the occurrence of Reye's syndrome, leading to seizure, coma, and death. Other toxicities associated with NSAIDs are hepatic, neuropsychiatric, and dermatologic.

REFERENCES

Bombardier C: An evidence-based evaluation of the gastrointestinal safety of coxibs. *Am J Cardiol* 2002;89:3D–9D.

FDA: Acetaminophen hepatotoxicity and NSAIDs related gastrointestinal and renal toxicity. Letter to state boards of pharmacy, posted on January 22, 2004. http://www.fda.gov/cder/drug/analgesics/letter.htm

FDA: Safety notices. FDA issues NSAID health advisory pending further evaluation. www.fda.gov (December 28, 2004).

Fitzgerald G: Cardiovascular pharmacology of nonselective nonsteroidal anti-inflammatory drugs and coxibs: clinical considerations. *Am J Cardiol* 2002;89:(6A)26D–32D.

NONSTEROIDAL ANTIINFLAMMATORY DRUGS

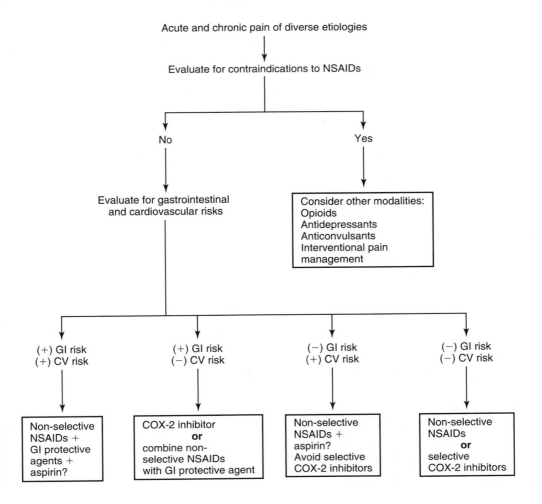

Steroids

SOMAYAJI RAMAMURTHY AND EULECHE ALANMANOU

Corticosteroids are very commonly used for the management of pain, mainly for their antiinflammatory action. They are very powerful inhibitors of the enzyme phospholipase A2, thereby reducing the arachidonic acid metabolites.

Steroids reduce ectopic discharge from injured nerve segments by exerting membrane stabilizing effect on the nociceptive C fibers. This, however, is a transient effect and therefore does not fully explain the long-term pain relief obtained with the use of steroids. Also, euphoric effect of steroids can be beneficial.

ORAL STEROIDS

Oral steroid preparations referred to as "steroid dose pack" are commonly used in the management of acute arthritis, acute herpes zoster and acute radiculopathy. Larger doses and longer therapy are employed in the management of rheumatic and collagen disorders, such as rheumatoid arthritis, lupus erythematosis, and ankylosing spondylitis.

Long-term use of steroids can be associated with side effects including fluid and electroytes disturbances, musculoskeletal problems including osteroporosis and fractures, immunosuppression and increased susceptibility to infections, cushingoid changes, increased blood sugar, and bleeding gastric ulcer. Their chronic use also produces suppression of the pituitary adrenal axis. Therefore, during the period of stresses such as surgical procedures, additional steroids may have to be administered. Tapering before discontinuation is mandatory to avoid adrenal crisis.

PARENTERAL STEROIDS

Intravenous and intramuscular use of injectable steroid preparations is not very common in the pain management setting. Preparations with prolonged action are preferred. Methylprednisolone in a depot form (depomedrol), triamcinolone (aristocort, and kenalog) and betamethasone (celestone) are commonly used. The long-acting preparations have other compounds to facilitate solubility and are usually in the form of a suspension. Depomedtrol has a tendency to precipitate when mixed with a local anesthetic or saline. The other preparations stay in the solution for a longer period when mixed with local anesthetic or saline, and consequently are more likely to provide uniform distribution when large volume of the mixture is injected subcutaneously or into a scar.

Long-acting steroid preparations are also injected into the joints and bursae such as hip, knee, facet, and sacroiliac. Because repeated injections into a joint can produce weakening of the underlying bone, many clinicians limit the number of injections to less than three per year.

Intradermal injection of high concentration steroid can produce skin breakdown and ulcers requiring skin graft. The authors prefer the use of triamcinolone 1 to 2 mg per milliliter for scar and subcutaneous injections.

EPIDURAL STEROIDS

Epidural steroid injection is one of the most commonly performed techniques for pain management. Epidural steroids are useful only in the presence of inflammation of the nerve root. Patients having pain due to other causes such as facet joint, myofascial, or disc pain are not likely to benefit from epidural steroid injection. Patients with diabetic radiculopathy also do not benefit, and their diabetes can significantly worsen.

There is no need to give a series of three injections in every patient, especially if the patient gets significant benefit from only one or two injections. Long-acting steroids remain in the epidural space for two or three weeks. Repeated injections at short intervals, such as once per week, can lead to systemic problems. Suppression of the pituitary adrenal axis can last six weeks or longer. Large sized particles of depomedrol or triamcinolone injected into radicular arteries have produced spinal cord infarction and paralysis. Betamethasone has the smallest particulate size and is usually preferred for transforaminal epidural injections, where the risk of radicular arterial injection is greater.

INTRATHECAL STEROIDS

Intrathecal steroids are controversial due to concerns about the effect of preservatives and other compounds which are present in the long-acting preparations. However, significant benefit of this method has been reported in post-herpetic neuralgia patients.

REFERENCES

Devor M, Govrin-Lippmann R, Raber P: Corticosteroids suppress ectopic neural discharge originating in experimental neuromas. *Pain* 1985;22:127.

Koes BW, Rob JPM, Scholten M, et al: Epidural steroid injections for low back pain and sciatica: An updated systematic review of randomized clinical trials. *Pain Dig* 1999;9:241.

Wilkinson HA: Intrathecal Depo-Medrol: A literature review. *Clin J Pain* 1992;8(1):49.

Kumar V: Neuraxial and sympathetic blocks in herpes zoster and postherpetic neuralgia: an appraisal of current evidence. *Reg Anesth Pain Med* 2004; 29(5):454-461.

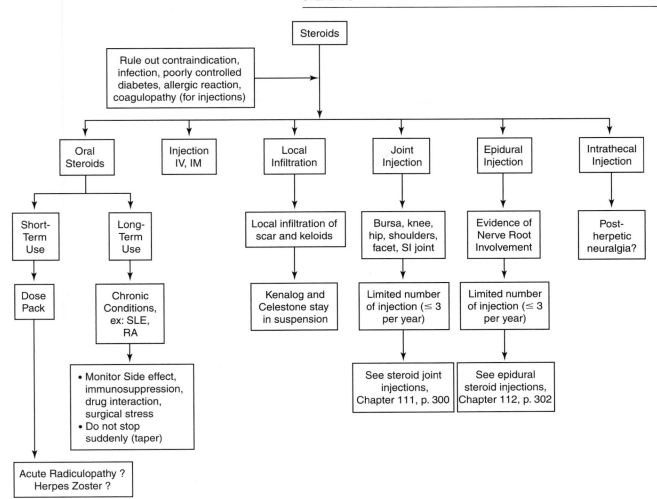

Antidepressants

SOMAYAJI RAMAMURTHY

Depression is present in the majority of chronic pain patients. Beck depression inventory or other depression scales demonstrate depression in 60% to 80% of these patients. Sixty percent of patients who have depression also have pain complaints even when they have no significant somatic etiology. The central nuclei and the pathways involved in the control of mood and pain utilize the same neurotransmitters such as norepinephrine and serotonin. Thus most chronic pain patients will require pharmacotherapy for the treatment of the associated depression. There has been a significant debate regarding whether the antidepressants act directly by decreasing the pain or indirectly by improving the depressed mood. There is significant evidence that many antidepressants, especially tricyclics, can decrease neuropathic pain even in the absence of associated depression. The doses of antidepressants used to manage chronic pain usually are much smaller than the usual antidepressant doses. The pain relief may be evident in 4 to 5 days while improvement in the depressed mood may require several weeks.

Antidepressant pharmacotherapy is one of the multiple modalities utilized in the management of chronic pain, after a thorough workup. There are numerous antidepressant medications to choose from. Tricyclic antidepressants are tried initially if a patient has neuropathic pain. Selective serotonin reuptake inhibitors (SSRIs) such as paroxetine or sertraline are preferred in the following situations: pain with no neuropathic component, tricyclics contraindicated, and in elderly patients.

TRICYCLIC ANTIDEPRESSANTS (TCAs)

Drug selection among TCAs depends on the individual circumstances such as the presence of insomnia, cardiovascular disturbances, elderly patients, or daytime sedation.

Tertiary amines such as amitriptyline, doxepin, and imipramine have significant sedative, antimuscarinic, and antihistaminic effects. Sedation is useful in patients with sleep disturbances. If daytime sedation is a problem, a secondary amine, such as desipramine, is chosen and can be administered even during daytime. The antihistaminic effect (H2) has been shown to heal peptic ulcers even better than cimetidine.

Sedation and postural hypotension leading to a fall are important causes of hip fracture in the elderly. It is preferable to start with small doses such as 10 mg of nortriptyline or desipramine if no sedation is needed. Nortriptyline, a metabolic breakdown product of amitriptyline, is reported to be better tolerated by the elderly because it produces less postural hypertension (alpha 1 effect).

The goal of pharmacotherapy is to arrive at the minimum effective dose. The end points are analgesia, intolerable side effects, or predetermined maximum dose. If analgesia is not achieved, a different antidepressant is chosen depending on the side effects and patient factors.

Numerous side effects, especially when used in large psychiatric doses, limit the usefulness of the tricyclics to smaller pain management doses. It is not uncommon to utilize the beneficial effects of small doses of tricyclics to treat the neuropathic pain and sleep disturbances, while treating the depression utilizing SSRIs or other drugs. The side effects of tricyclics are secondary to antimuscarinic and cardiovascular effects. Muscarinic side effects include dry mouth, constipation, difficult urination, and sexual dysfunction. Ocular effects contraindicate their use in patients with narrow-angle glaucoma. Cardiovascular side effects related to arrhythmias and postural hypotension limits their use in elderly individuals and in patients with cardiovascular disease. Amoxapine and maprotiline are not commonly used because of their poor side effect profile.

OTHER ANTIDEPRESSANTS

Trazodone in 50–100 mg doses is very useful in patients with sleep disturbances. There are very few cardiovascular side effects and no muscarinic side effects. This drug is preferred in elderly patients and also in patients who are on SSRIs and have sleep disturbances. There is a low incidence (1 in 10,000) of priapism when used in higher doses.

Nefazodone (which is structurally related to trazodone) does not have sedation and priapism as side effects. Trazodone and nefazodone do not have specific benefits in patients with neuropathic pain but are useful in the treatment of depression.

Venlafaxine (Effexor) has proven to be useful in the treatment of neuropathic pain because of its effects on norepinephrine in the central nervous system. Hypertension is a side effect.

Wellbutrin is an effective antidepressant with no specific analgesic effect. Its side effects include convulsions.

SSRIs are very useful because of their low side effect profile. In general, they are utilized in the treatment of depression, but do not have any particular analgesic effect except for paroxetine, which has been shown to have some benefit in diabetic neuropathy.

Monoamine oxidase (MAO) inhibitors are not commonly used because of their severe interaction with various food substances and other drugs.

REFERENCES

Magni G: The use of antidepressants in the treatment of chronic pain. *Drugs* 1991;42:730–748.

McQuay HJ, Tramer M, Nye BA, et al: A systemic review of antidepressants in neuropathic pain. *Pain* 1996;68:217–227.

Sindrup SH, Gram LF, Brosen K et al: The selective serotonin reuptake inhibitor paroxetine is effective in the treatment of diabetic neuropathy symptoms. *Pain* 1990;42:135–144.

ANTIDEPRESSANTS

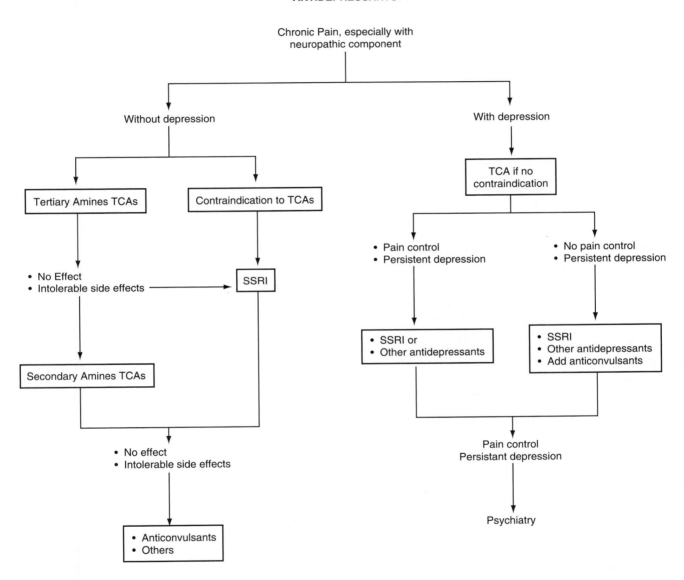

Anticonvulsants

SERGIO ALVARADO

The successful use of the antiepileptic drug carbamazepine for trigeminal neuralgia in a series of patients was reported in *Lancet* in 1962 by Blom. That remarkable success was confirmed by subsequent well-designed studies and led to the establishment of carbamazepine as the treatment of choice for trigeminal neuralgia and to the investigation of its use for other neuropathic conditions. Studies of carbamazepine in painful diabetic neuropathy (PDN) showed some benefit, but clinical experience was unsatisfactory. Results of the use of phenytoin in PDN were equivocal. Other older antiepileptic drugs (AEDs) failed to demonstrate any benefit in neuropathic pain or headache, with the exception of sodium valproate. Trials in patients with migraine in the early 1990s showed some benefit from valproic acid. At the same time a new generation of AEDs was introduced into practice with new mechanisms of action, better tolerability, and fewer drug–drug interactions owing to less effect on the cytochrome P450 enzyme system. This created excitement about their potential use as analgesics.

A. Pain syndromes that may benefit from therapy with AEDs include painful diabetic neuropathy, postherpetic neuralgia, trigeminal neuralgia, complex regional pain syndrome, radiculopathies, painful human immunodeficiency virus (HIV)-associated neuropathies, central poststroke pain, spinal cord injury, deafferentation syndromes such as phantom limb pain, and migraine headache.

B. Carbamazepine is an older AED that is structurally related to tricyclic antidepressants, blocks voltage-gated sodium channels, and inhibits voltage-dependent calcium channels. It has proven benefit in trigeminal neuralgia and remains first line treatment for that disorder at doses of 400 to 1000 mg/day. The main drawback is its hematologic and metabolic effects with need for monitoring of blood counts, liver enzymes, and serum levels. It has a significant number of drug–drug interactions, as do all the older AEDs. Adverse effects include ataxia, cognitive deficits, and weight gain. Phenytoin blocks sodium channels and inhibits the rapid excitatory sodium influx necessary for the formation of an action potential. Evidence for its efficacy in neuropathic pain is weak, although a recent trial suggests benefit in an acute flare-up of chronic neuropathic pain when given as an intravenous infusion of 15 mg/kg over 2 hours. Intravenous infusion may also be considered for rapid treatment of trigeminal neuralgia while titrating dosage of another AED. Valproic acid and the alternative preparation divalproex sodium have demonstrated benefit in treatment of migraine. Their use has been limited by high rates of adverse effects including nausea, weight gain, and tremor, as well as the need for regular monitoring of blood counts, liver enzymes, and drug levels. Their efficacy, however, has led to interest in use of the newer AEDs for migraine.

C. Oxcarbazepine is a structural analog of carbamazepine with the same mechanism of action and a much better safety profile. It does not appear to have the risk of hematologic and hepatic effects of carbamazepine and serum monitoring is not required, making it a desirable alternative for treatment of trigeminal neuralgia. The initial dose is 150 to 300 mg at bedtime with increases of 150 to 300 mg/day every 3 to 5 days and a target range of 900 to 1800 mg/day b.i.d. It has the greatest incidence of adverse effects of the new AEDs, with dizziness, somnolence, ataxia, nystagmus, diplopia, visual abnormalities, vertigo, nausea, vomiting, fatigue and hyponatremia reported.

D. Gabapentin has emerged as front-line treatment for neuropathic pain because of its favorable safety profile with minimal concern for drug interactions and interference with liver enzymes. It does not appear to affect γ-aminobutyric acid (GABA) receptors and is believed to bind to the alpha-2-delta subunit of N-type calcium channels, suppressing neuronal hyperexcitability by preventing calcium influx and the release of various neurotransmitters from presynaptic terminals. The initial dose should be 300 mg/day to 300 mg t.i.d. with increase by 300 mg/day while maintaining t.i.d. dosing. Effective dosages range from 1800 mg/day to 4800 mg/day. Gabapentin has gained popularity because of its tolerability, with common adverse effects limited to somnolence, dizziness, ataxia, and fatigue, which are dose dependent. Dosage adjustment is necessary in renal impairment.

E. Lamotrigine is a promising AED for treatment of pain because of its antinociceptive effects resulting from sodium channel blockade and inhibition of release of the excitatory neurotransmitters glutamate and aspartate. The initial dose is 25 mg/day with gradual titration to 25 mg b.i.d. for 2 weeks, then to 50 mg b.i.d. for 2 weeks, then increased by 100 mg/week. The effective dose ranges from 200 to 500 mg/day with greater efficacy at doses above 300 mg/day. Adverse effects include dizziness, somnolence, headache, ataxia, nausea, and rarely serious skin rashes. Topiramate is another new AED shown to be effective for neuropathic pain. It blocks sodium channels, enhances GABA effects, and blocks glutamate receptors. The starting dose is 25 to 50 mg/day with increases by 25 to 50 mg/week and target dose of 50 to 500 mg/day b.i.d. Adverse effects are somnolence, dizziness, ataxia, confusion, speech disorders, and weight loss. The dose may need to be adjusted in renal failure. Zonisamide is another novel AED that may be useful for treatment of chronic pain. It has several mechanisms including sodium and calcium channel blockade, scavenging of free radicals, enhancement of serotonergic transmission, and inhibition of nitric oxide formation. Treatment is initiated at 100 mg/day with an increase to 200 mg/day after 2 weeks, then increased by 300 mg/day for 2 weeks, then increased by 100 mg/week with target dose of 100 to 500 mg/day administered b.i.d. or q.h.s. It is a sulfonamide and thus poses a risk for serious hematologic and dermatologic reactions. The incidence of these effects has so far been extremely low. It is structurally different from sulfonamide antibiotics and no cross-reactivity has been seen. Rash occurs at a background rate of 2%, with the most common side effects being somnolence, dizziness, and weight loss. Levetiracetam is another new AED that is not well studied, but in a few case reports has demonstrated improvement in pain symptoms and sleep with few side effects. Doses ranged from 500 to 3000 mg/day usually dosed b.i.d. with greater efficacy in the higher end of the range.

Selection of a particular AED is usually a result of careful consideration of multiple factors including proven efficacy, adverse effects, potential drug interactions, and cost. Serious thought must be given to whether or not a particular AED has been tried previously, and if an appropriate dosage administered and time interval for evaluation of efficacy allowed. Mechanism of action of the agent used must be considered, especially when switching or adding AEDs. Intravenous testing with local anesthetic may predict response to therapy of AEDs, especially those that block sodium channels, and is described in detail in Chapter 16, p. 34.

REFERENCES

Namaka M, Gramlich CR, Ruhlen D, et al: A treatment algorithm for neuropathic pain. *Clin Ther* 2004;26:951–979.

Pappagallo M: Newer antiepileptic drugs: Possible uses in treatment of neuropathic pain and migraine. *Clin Ther* 2003;25:2506–2538.

Patients requiring ANTICONVULSANTS

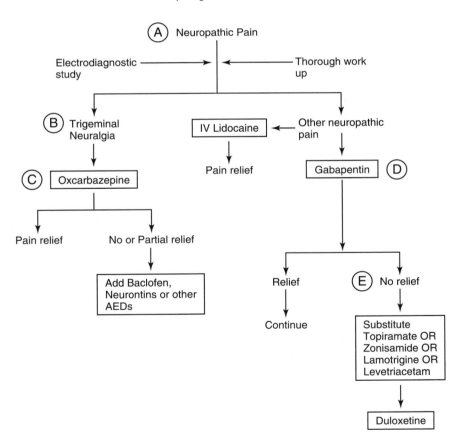

Opioids

EULECHE ALANMANOU

Opioid drugs are frequently used in the treatment of acute pain and pain of malignant origin. It is in the area of chronic noncancer pain that controversies persist. Opioids produce analgesia by binding to opioid receptors both within and outside the central nervous system. Opioid receptors include mu, kappa, and delta receptors. Mu receptors mediate supraspinal analgesia, euphoria, depressed respiration, and physical dependence. Kappa receptors mediate spinal analgesia, miosis, and sedation. Delta receptors mediate spinal analgesia and modulate mu receptor activity. Opioid analgesics are classified as full agonists and mixed agonist/antagonists, depending on the manner in which they interact with opioid receptors. Methadone was shown to also block N-methyl-D-aspartate (NMDA) receptor (involved in nociceptive processing and the phenomenon of wind-up).

A. Oral administration with immediate or sustained release of opioids remains the method of choice. The use of alternative routes of administration (transdermal, transmucosal, parenteral, neuraxial) depends on individual patient circumstances. Opioids undergo biotransformation, and most of their metabolites are excreted by the kidneys. Morphine's metabolite, M6G, accumulates after morphine administration to patients with renal insufficiency. Normeperidine, which is a metabolite of meperidine, also accumulates in patients with poor renal function. This is why hydromorphone, fentanyl, and methadone are preferred to morphine in chronic pain patients with poor renal function.

   Before prescribing opioids, it is important to classify the pain as acute or chronic, nociceptive or neuropathic. Age, gender, and renal and hepatic function must be taken into account. A precise diagnosis of the cause of pain is preferred. A psychiatric evaluation should precede the initiation of opioid therapy when a patient has a history of psychiatric illness. It is important to remember that a patient with a history of drug or alcohol abuse can suffer from chronic pain just like anybody else. This patient should be referred to a multidisciplinary clinic (ideally including an addiction specialist).

B. The correct dose of an opioid is that which effectively relieves pain without inducing unacceptable side effects. Opioids are administered around the clock, and additional doses are available for breakthrough pain. Constipation is a common side effect in patients undergoing opioid therapy. These patients should receive prophylactic therapy with stool softener, often in combination with bulk-forming agents, osmotic laxatives, or stimulant cathartics.

C. Other side effects of opioids, including sedation, respiratory depression, nausea and vomiting, cognitive impairment, myoclonus, pruritus, and urinary retention, should be treated when they occur. Prophylaxis is not indicated. When tolerance to an opioid develops, another opioid may be substituted to provide better analgesia because the cross-tolerance among opioids is incomplete. It is recommended, however, that the calculated dose be reduced by 25% to 50% to account for that incomplete cross-tolerance when converting between opioids (based on clinical studies the methadone dose should be reduced by 75% to 90%). If switching to transdermal fentanyl, reducing the equianalgesic dose is not necessary because a safety factor has been incorporated in the conversion guidelines during the development of this formulation.

D. To reduce opioid requirements, nonopioid analgesics (acetaminophen, nonsteroidal anti-inflammatory drugs), adjuvant analgesics (antidepressants, α_2-adrenergic agonists, NMDA receptor blockers, anticonvulsants, topical analgesics), or both could be added. Neuropathic pain may be the most common target of adjuvant analgesic therapy.

E. Findings indicate that opioid therapy for chronic noncancer pain does not necessarily lead to problematic drug use. An opioid agreement is recommended before an opioid trial, which could last 3 months. Assessment during opioid use includes the analgesic effect, level of function, side effects, and aberrant behavior. Factors that tend to decrease opioid responsiveness include a neuropathic mechanism, the presence of severe breakthrough pain, psychological distress, and any factor that predisposes the patient to side effects (e.g., advanced age, major organ failure). More research is needed to help predict which individual is best suited for opioid therapy of chronic noncancer pain.

REFERENCES

Bruera E, Schoeller T, Wenk R, et al: A prospective multicenter assessment of the Edmonton staging system for cancer pain. *J Pain Symptom Manage* 1995;10:348–355.

Cherny NI, Thaler HT, Friedlander-Klar H, et al: Opioid responsiveness of cancer pain syndromes caused by neuropathic or nociceptive mechanisms. *Neurology* 1994;44:857–861.

Gourlay GK: Clinical pharmacology of opioids in the treatment of pain. In: Giamberardino MA (ed) *Pain 2002—An Updated Review: Refresher Course Syllabus.* Seattle, IASP Press, 2002.

Kalso E, Allan L, Dellemihn PL, et al: Recommendations for using opioids in chronic non-cancer pain. *Eur J Pain* 2003;7:381–386.

Portenoy RK: Clinical strategies for the management of cancer pain poorly responsive to systemic opioid therapy. In: Giamberardino MA (ed) *Pain 2002—An Updated Review: Refresher Course Syllabus.* Seattle, IASP Press, 2002.

OPIOIDS

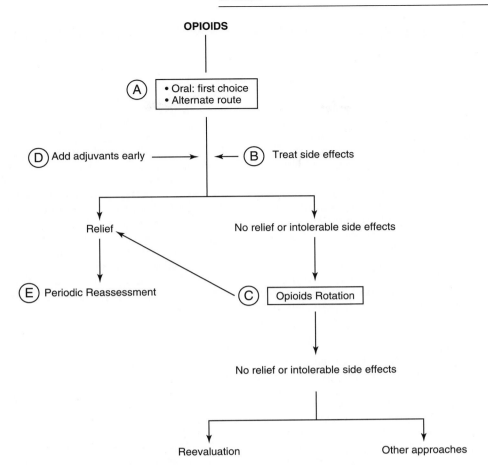

Botulinum Toxin—Pharmacology

NIKESH BATRA

Clostridium botulinum produces a potent neuromuscular toxin, with seven distinct serotypes, A through G. The serotypes currently available in the market are A and B. Serotype A is U.S. Food and Drug Administration (FDA)-approved for treating cervical dystonia, strabismus, blepharospasm, and facial nerve disorders. Serotype B is approved for treating cervical dystonia only.

Although more than 60 uses of botulinum toxin have been reported, few are supported by level-one research. Among the uses for botulinum toxin found in the literature are treatment for focal dystonias, spasticity, nondystonic disorders of involuntary muscle activity (e.g., tremors, tics, myoclonus, strabismus, nystagmus), disorders of localized muscle spasm, low back pain, myofascial pain syndrome, headaches, smooth muscle hyperactive disorders (e.g., detrusor sphincter dyssynergia, achalasia cardia, Hirschsprung's disease), proctalgia fugax, hyperkinetic facial lines, brow wrinkles, and sweating disorders.

Among the seven serotypes of botulinum toxin, human botulism consists mainly of serotypes A, B, and E and of F and G in rare cases. Serotypes C and D are found to cause toxicity in animals only. The seven botulinum serotypes are produced as single-chain polypeptides, with a total molecular weight of approximately 150 kDa. During fermentation, endogenous bacterial proteases nick the serotype structure to form two chains: a heavy chain (~100 kDa) and a light chain (~50 kDa), linked by a disulfide bond.

The heavy chain from each serotype functions as a unique receptor recognition and binding site on the motor nerve terminal, allowing transport into the motor neuron. The regions of these heavy chains are sufficiently different to prevent competitive binding. The light chain from each serotype targets the docking proteins and contains the catalytic domain that results in the inhibition of acetylcholine release.

These docking proteins, also known as the SNARE complex, are an acronym for "SNAP (soluble *n*-ethylmaleimide sensitive factor *attachment protein) receptor complex.*" This group of proteins controls the docking and fusion of the neurotransmitter vesicle with the presynaptic membrane as well as the release of acetylcholine. All the botulinum serotypes share the same mechanism of action, with the net result of inhibiting acetylcholine release into the synaptic cleft. There are three steps in this process: binding, internalization, and toxic action.

A. Binding: (1) heavy-chain-mediated neurospecific binding of the toxin; and (2) toxin binding to specific receptors on the cholinergic neuron

B. Internalization: internalization of the toxin by receptor-mediated endocytosis

C. Toxic action: ATP- and pH-dependent translocation of the light chain to the neuronal cytosol, where the light chain functions as a zinc-dependent endoprotease, cleaving polypeptides essential for neurotransmitter release

Each serotype of the botulinum toxin acts at a specific cleavage site on the SNARE complex. Serotypes A and E cleave the SNAP 25 molecule. Serotypes B, D, F, and G cleave synaptobrevin (vesicle-associated membrane protein, or VAMP) at specific sites. Serotype C_1 cleaves syntaxin and SNAP 25, acetylcholine release is inhibited, the nerve impulses no longer cause the muscles to contract. Over time, the nerve creates new extensions; this phenomenon is called "sprouting." The effect of botulinum toxin "wears off" when these new nerve terminals establish contact with the muscles. Botulinum toxin injections typically result in a dose-dependent reduction of hyperactive muscle contraction. The onset of clinical effect is 3 to 10 days; it peaks in 2 weeks and lasts for 3 to 6 months.

Several animal studies have shown an association between abnormal spindle physiology and painful muscular conditions. Botulinum neurotoxins delivered at doses smaller than the doses used to treat hypertonia may be sufficient for weakening and resetting the intrinsic (spindle) fibers. This method is effective for pain relief associated with spasticity or dystonia by creating a combination of local muscle paralysis and decreased muscle tone.

In cases of head and neck pain, botulinum toxin may be injected into the temporalis, splenius capitus, levator scapulae, and paravertebral muscles of the neck. In cases of low back pain, lumbar strain, and spasm of muscular origin, the toxin may be injected into the localized trigger points and the piriformis, psoas, quadratus lumborum, gluteal, and paravertebral muscles. However, conventional trigger point injections with botulinum toxin provide pain relief for only a brief period. Botulinum toxin therefore should never be the first line of treatment; it should be utilized only after conservative treatment (including physical therapy and appropriate medications) have been tried without success.

Botulinum toxins are usually injected in a tuberculin syringe with a 25- to 30-gauge needle. For most muscles, the use of electromyography or motor point stimulation is recommended. Side effects with botulinum toxin injections are usually transient, well tolerated, and amenable to treatment. Most complications are related to diffusion or inadvertent injection (e.g., dysphagia or neck weakness following treatment of cervical dystonia; hoarseness and aspiration following treatment of spasmodic aphonia). Generalized weakness mimicking botulism is rare. Pain on injection and a flu-like syndrome, especially after the first injection, has been reported. Brachial plexopathy is a rare complication. Development of antibodies is a problem that leads to therapeutic failure, especially in patients who were initially responsive to botulinum toxin therapy. Antibodies usually develop if later doses of the toxin are used within short intervals. They can be detected by an enzyme-linked immunosorbent assay or an in vivo neutralization assay in mice, which is a more reliable method. Patients with antibodies to one type of botulinum toxin may be responsive to the other types.

Contraindications are hypersensitivity to botulinum toxin or infection at the site of the injection. Relative contraindications include pregnancy: It is a pregnancy class C drug, and abortion or fetal malformation have been reported in rabbit studies. It is also contraindicated in lactating patients, those with coexisting neuromuscular diseases, and in the presence of profound atrophy of the contractors. Botulinum toxin may interact with aminoglycosides and other drugs that interfere with neuromuscular transmission.

REFERENCES

Coffield JA, Considine RV, Simpson LL: The site and mechanism of action of botulinum neurotoxin. In: Jankovic J, Hallett M (eds) *Therapy with Botulinum Toxin.* New York, Marcel Dekker, 1994, pp 3-13.

Das Gupta BR: The structure of botulinum neurotoxin. In: Simpson LL (ed) *Botulinum Neurotoxins and Tetanus Toxin.* San Diego, Academic Press, 1989, pp 53–67.

Martin K, Childers DO: Botulinum toxin in pain management. *eMed J* 2001;2(5).

Raj PP: Botulinum toxin in the treatment of pain associated with musculoskeletal hyperactivity. *Curr Rev Pain* 1997;1:403–416.

Van den Bergh P, Francart J, Mourin S, et al: Five-year experience in the treatment of focal movement disorders with low dose Dysport botulinum toxin. *Muscle Nerve* 1995;18:720–729.

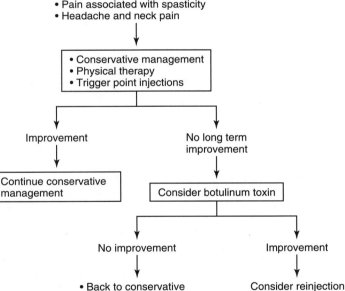

BOTULINUM TOXIN IN PAIN MANAGEMENT

Neurolytic Agents

SERGIO ALVARADO

The use of neurolytic agents in the treatment of pain was first described in 1863 by Luton, who injected irritants subcutaneously into painful areas that produced analgesia for sciatic neuralgia. Dogliotti described subarachnoid chemical neurolysis with alcohol for sciatica in 1931. Maher described use of hyperbaric phenol and silver nitrate for intrathecal neurolysis in 1956. As a result of an increased understanding of pain mechanisms; development of novel pharmacologic agents; and widespread use of opioids, anticonvulsants, antidepressants, and other adjunctive analgesics, neurolytic blocks are less commonly used. Chemical neurolysis is reserved for a small percentage of cancer patients via subarachnoid block (SAB) and sympathectomy with primarily two agents: alcohol and phenol. Cryoablation and radiofrequency lesioning are two forms of physical neurolysis that have evolved recently, with radiofrequency gaining increasing popularity. Surgical lesioning, especially for sympathectomy, and stereotactic radiosurgery for trigeminal neuralgia are other physical techniques in use.

A. Chemical neurolysis is most useful in cancer pain, especially visceral and somatic pain. It appears to be less effective for neuropathic pain. Intrathecal neurolysis in particular is more useful for somatic pain such as chest wall and peritoneum in comparison to visceral sources including pancreatic, gastric, and rectal. Chemical agents are also effective for neurolysis of the Gasserian ganglion in trigeminal neuralgia. Pain due to ligaments, graft donor sites, peripheral nerves, cervical and lumbar facet joints, and radicular pain can be treated with cryoneurolysis, while central nervous system (CNS) lesions, cranial nerves, sympathetically mediated pain, facet pain of any spinal level, radicular pain, and sacroiliac pain may be more amenable to radiofrequency lesioning. More conservative treatments should be tried before considering neurolysis. Significant pain relief with diagnostic small-volume local anesthetic blocks should be documented. Absolute contraindications include coagulopathy and local infection of the area.

B. Cryoneurolysis involves neurodestruction by exposing nerves to extremely low temperatures via placement of a cryo probe into the area. Modern machines include a nerve stimulator function to localize the site of intended effect. Two or three 2-minute cycles are usually sufficient. Most commonly a 1.3-mm probe is passed via a 16-gauge catheter. Prolonged conduction block occurs when the nerve is frozen at $-5°$ to $-20°$C. This causes axonal disintegration and breakdown of myelin sheaths. Wallerian degeneration occurs with the perineurium and epineurium remaining intact. Regeneration is accurate and complete. Recovery depends on the rate of axonal regeneration (1 to 3 mm/day) and the distance of the cryolesion from the end organ.

C. Radiofrequency (RF) technology offers potential advantages for lesioning the CNS as well as peripheral structures. Precise temperature control and lesion size, stimulation of sensory and motor nerves, monitoring of impedance, and recording of these parameters are all important factors. The traditional RF process involves applying RF current to tissue via an active electrode tip with heating being primarily an ionic process. In essence, the tissues adjacent to the electrode tip heat the electrode as the current moves through body tissues and exits the grounding system. A broad range of temperatures has been advocated, with the most common between $67°$C and $80°$C. It is thought that temperatures above $45°$C produce tissue damage. Alternatively, pulsed RF, a relatively recent development by Sluijter, can be used without destruction of tissue. It involves the application of two 20-millisecond RF cycles delivered each second, allowing for the electromagnetic process of RF current to take effect while temperatures remain below $42°$C. The prevailing explanation for the beneficial effects is that the electromagnetic field created by the RF current induces antinociceptive metabolic changes as opposed to the thermal effects with traditional RF. At this time there are no studies comparing the two modalities.

D. Phenol is a neurolytic agent with local anesthetic properties. It is prepared as a 3% to 12% solution, with concentrations greater than 6.7% requiring addition of glycerin. There is a direct relationship between concentration and destruction. Injection produces a biphasic action with initial warmth and numbness followed by nonselective destruction. The full effect is noted on the first day with the quality and extent of analgesia diminishing over the first 24 hours. Phenol is directly neurotoxic. The duration of the effect is variable but is usually at least 2 months. It can cause CNS depression and ultimately cardiovascular collapse; however, clinical doses of 10 ml of 10% solution rarely produce serious systemic toxicity. Potential advantages over alcohol are its compatibility with contrast dyes and its comparatively rapid onset, allowing assessment of analgesia within 24 hours.

E. Alcohol is commercially available as a 100% solution and can be combined with local anesthetic. It has been suggested that at least a 35% to 50% concentration is needed for destruction. In contrast to phenol, it is hypobaric in comparison to cerebrospinal fluid (CSF) with a specific gravity of 0.789 to 0.807. This will determine positioning of the patient when performing subarachnoid injection. A 40% alcohol has neurolytic potency approximately equivalent to that of a 3% phenol solution. It produces a burning sensation on injection that can be useful to localize dermatomal level when used intrathecally. Alternatively, local anesthetic can be given prior to alcohol to minimize the burning, which may be useful for celiac blocks. It exerts its effects

NEUROLYTIC AGENTS

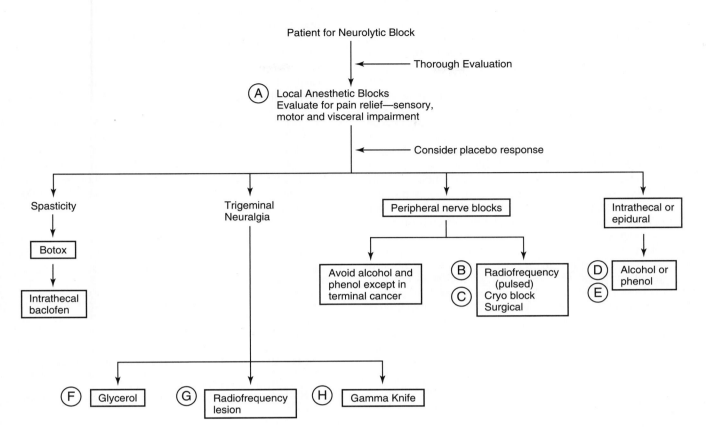

via dehydration with resultant sclerosis of nerve fibers and myelin sheaths. It may spare the neural tube allowing for regeneration along the axonal course, enabling return of neural function and thus pain. After intrathecal injection, the patient should remain in the same position for 1 hour. The full onset of effect is 3 to 5 days with duration variable and one series reporting relief of at least 6 months in 50% of 57 patients. There are no studies directly comparing alcohol and phenol that support the use of one over the other. Ability of the patient to be positioned may determine which agent is used based on baricity for neurolytic SAB. Complications are discussed elsewhere, with the most serious ones being loss of bowel, bladder, or motor function. Cancer patients may be willing to accept those effects if they are rendered pain-free and thorough discussion must precede any injection.

F. Glycerol is a mild neurolytic alcohol that appears to have unique properties suited to trigeminal ganglion block. Its mechanism of action is not well understood. Bennett and Lunsford hypothesized that glycerol preferentially affects the damaged myelinated axons responsible for the symptoms of trigeminal neuralgia. One hundred percent glycerol is used for neurolytic Gasserian rhizotomy, although radiofrequency techniques are gaining popularity. There are no long-term data supporting one over the other; however, there appears to be a lower complication rate with glycerol.

G. Surgical lesioning, including dorsal root entry zone (DREZ) lesioning and cordotomy, can be effective therapy. However, with the advent of less invasive physical methods, surgery is often reserved for refractory cases.

H. Stereotactic radiosurgery, or Gamma Knife radiosurgery, is an effective treatment for trigeminal neuralgia, and is associated with the lowest incidence of complications of any of the neurolytic treatments.

Neurolytic agents can provide prolonged analgesia in many pain syndromes. Chemical agents offer predictable and reliable efficacy with a greater potential for complications since there is less control of the lesion in comparison to physical techniques. A thorough discussion of the potential risks and benefits of any neurolytic procedure should occur prior to proceeding.

REFERENCES

Candido K, Stevens RA: Intrathecal neurolytic blocks for the relief of cancer pain. *Best Pract Res Clin Anesthesiol* 2003;17:407–428.

de Leon-Casasola OA, Ditonto E: Drugs commonly used for nerve blocking: Neurolytic agents. In: Raj PP (ed) *Practical Management of Pain*, 3rd ed. St. Louis, Mosby, 2000, pp. 575–578.

Lopez BC, Hamlyn PJ, Zakrewska JM: Systematic review of ablative neurosurgical techniques for the treatment of trigeminal neuralgia. *Neurosurgery* 2004;54:973–983.

Saberski L, Fitzgerald J, Ahmad M: Cryoneurolysis and radiofrequency lesioning. In: Raj PP (ed) *Practical Management of Pain*, 3rd ed. St. Louis, Mosby, 2000, pp. 753–767.

Sluijter M: Radiofrequency, Part I: Flivopress SA. Switzerland, Meggan (LU); 2001.

Topical Agents

LEY L. TAYLOR-JONES AND EULECHE ALANMANOU

Numerous topical agents are used in the pain management setting. When determining which product(s) to use, one needs an accurate diagnosis, familiarity with the currently available agents, and knowledge about their mechanisms of action. The most common pain syndromes managed with these products include herpes zoster, postherpetic neuralgia, diabetic neuropathies, human immunodeficiency virus neuropathies, scar pain, and muscle and joint pain.

A. The most commonly used topical agents can be categorized into five groups. Local anesthetics comprise the largest group, with a large variety of forms and routes of administration. They are divided into ester and amide classes; both classes produce a conduction blockade of the sodium channels in the resting state. Other groups include capsacin, aspirin mixed with a vehicle for delivery, clonidine, and over-the-counter balms and ointments.

   1. Ester anesthetics include cocaine, benzocaine, cetacaine, and tetracaine. Cocaine blocks the reuptake of norepinephrine, giving it unique vasoconstrictive properties. Although the vasoconstrictive properties of this drug are useful in the oral and nasal mucosa, cocaine is not without drawbacks, including its high toxicity and addictive properties. Benzocaine exists as a nonionized base, with an acid ionization constant well below the physiologic range. This property makes it nearly insoluble in water, which limits its use to topical anesthesia. It has a rapid onset and short duration of action. Cetacaine is a combination product of two ester local anesthetics: 14% benzocaine and 2% tetracaine. This spray has a rapid onset and a short duration of action and is indicated for anesthesia of any mucous membrane except the eyes. Tetracaine can also be found in other preparations, usually in a 2% mixture. Side effects include those limited to local anesthetics.

   2. Lidocaine is a widely used amide anesthetic; it provides analgesia by blocking neuronal sodium channels. It is found in 4%, 5%, and 10% concentrations and can be applied to mucous membranes. Lidoderm, available in a patch form, contains 5% lidocaine (700 mg) and is often used for postherpetic neuralgia. It is applied to the skin over areas of chronic pain. Lidocaine EMLA is a eutectic mixture of local anesthetics, containing 2.5% prilocaine and 2.5% lidocaine in a cream or a disk form. It is commonly applied to the skin before intravenous cannulation and dermal procedures. The cream provides dermal analgesia by releasing prilocaine and lidocaine into the epidermal and dermal layers of the skin, which then accumulates in the vicinity of dermal pain receptors and nerve endings. There are ongoing studies examining the efficacy of EMLA for postherpetic neuralgia. Side effects are limited to those common to all local anesthetics.

   3. Capsaicin is believed to deplete substance p from nociceptive primary afferents leading to a local desensitization; and therefore it can be used for a variety of painful states including postherpetic neuralgia, painful diabetic neuropathy, Guillain-Barré syndrome, postsurgical pain states, and painful joints and muscles. Capsaicin does have a number of adverse side effects, including a burning sensation upon application, itching, rash, and irritation of mucous membranes. If the cream is aerosolized, it may elicit bronchospasm.

   4. Topical aspirin, mixed in chloroform or diethyl ether, is another formulation that has been used successfully for treating herpes zoster, postherpetic neuralgia, and musculoskeletal pain. Its mechanism of action is inhibition of prostaglandin synthesis. Systemic poisoning can occur from a topical application to large areas of skin.

   5. Clonidine is an α_2-adrenergic partial agonist. A peripheral neuropathic pain state has been suggested to present abnormal adrenergic sensitivity. Topical clonidine may help decrease the ectopic impulses by reducing the release of norepinephrine from sympathetic nerve terminals.

B. There are numerous over-the-counter balms, ointments, and creams used topically for pain relief. Many of these drugs contain menthol or local anesthetics.

REFERENCES

Goodman & Gilman's The Pharmacological Basis of Therapeutics. 9th ed. New York, McGraw-Hill, 1996;680–689.

King RB: Concerning the management of pain associated with herpes zoster and of postherpetic neuralgia. *Pain* 1988;33:73–78.

Minami T, Bakoshi S, Nakano H, et al: The effects of capsaicin cream of prostaglandin-induced allodynia. *Anesth Analg* 2001;93; 419–423.

Raj PP (ed): *Practical Management of Pain,* 3rd ed. St. Louis, Mosby, 2000, p 924.

TOPICAL AGENTS

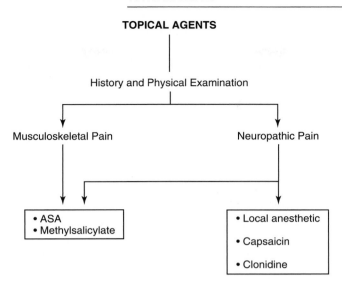

THERAPEUTIC MODALITIES

Physical Therapy

Transcutaneous Electrical Nerve Stimulation

Occupational Therapy

Vocational Rehabilitation

Evaluation and Preparation for Regional Anesthesia

Peripheral Nerve Stimulators

Peripheral Nerve Blocks

Pediatric Extremity Blocks

Epidural Block

Subarachnoid Block

Cranial Nerve Block

Sympathetic Blocks

Continuous Neural Block

Intravenous Regional Block

Steroid Joint Injections

Epidural Steroid Injections

Radiographic Contrast Media

Intradiscal Therapies

Epidural Endoscopy

Intravertebral Analgesics

Complications of Neurolytic Blocks

Cryoanalgesia

Radiofrequency Ablation

Spinal Cord Stimulation

Neurosurgical Procedures for Pain

Prosthetic Support

Psychological Interventions

Biofeedback

Hypnosis

Acupuncture

Weaning Opioid and Sedative Hypnotic Drugs

Physical Therapy

JAMES G. GRIFFIN

There are a variety of physical modalities used by therapists for treating pain. The following is a brief description of some of those that are more commonly used, the indications for their use, and recommended precautions.

A. *Superficial heat.* Heat is probably the most commonly used physical therapy modality. Heat increases blood flow and tissue distensibility. Heat decreases muscle spasm and produces analgesia, apparently through the action of cutaneous receptors. Heat is indicated in cases of chronic stiffness, spasm, and pain. By increasing blood flow and tissue distensibility, heat is generally helpful before stretching or exercise. Hot packs, heating pads, paraffin baths, or whirlpools can be used to deliver heat. A modality called "fluidotherapy" uses particles of finely ground cellulose suspended in hot air (120°F) circulating through a cabinet. The limb is inserted in the cabinet, and range-of-motion exercise may be done during treatment. Chronic use of a heating pad often results in a nonreversible mottling of the skin (erythema ab igne), which is seen in persons who use heat many hours a day.

Contraindications for the use of heat are sensory impairment, circulatory insufficiency, malignancy, and infection. Care should also be taken with elderly patients whose sensation and judgment may be suspect (Michlovitz 1986).

B. *Deep heat.* Ultrasound is produced by electrical stimulation of a quartz or artificial crystal, which vibrates in response. At 1 MHz, the most commonly used frequency, tissue penetration to 5 cm occurs. The rapid vibration of the tissue by the sound waves produces heat, with the maximum effect occurring at the junction of bone and muscle. Clinical studies have shown ultrasound to be effective for treating the following: frozen shoulder, postamputation pain, decubitus ulcer healing, and complex regional pain syndrome. Ultrasound is safe for use with implants and does not increase their temperature. Contraindications for the use of ultrasound include malignancy, circulatory impairment, pregnancy, impaired sensation, and infection; it also may not be used over the eye (Griffin and Karselis 1982).

Shortwave and microwave diathermy produce heating of the tissue to a depth of 3 to 4 cm. Shortwave diathermy produces a high-frequency alternating signal at 27.12 MHz, whereas microwave diathermy is produced at 2450 MHz with a magnetron tube. Both types are nonionizing electromagnetic radiation, and they have no effect on nerves or contractile tissue. Indications for use are those for any other form of thermotherapy. The advantage of diathermy is the depth of penetration it provides. Care must be taken to keep metal out of the electromagnetic field during treatment; moreover, patients with any metallic implant should not be treated. Areas of high fluid volume, such as the eyes or joint effusions, can potentially overheat. Pregnancy, ischemic tissue, and pain or sensory deficit are other contraindications (Kloth 1986).

C. *Cold.* Cold decreases pain, spasm, and swelling; it also decreases nerve conduction velocity. Cold is generally used to treat acute injury or acute exacerbation of chronic injuries. Many chronic pain patients who have not tried cold may find it effective for their pain or for a temporary exacerbation following activity or exercise.

Ice bags, ice massage, or reusable cold packs are most commonly used for cold application. Treatment time for cold application is 10 to 20 minutes or until the area is numb. Following treatment, the area should be red or pink, insensitive to touch, and cool. Care must be taken when treating extremities or tissue over superficial nerves, such as the ulnar or peroneal nerves. Precautions include impaired sensation or circulation and cold intolerance (Griffin and Karselis 1982). Cold spray, such as ethyl chloride or fluromethane, is used in conjunction with stretching for treatment of myofascial pain (Travell and Simmons 1983).

Contrast baths, using two containers or whirlpools is advocated for treating the extremities for sprains, strains, arthritis, and some cases of peripheral vascular disease. The extremity is immersed alternately in warm water (40°C) and then cool water (15°C) at a time ratio of 3:1 or 4:1 for 30 minutes, finishing in the warm water. In theory, this increases circulation in the extremity, although no adequately performed studies are in the literature (Walsh 1986).

D. *Electrical stimulation.* Electrical stimulation is provided with either direct current or alternating current. Direct-current devices are now commonly used only for stimulation of denervated muscle and to drive medication subcutaneously (iontophoresis). Most of the devices on the market use some form of alternating current (AC), with the waveform electronically modified to the desired parameters. AC devices produce low total current (milliamps) and do not produce thermal or chemical effects. Most AC devices produce high-voltage output (designated as >150 volts) with a monophasic waveform and allow adjustment of intensity, pulse rate and pulse width. Clinical guidelines for high-voltage stimulation are available for treating acute and chronic conditions, including pain, joint effusion, muscle spasm, muscle disuse atrophy, circulatory disorders, and wound healing (Alon 1987). "Interferential current" supposedly avoids the cutaneous discomfort of traditional electrical stimulation by using a high-frequency carrier current that cannot be felt on the skin and is canceled out at the site of treatment, leaving a lower therapeutic frequency. There are clinical guidelines for treatment of acute and chronic pain conditions, including orthopedic and vascular disorders, peripheral neuritis, and urinary incontinence. Contraindications for electrical stimulation include use of a pacemaker, directing it across the pregnant uterus, stimulating the carotid sinus, systemic infection, and malignancy (Travell and Simmons 1983).

Transcutaneous electrical nerve stimulation (TENS) is considered a special form of electrical stimulation, but any electrical stimulation is TENS (Alon 1987). Two mechanisms may explain TENS' effect. Melzack and Wall proposed the "gate theory," where stimulation of the larger nerve fibers overwhelms the input of the smaller "C" fibers at the spinal level. TENS' effects have been shown to be reversible with opiate and serotonin antagonists, suggesting that it stimulates the body's endogenous opiates. TENS has been shown to be effective for alleviating acute pain, postoperative pain, and numerous chronic pain conditions. Numerous clinical usage guides are available (Klein and Pariser 1987; Ottoson and Lundberg 1988).

E. *Phonophoresis/iontophoresis.* Phonophoresis is the use of ultrasound to drive medication through the skin. Iontophoresis is the use of direct current to achieve the same purpose. Any ultrasound device may be used for this purpose, and battery-powered commercial devices are available for performing iontophoresis. Local anesthetic and steroid medications (lidocaine, salicylate, cortisone) are typically used for painful inflammatory conditions. Both of these methods have shown to be clinically effective for treating superficial bursitis, tendinitis, ligamentous strain, and painful trigger points; they may also be useful when an injection would not be tolerated. Precautions are necessary regarding drug allergies and side effects as well as any of the precautions assumed for the use of ultrasound or electrical stimulation (Cummings 1987; Greenman 1989).

F. *Traction.* Traction, in various modes, has been shown to be effective for treating cervical and lumbar disc disorders, muscle spasm, hypomobility, and osteoarthritis of the lumbar and cervical spine. Continuous traction is often used with bed rest, primarily to keep patients immobile, as the amount of weight commonly used is insufficient to cause any sort of physical distraction of the cervical or lumbar vertebrae. Positional traction can be achieved by specific self-positioning by the patient to relieve pain. Gravity traction for the low back can achieve distraction forces of up to 40% of the individual's body weight. Manual traction can be done for both the cervical and lumbar spine to determine the effectiveness of treatment or in cases where the patient does not tolerate mechanical traction. Autotraction is a modality developed in Sweden that utilizes gravity traction and three-dimensional positional traction to treat lumbar disc problems (Saunders 1986).

Intermittent mechanical traction is most commonly used and is typically done on an outpatient basis using a special pelvic or cervical harness. Lumbar traction requires a pull of 50% or more of body weight to achieve vertebral distraction. Lumbar traction can be administered supine or prone with varying degrees of flexion and utilizing a bilateral or unilateral pull (Saunders 1986).

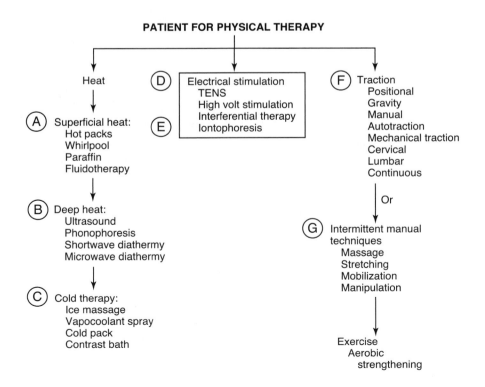

Cervical traction requires a minimum pull of 25 pounds to achieve separation of the posterior elements of the cervical spine with the neck in 25 to 30 degrees of flexion. Distraction of the atlanto-occipital and atlanto-axial joints requires only 10 pounds of pull in a neutral position. Symptomatic relief may be achieved at lower levels. Cervical traction has traditionally used a harness that fits on the head and can be administered in the sitting or supine position. The Saunders harness is more comfortable and applies no pressure on the chin or temporomandibular joint. This apparatus requires the patient to be supine and allows traction to be done with a straight pull or in flexion or side bending (DeLacerda 1986).

Contraindications for traction are instability secondary to tumor, disease, or infection; vascular compromise; and situations in which movement is contraindicated. Relative contraindications are recent sprain or strain, osteoporosis, hiatal hernia, and pregnancy; another contraindication is if the patient exhibits any increase in neurologic symptoms with treatment. Patients with claustrophobia may not tolerate the restrictive nature of this treatment (DeLacerda 1986; Saunders 1986).

G. *Manual therapy*. A variety of manual techniques can be applied as part of the treatment of pain. Massage, in its many forms, can be useful for encouraging circulation and promoting venous and lymphatic return. Cross-friction massage is used to break down soft tissue adhesions and restore mobility to fascia, muscle, tendons, and ligaments. Specific manual techniques (myofascial release) can stretch the skin, fascia, and connective tissues to increase motion and pliability and to treat pain (accupressure) (Deyo et al. 1990). Stretching, whether performed manually or done by the patient, is important when treating muscle and connective tissue shortening of primary musculoskeletal injury or secondary myofascial pain (Travell and Simmons 1983).

Joint hypomobility can be assessed and treated with manual techniques. Repetitive oscillation of a joint can be used to increase range and improve the "quality" of a joint's motion. Specific mobilizing motions or contract–relax stretching (muscle energy techniques) can be used to improve joint range of motion. Such techniques exist for most of the synovial joints of the body. Manipulation is mobilization with impulse, where the motion barrier is met and thrust through to achieve more normal joint motion (Deyo et al. 1990). Manipulation is possible in many joints of the body

and is advocated as the treatment for specific musculoskeletal disorders in such disparate areas such as the low back and foot (Kirkkaldy-Willis 1988; Newell and Woodle 1981).

The manual techniques represent a continuum of treatment techniques that are indicated for musculoskeletal pain. Precautions for soft tissue techniques include open wounds, recent surgery, and infection. For joint mobilization and manipulative techniques, the precautions also include osteoporosis, pregnancy, and active inflammatory processes in the joint. Contraindications for manipulation are tumor, malignancy, segmental instability, and neurologic deficit.

REFERENCES

Alon G: Principles of electrical stimulation. In: Nelson R, Currier D (eds) *Clinical Electrotherapy*. Los Altos, CA, Appleton & Lange, 1987.

Cummings J: Iontophoresis. In: Nelson R, Currier D (eds) *Clinical Electrotherapy*. Los Altos, CA, Appleton & Lange, 1987.

DeLacerda FG: Cervical traction. In: Grieve GP (ed) *Modern Manual Therapy of the Vertebral Column*. New York, Churchill Livingstone, 1986.

Deyo RA, Walsh NE, Martin DC, et al: A controlled trial of transcutaneous electrical nerve stimulation (TENS) and exercise for chronic low back pain. *N Engl J Med* 1990;322:1627–1634.

Greenman PE: *Principles of Manual Medicine*. Baltimore, Williams & Wilkins, 1989.

Griffin J, Karselis P: *Physical Agents for Physical Therapists*. Springfield, IL, Charles C Thomas, 1982.

Kirkkaldy-Willis WH: A comprehensive outline of treatment. In: Kirkaldy-Willis (ed) *Managing Low Back Pain*, 2nd ed. New York, Churchill Livingstone, 1988.

Klein J, Pariser D: Transcutaneous electrical nerve stimulation. In: Nelson R, Currier D (eds) *Clinical Electrotherapy*. Los Altos, CA, Appleton & Lange, 1987

Kloth L: Shortwave and microwave diathermy. In: Michlovitz S (ed) *Thermal Agents in Rehabilitation*. Philadelphia, Davis, 1986.

Michlovitz S: Biophysical principles of heating and superficial heat agents. In: Michlovitz S (ed) *Thermal Agents in Rehabilitation*. Philadelphia, Davis, 1986.

Newell SG, Woodle A: Cuboid syndrome. *Physician Sports Med* 1981; 1:71–76.

Ottoson D, Lundberg T: *Pain Treatment by Transcutaneous Electrical Nerve Stimulation*. New York, Springer-Verlag, 1988.

Saunders D: Lumbar traction. In: Grieve GP (ed) *Modern Manual Therapy of the Vertebral Column*. New York, Churchill Livingstone, 1986.

Savage B: *Interferential Therapy*. Boston, Faber & Faber, 1984.

Travell JG, Simmons DG: *Myofascial Pain and Dysfunction*. Baltimore, Williams & Wilkins, 1983.

Walsh M: Hydrotherapy: the use of water as a therapeutic agent. In: Michlovitz S (ed) *Thermal Agents in Rehabilitation*. Philadelphia, Davis, 1986.

Transcutaneous Electrical Nerve Stimulation

JAMES G. GRIFFIN

As a modality for treatment of pain, transcutaneous electrical nerve stimulation (TENS) can be used for a wide variety of acute and chronic conditions, including but not limited to acute and chronic musculoskeletal pain, postoperative pain, dental pain, headaches, peripheral neuropathies, complex regional pain syndrome, postherpetic neuralgia, and cancer pain. TENS works by inhibiting C-fiber activity in the dorsal horn neurons through stimulation of large cutaneous A fibers. TENS may also access the body's endogenous opioids, as the analgesia produced by some forms of TENS stimulation has been shown to be reversible by naloxone, an opioid antagonist, and by serotonin antagonists. TENS is safe and non-addictive. Contraindications include pregnancy and use over the carotid sinus. Use of a cardiac pacemaker may not be an absolute contraindication, as there are case reports of the safe use of TENS with a pacemaker. TENS' immediate effectiveness in pain control has been shown to be up to 60% to 80% in some studies, but this falls off over time. At 1 year, estimates of TENS' effect on chronic conditions falls to 25% to 30%.

Modern TENS units are small, portable devices powered by a 9-volt battery. Most units have two channels, each controlling a pair of electrodes that are affixed to the body at the desired locations. The output of each channel, except for intensity, is identical and can be altered by varying the stimulation parameters of the unit. Commercial units allow the clinician to alter intensity, pulse width, and pulse rate; and they may offer any or all such features as an automatic modulation mode, a dedicated burst or acupuncture mode, automatic timer, battery life indicator, and other stimulation or convenience options. Given the cost of such devices (more than $600 retail), a 5-year or lifetime warranty is desirable and available from some manufacturers.

The TENS units produce a small electrical current ranging up to 120 mA, depending on the TENS unit selected. Most commercial devices automatically alter the voltage output to account for variations in skin resistance and produce a constant current. Depending on the unit, the pulse rate can be altered between 2 and 200 pulses per second, and the pulse width can be varied from 9 to 500 μsec. Most TENS units now offer a modulation setting that automatically alters pulse rate, pulse width, and intensity around previously selected parameters. This feature is said to diminish the body's tendency to accommodate to a constant stimulus—one reason the effect of TENS is theorized to fall off over time. The waveform varies with the TENS unit selected and is generally not an adjustable parameter. There is no consensus on an optimal waveform, and there may be little difference in waveforms once they have penetrated the tissue.

A. Microcurrent TENS devices are being marketed that purport to use microamperage current to produce pain relief for conditions treated with traditional TENS. Numerous anecdotal claims are made for these devices, but no research exists at this time to validate their effectiveness. Stimulation of peripheral nerves can be achieved at their most superficial site to obtain analgesia distally. Electrodes can be placed paraspinally and distally in the corresponding dermatome to treat radicular pain. Electrodes may be placed contralaterally in appropriate stimulus sites if the ipsilateral side is too irritable to allow electrode placement, as in the case of reflex sympathetic dystrophy.

B. Successful electrode placement can be achieved using a number of methods shown by research to be effective. It is most common to place the electrodes on or bracketing the painful site. Both electrodes from each channel may be on one side of the painful area or in a crisscross pattern.

C. Electrodes may be placed in the dermatome, myotome, or sclerotome in which the painful site is located. Specific sites in a region may be targeted (e.g., a trigger point), or placement may be on the anterior and posterior of the dermatome, as in the thoracic region.

D. Acupuncture points, trigger points, or motor points may be effective stimulation sites. There is a high percentage of correlation between acupuncture points and trigger points and between acupuncture points and the superficial areas of peripheral nerves. Acupuncture and trigger point charts are available to guide the clinician. Acupuncture points may be located with a probe indicating areas of decreased tissue resistance. They may also be located by the clinician using himself or herself in the circuit to locate them.

E. If pain with motion is a major difficulty, the clinician may wish to try a series of electrode locations with the patient performing the offending action(s) by stimulating selected points. Stimulus sites may be any combination of the points described above. This method can be time-consuming but is of great functional significance to the patient.

F. High-frequency or conventional TENS is the stimulation mode most commonly used. It employs a pulse rate of 50 to 100 Hz and a short pulse width of 20 to 60 μsec. Treatment time may vary from 30 minutes to several hours per day at a perceptible, comfortable level of stimulation. Studies on a clinical pain population have shown that a subthreshold stimulus is also effective for initial TENS trials. Conventional TENS has been shown to be effective with a wide variety of conditions; it is the method of choice for use in acute or postsurgical situations and a starting point for treating chronic pain conditions.

PATIENT FOR TRANSCUTANEOUS ELECTRICAL NERVE STIMULATION TRIAL

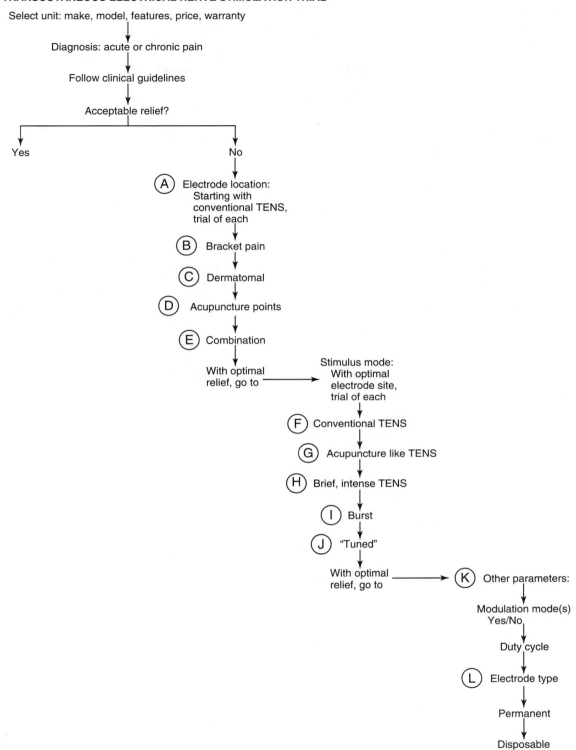

Select unit: make, model, features, price, warranty

Diagnosis: acute or chronic pain

Follow clinical guidelines

Acceptable relief?

Yes

No

(A) Electrode location:
Starting with
conventional TENS,
trial of each

(B) Bracket pain

(C) Dermatomal

(D) Acupuncture points

(E) Combination

With optimal
relief, go to

Stimulus mode:
With optimal
electrode site,
trial of each

(F) Conventional TENS

(G) Acupuncture like TENS

(H) Brief, intense TENS

(I) Burst

(J) "Tuned"

With optimal
relief, go to

(K) Other parameters:

Modulation mode(s)
Yes/No

Duty cycle

(L) Electrode type

Permanent

Disposable

G. Other stimulus modes may be more effective for chronic pain conditions. Acupuncture-like TENS uses a low frequency (1 to 4 Hz) and wide pulse (150 to 250 μsec). Intensity is at a level that produces a strong, visible muscle contraction in the related myotome. Treatment time is 20 to 30 minutes once or twice a day. Analgesia takes longer to produce but is of longer duration than conventional TENS.

H. Similar to this is burst, or pulse train, TENS. This technique employs a series of 4 to 10 high-frequency pulses (70 to 100 Hz) delivered one to four times per second. Stimulation intensity is to the point of muscle contraction.

I. Brief, intense TENS employs a high frequency (> 100 Hz) and a wide pulse width (150 to 250 μsec) at the highest intensity the patient can tolerate for 1 to 15 minutes. It is hypothesized that this stimulus mode may disrupt the "pain memory" or act centrally in some other way.

J. If none of the above modes produces acceptable analgesia, the clinician may try to "tune in" an optimal setting by first holding the pulse width constant at about 100 μsec and sweeping through the pulse rate in small increments to find an optimal setting. The process is then repeated for the pulse width with the pulse rate at the previously determined level.

K. Authorities differ in their recommendations of duration and frequency of stimulation during the day. Relief has been obtained experimentally with treatment ranging from 30 minutes twice a week to constant stimulation. As TENS stimulation has a carryover effect, a treatment cycle that gives relief with scheduled on and off periods should be established. By avoiding constant use, it is theorized that accommodation to TENS may be delayed or prevented. Intermittent use may also slow or prevent depletion of endogenous pain-relieving substances accessed by TENS stimulation.

L. Several types of TENS electrodes are available. Carbonized silicon electrodes are durable and inexpensive but require the use of a conductive gel and an adhesive gel or patch. Single and multiuse disposable electrodes are available that are pregelled, self-adhering, sterile (for postoperative pain), and available in a variety of sizes and shapes. These electrodes are convenient but more expensive. Any of the electrodes may cause skin irritation. An individual's skin chemistry or strenuous activity may result in failure to maintain a good bond. Different electrodes may have different conduction properties. A trial of several electrodes may be necessary to find the optimal brand.

Successful use of TENS requires skill and perseverance on the part of the clinician and the patient. Initially, pain relief may require several hours or days of TENS application, as some individuals respond in a cumulative fashion. Long-term studies of patients who have used TENS successfully indicate that, for chronic conditions, optimum results with TENS is a question of individualizing the electrode type and placement, stimulation parameters, and stimulation time to the patient's requirements.

REFERENCES

Barr JO: Transcutaneous electrical nerve stimulation for pain management. In: Nelson RM, Currier DP (eds) *Clinical Electrotherapy*. Appleton & Lange, Norwalk, CT, 1991, pp 261–316.

Barr JO, Nielsen DH, Soderberg GL: Transcutaneous electrical nerve stimulation characteristics for altering pain perception. *Phys Ther* 1986;66:1515–1521.

Berlant SR: Method of determining optimal stimulation sites for transcutaneous electrical nerve stimulation. *Phys Ther* 1984;64:924–928.

Gersh MR: Microcurrent electrical stimulation: putting it in perspective. *Clin Manage* 1989;9:51–54.

Gersh MR, Wolf SL: Applications of transcutaneous electrical nerve stimulation in the management of patients with pain. *Phys Ther* 1985;65:314–336.

Johnson MI, Ashton CH, Thompson JW: An in-depth study of long term users of transcutaneous electrical nerve stimulation (TENS): implications for clinical use of (TENS). *Pain* 1991;44:221–229.

Johnson MI, Ashton CH, Thompson JW: The consistency of pulse frequencies and pulse patterns of transcutaneous electrical nerve stimulation (TENS) used by chronic pain patients. *Pain* 1991;44:231–234.

Lamm K: *Optimal Placement Techniques for TENS: A Soft Tissue Approach*. Tucson, AZ, Kenneth E. Lamm, 1986.

Leo KC, Dostal WF, Bossen DG, et al: Effect of transcutaneous nerve stimulation characteristics on clinical pain. *Phys Ther* 1986;66:200–205.

Nolan MF: Conductive differences in electrodes used with transcutaneous electrical nerve stimulators. *Phys Ther* 1991;71:746–751.

Ottoson D, Lundeberg T: *Pain Treatment by Transcutaneous Electrical Nerve Stimulation*. New York, Springer-Verlag, 1988.

Shade SK: Use of transcutaneous electrical nerve stimulation for a patient with a cardiac pacemaker. *Phys Ther* 1985;65:206–208.

Woolf CF, Thompson JW: Stimulation-induced induced analgesia: transcutaneous electrical nerve stimulation (TENS) and vibration. In: Wall PD, Melzack R (eds) *Textbook of Pain*, 3rd ed. New York, Churchill Livingstone, 1994.

Occupational Therapy

STEPHEN W. DINGER

Work-related injuries are an inevitable part of industry. While employers have become proactive in preventing the number of injuries sustained while on the job in recent years, accidents still occur. Preventative measures that have shown to be effective in decreasing employee injuries include back school, physical conditioning, healthy lifestyle, regular exercise, and ergonomic modifications. Industrial injuries are costly in several respects, affecting the employer in terms of lost productivity and the injured employee in terms of lost wages and expenses for health care and rehabilitation. Heavy lifting, repetitive vibratory stresses, and cumulative trauma disorders account for the majority of work-related injuries resulting in contusions, lacerations, fractures, low back pain, tendonitis, compression neuropathies, muscle strains, bursitis, disk disease, ligamentous injury, and cartilage damage. Chronic low back pain is the leading cause of disability in individuals between 19 and 45 years of age, and has significant economic and personal implication. Occupational rehabilitation aids the workers' recovery process and is an integral component in assisting patients to regain lost or impaired function.

A. Evaluation of the injured worker takes place in either an emergent or urgent setting without delay. Evaluation consists of a detailed history of present illness, past medical history, and physical examination consisting of a general assessment and comprehensive musculoskeletal exam. It is important to obtain information on nonorganic findings, symptom magnification, the overall job task, precipitating events, duration at a specific task, work satisfaction, pending litigation, and outlook for the future. This is essential to conclude if indeed a work-related problem did occur. Studies show that workers who do not enjoy their jobs or who are involved in pending litigation show slower recovery and less response to treatment.

B. A working diagnosis is formulated based on the history and physical. It is important to inform patients about the diagnosis, educate them about their condition, and discuss the prognosis and time frame for return to work.

C. The appropriate treatment regimen is now implemented. The majority of workers will respond well to the initial treatment and return to work relatively quickly. Pain is the major symptom of most acute injuries, and the cornerstone of therapy is RICE (rest, ice, compression, and elevation), proper analgesic medication, and modalities.

D. About 10% of workers will not respond well to the acute treatment and will go on to have pain symptoms and disability which prevents them from returning to productive employment. The longer that the worker is away from work the less likelihood that the worker will return to work. If the worker is out of work for 6 months, there is a 50% chance that he or she will return, if out for 1 year only a 25% chance, and if greater than 2 years almost 0% chance of return.

E. Functional capacity evaluations are performed, usually by a trained therapist, to assess the patient's ability to perform job tasks efficiently and safely. Functional status aids in determining when the patient is able to return to work.

F. If the injured worker does not return to work in the first several weeks, then enrollment into a more structured program that prepares the worker for return to his job may be needed. Work conditioning provides active participation of the worker to regain physical conditioning, address functional deficits, and prepare the worker physically to return to the job.

G. If the worker has been off of the job for several months, then a more intense and comprehensive work hardening program should be utilized. Work hardening consists of physical, psychologic, and vocational conditioning. Both general and job-specific physical conditioning are incorporated into the program. Most work hardening programs are scheduled 5 days a week for about 6 weeks. Approximately 80% to 85% of workers who are carefully selected and participate in work hardening programs will return to work.

H. Vocational rehabilitation programs have been established to return patients with physical disabilities to work at some capacity. The patient works closely with his or her counselor, and undergoes evaluation, education, retraining, and placement in an appropriate position (see the chapter on Vocational Rehabilitation).

I. A small percentage of workers will have resulting chronic pain syndromes. Chronic pain management includes a multifaceted treatment approach including modalities, physical therapy, oral medications, injections, and pumps. Psychologic factors, such as depression, anxiety, medication dependence, and somatization are important factors in overall treatment.

J. After the patient's functional status has reached a plateau, and there is no expected change, then an impairment evaluation is performed.

REFERENCES

Delisa JA (ed): Rehabilitation Medicine: Principles and Practice, 3rd ed. Philadelphia, Lippincott, 1998.
Randall L, Braddom R, Buschbacher RM (eds): Physical Medicine and Rehabilitation, 2nd ed. Philadelphia, WB Saunders, 2000.

OCCUPATIONAL REHABILITATION

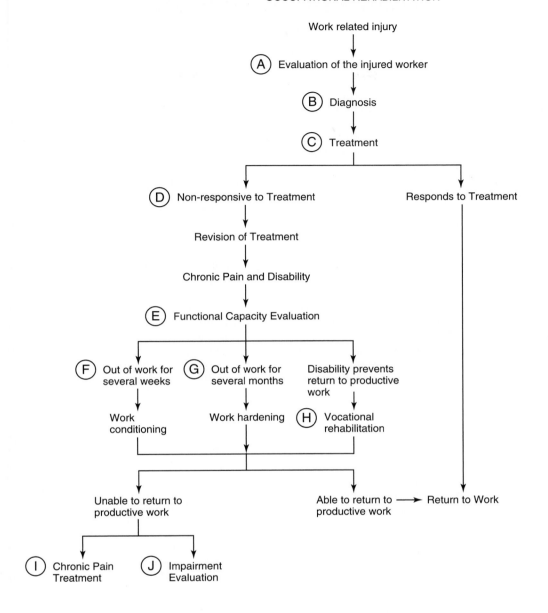

Vocational Rehabilitation

STEPHEN W. DINGER

Many patients seen for treatment in the pain management system have sustained injuries resulting in unresolved pain and physical disability; several of these injuries are work related. Vocational rehabilitation involves not only treating the injury with the goal of preventing long-term disability, but also providing those patients with inevitable disability the assistance and resources for returning to the workforce. Employment of patients with disability promotes autonomy, productivity, and an overall better quality of life. Comparatively, the development of chronic disability and inability to return to work has significant socioeconomic consequences for both the patient and for society. Therefore, federal, state, and private agencies have been formed to help facilitate returning the injured/disabled patient to a productive work environment. These agencies include vocational evaluation, functional assessment, work hardening and reconditioning, work capacity evaluations, job site analysis, job accommodations, skill training, job placement, and follow-up service. The overall goal of the vocational rehabilitation process is to improve the patient's physical, social, financial, and psychologic function.

A. Referral of a patient with a particular disability to the appropriate vocational rehabilitation organization, for assessment and evaluation.

B. Vocational rehabilitation evaluation helps identify the need for services, vocational interests, expectations, strengths and weaknesses, needs, and potential.

C. After the patient is deemed an appropriate candidate for vocational rehabilitation services, a complete medical evaluation is performed. This consists of a complete medical and employment history, specialized skills, financial needs, expectations, educational background, and transportation needs. A written test can help to identify current aptitude, abilities, and work interests.

D. Functional assessment helps to place individuals in a functional category, based on the patient's abilities. The patient's mobility, interpersonal communication skills, emotional stability, endurance, and learning ability are also assessed, which helps develop the rehabilitation plan for the patient.

E. An Individualized Written Rehabilitation Plan is composed with the patient's assistance. The document includes long-term vocational goals, intermediate objectives, services provided, designated counselor and patient responsibilities, criteria for evaluation of the patient, and an annual review while the case is open.

F. After a plan is devised, the patient must be trained appropriately to perform the necessary tasks to meet his objectives and goals. This may be achieved by taking secondary or college courses or by concentrating on a specific occupational skill. The level and choice of training will be influenced by the patient's abilities, interests, performance on prior testing, previous strengths and skills, and consideration of physical disabilities.

G. Assessing family support, community resources, and employment readiness are instrumental in facilitating a positive experience and outcome. Availability of help and support from family members and caregivers is extremely important. The patient must be psychologically prepared, motivated, and confident to return to work, and should have realistic expectations. Transportation is also paramount, and the patient may need to rely on alternative modes of transportation if he or she is unable to drive as this may be an obstacle to success.

H. Once training is completed, the patient is prepared for placement into the workforce. The patient, along with the help of the counselor, will analyze prospective jobs in order to determine the most appropriate potential placement. The patient may be able to return to his or her previous occupation or an alternative occupation in which he or she received appropriate training. It is important to note that the employer is required to make reasonable accommodation for the patient, including modifications to job facilities and equipment, job design, training, and support. Some patients will not be able to return to the competitive labor market even after extensive rehabilitation. For these individuals other options exist. These include transitional or supported employment, such as government-sponsored programs or Goodwill Services, and numerous volunteer positions. For some patients, the goal of rehabilitation is limited to increased independence in activities of daily living.

I. Follow-up services address any problems that are present, as well as any further modifications that are needed.

REFERENCES

Delisa JA (ed): *Rehabilitation Medicine: Principle and Practice*, 3rd ed. Philadelphia, Lippincott, 1998.

Ingmundson PT: Vocational rehabilitation. In: Ramamurthy S, Rogers J (eds) *Decision Making in Pain Management*. Chicago: Mosby Year Book, 1993, pp. 192–193.

Randall L, Braddom RL, Buschbacher RM: *Physical Medicine and Rehabilitation*, 2nd ed. Philadelphia, WB Saunders, 2000, pp. 731–735.

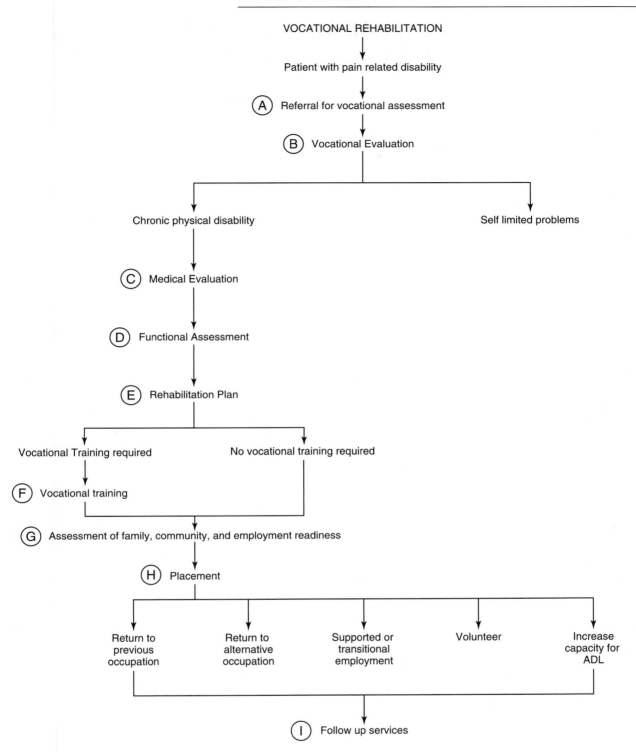

VOCATIONAL REHABILITATION

Patient with pain related disability

(A) Referral for vocational assessment

(B) Vocational Evaluation

Chronic physical disability

Self limited problems

(C) Medical Evaluation

(D) Functional Assessment

(E) Rehabilitation Plan

Vocational Training required

No vocational training required

(F) Vocational training

(G) Assessment of family, community, and employment readiness

(H) Placement

Return to previous occupation

Return to alternative occupation

Supported or transitional employment

Volunteer

Increase capacity for ADL

(I) Follow up services

Evaluation and Preparation for Regional Anesthesia

DOUGLAS M. ANDERSON AND JERRY A. BEYER

The principles of preoperative evaluation of a patient for regional anesthesia are similar to those applied to evaluation for other anesthetics (Bridenbaugh and Crews 1998; Buckley 2001). Regional techniques are generally safe and effective but are not without risks and failures; the emergent induction of general anesthesia is sometimes necessary. The potential risks, benefits, and limitations of the proposed regional techniques must be discussed with the patient. Always attempt to minimize risks and be prepared to manage all potential complications or side effects.

A. Acquire a thorough understanding of applied anatomy and local anesthetic pharmacology. This knowledge is necessary when choosing the most suitable technique and medications to be used. Review the patient's medical history, allergies, anatomy, physiologic state, and psychological profile. Be familiar with the duration and extent of the surgical procedure when caring for surgical patients. Speak with the surgeon to ensure that the proposed anesthetic plan will provide the operating conditions necessary to perform the surgical procedure.

B. Consider the side effects and potential complications of any regional technique you plan to administer. Pathophysiologic considerations are extremely important for guiding the practitioner to the safest anesthetic plan. Problems such as trauma, infection, anatomic abnormalities, burns, dressings, splints, and casts can interfere with safe performance of a regional block. Do not ignore systemic problems [e.g., hypovolemia, liver disease, coagulopathy, chronic obstructive pulmonary disease (COPD), and cardiovascular disease], which could result in potentially devastating complications. A patient having a contraindication for one particular regional technique may be well suited for another. For example, an elderly patient with a distal radius fracture and severe COPD may not be a good candidate for an interscalene block (because of the risk of a unilateral phrenic nerve block) but would benefit from an axillary or infraclavicular block (avoiding the risks associated with endotracheal intubation and general anesthesia).

C. Evaluate the psychological profile of the patient. When a patient is combative, uncooperative, or extremely anxious, it is exceedingly difficult and potentially dangerous to perform almost any regional technique. Likewise, an extremely anxious patient may not tolerate a regional technique as the sole anesthetic for an operation given the difficulty encountered in blocking proprioception. Not all patients are good candidates for regional anesthesia.

D. Many patients are reluctant to have regional anesthesia because they do not want to be aware of what is happening in the operating room. Explain to such a patient that medications will be administered to help with relaxation and sleep and that there will be no surgical pain. Reassure him or her that general anesthesia is still available after the block has been placed. Some patients request that blocks be placed after induction of general anesthesia because they fear needles and pain during block placement. This technique is not recommended and can be potentially dangerous.

E. Before sedating a patient for placement of a regional block, recognize that this practice is controversial. Some believe that sedating medications (e.g., benzodiazepines, opioids) prevent early recognition of local anesthetic toxicity and may mask paresthesias. Most practitioners, however, do provide sedation and analgesia during the performance of regional blocks. Midazolam and opioids are commonly used for this purpose. Midazolam is a popular choice because of its short half-life and profound amnestic qualities. Midazolam, as all benzodiazepines, raises the seizure threshold and serves to protect patients from central nervous system toxicity. Benzodiazepines offer no protection from cardiovascular toxicity.

F. Do not assume that a patient inadequately prepared for an elective procedure under general anesthesia (e.g., untreated systemic disease) can be safely anesthetized with "just a block." A patient scheduled for an elective procedure must be a candidate for general anesthesia before being considered for regional anesthesia. Any regional anesthetic may require conversion to a general anesthetic when toxicity or incomplete anesthesia is encountered. Therefore, have emergency drugs and airway equipment immediately available when performing any regional technique.

REFERENCES

Bridenbaugh PO, Crews JC: Perioperative management of patients for neural blockade. In: Cousins MJ, Bridenbaugh PO (eds) Neural Blockade in Clinical Anesthesia and Management of Pain, 3rd ed. Philadelphia, Lippincott-Raven, 1998, pp 179–199.

Buckley FP: Regional anesthesia with local anesthetics. In: Loeser JD (ed) Bonica's Management of Pain, 3rd ed. Philadelphia, Lippincott Williams & Wilkins, 2001, pp 1893–1952.

PREOPERATIVE EVALUATION AND PREPARATION FOR REGIONAL ANESTHESIA

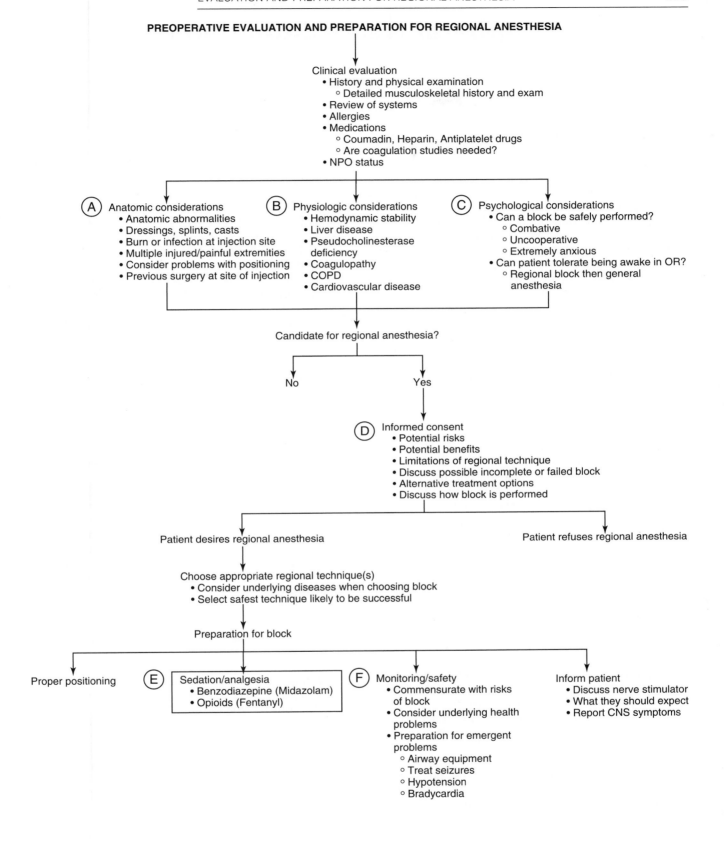

Peripheral Nerve Stimulators

JAY ELLIS

Peripheral nerve stimulators are a valuable aid for regional anesthesia. They are not a substitute for knowledge of anatomy and sound technique, but they do allow for more precise localization of peripheral nerves. It is useful to consider nerve stimulators as to what they can do, cannot do, and areas of use that remain controversial before discussing the elements of successful stimulator use.

Peripheral nerve stimulators can offer the option of seeking multiple nerves during a block, which in some studies increased the overall success of the procedure, provided more complete anesthesia of the affected area, and hastened the onset of anesthesia (Fanelli et al. 1999). Using a peripheral nerve stimulator can eliminate the need for paresthesias, although paresthesias still occur incidentally. Reducing paresthesias may reduce the incidence of nerve injury, although there are no prospective trials to confirm that nerve stimulators reduce nerve injury. While the use of peripheral nerve stimulators may reduce the incidence of nerve injury, it by no means eliminates them. The literature contains case reports of severe long-lasting nerve injury associated with the use of peripheral nerve stimulators (Auroy et al. 2002).

Other areas in the use of peripheral nerve stimulators remain more controversial. The exact amount of current needed to optimally stimulate the nerve for a successful block varies from study to study, with current levels from 0.3 mA to 1.0 mA recommended. The advantage of higher current levels is ease of localization of the nerve. The disadvantage is that higher current levels may stimulate the nerve at a distance not sufficient for local anesthetic to spread and provide a complete nerve block. Use of lower current amounts should provide more precise localization, but may actually increase the risk of nerve injury if the needle tip is so close that it results in intraneural injection. Another potential source of error in determining adequate current levels is that there is considerable variation in current output between different types of nerve stimulators, especially at current levels less than 0.5 mA (Hadzic et al. 2003). Further confounding the debate is the observation that at times a needle will elicit a paresthesia yet not result in any nerve stimulation (Mulroy and Mitchell 2002; Urmey and Stanton 2002). Injection of the local anesthetic after the paresthesia results in a nerve block, despite the lack of stimulation. What may be most important about the nerve stimulation is not so much the amount of current required for minimal stimulation, but the type of motor response elicited (Franco et al. 2004). An upper extremity stimulation that causes a motor response in the fingers and hand is more likely to result in a successful block than stimulation of more proximal muscle groups. The same is true of a lower extremity block that results in inversion or plantar flexion of the foot instead of the more proximal muscles (Sukhani et al. 2004). Stimulation of more proximal muscles may result in successful block, but introduce two sources of error: (1) the nerve may be stimulated outside the fascial boundary of the plexus, such as direct stimulation of the suprascapular nerve outside the brachial plexus sheath or (2) there may be direct muscle stimulation, such as direct stimulation of the triceps during axillary block or the hamstring muscles during sciatic block. The net result is that current levels of 0.5 to 1.0 mA are adequate for localization of most nerves, as long as the motor response to stimulation is consistent with nerve stimulation within the target area. Using current levels less than 0.5 mA may permit more precise localization, but could conceivably increase the risk of nerve injury.

Using nerve stimulation to perform nerve blocks on anesthetized patients is another area of controversy. A review of complications of interscalene block on anesthetized patients reported serious neurologic complications caused by apparent injections of local anesthetic into the spinal cord (Benumof 2000). Use of a nerve stimulator in the anesthetized patient, especially for nerve blocks near the neuraxis, could result in inadvertent stimulation of the spinal cord which is mistaken for peripheral nerve stimulation. Injection into the spinal cord can result in catastrophic injury. Some situations require general anesthesia for the performance of nerve blocks. Children and patients unable to cooperate are examples of situations where general anesthesia may be necessary to perform the procedure safely. However, the risk of serious nerve injury with the procedure must be justified by the benefit to the patient.

Many adequate peripheral nerve stimulators are commercially available. The device should deliver voltages over a range of 1 to 10 V. The current output should have a variable setting allowing for outputs ranging from 0.1 to 10 mA. Most of the devices allow for easy connection with insulated needles. Such needles allow for maximum current density at the needle tip and are specifically designed for regional analgesia. It is possible to use noninsulated needles, but current density is not maximal at the needle tip, making nerve localization less precise.

A. Prepare the patient for nerve block as usual. Sedation may be used, but should be weighed against the advantages of having an alert cooperative patient who can respond to inadvertent intraneural injection or signs of local anesthetic toxicity. Decide beforehand on the optimal muscle stimulation needed to elicit a successful block and plan the needle approach to stimulate the appropriate nerve.

B. Attach the ground, or anode (+) lead to the patient. Location of the ground is not critical, but it is best placed on the patient where good contact is ensured. The lead should be close enough to the site of injection to facilitate good current flow, but need not be so close as to interfere with performance of the block. The cathode (−) lead is attached to the needle. This arrangement minimizes the amount of current required for stimulation.

C. Puncture the skin and turn the nerve stimulator to a setting of 5 mA of current or less. Lower current levels are better tolerated by patients.

PERIPHERAL NERVE STIMULATOR

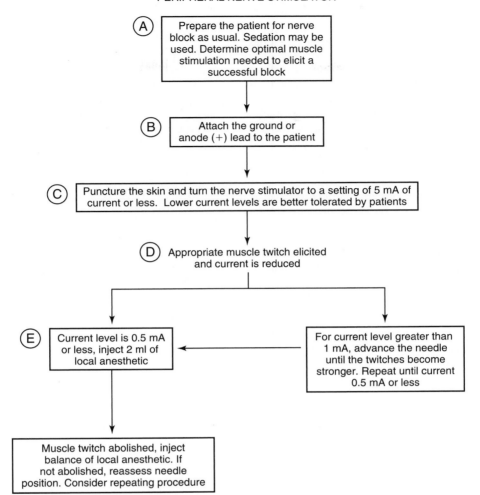

(A) Prepare the patient for nerve block as usual. Sedation may be used. Determine optimal muscle stimulation needed to elicit a successful block

(B) Attach the ground or anode (+) lead to the patient

(C) Puncture the skin and turn the nerve stimulator to a setting of 5 mA of current or less. Lower current levels are better tolerated by patients

(D) Appropriate muscle twitch elicited and current is reduced

(E) Current level is 0.5 mA or less, inject 2 ml of local anesthetic

For current level greater than 1 mA, advance the needle until the twitches become stronger. Repeat until current 0.5 mA or less

Muscle twitch abolished, inject balance of local anesthetic. If not abolished, reassess needle position. Consider repeating procedure

D. Advance the needle toward the target area. Once muscle twitches begin, determine if they are local muscle contractions or the result of nerve stimulation. Local muscle twitches due to direct muscle stimulation should be ignored and will subside as the needle transits the muscle. If the twitches are from nerve stimulation then reduce the current until the twitches are barely perceptible. If the current level is greater than 1 mA then advance the needle until the twitches become noticeably stronger. Continue the process of advancing the needle and reducing the current until the current level reaches 0.5 mA or less (current levels of 0.5 to 1.0 mA are also acceptable if muscle twitch is thought to be optimal). If advancing the needle does not result in a return of the muscle twitch then the needle has traveled past the nerve and should be withdrawn and redirected to elicit the muscle twitch.

E. Once the current level is 0.5 mA or less, inject 2 ml of local anesthetic. This should abolish the muscle twitch. If twitch is not abolished consider the possibility of muscle twitch due to direct muscle stimulation and repeat the procedure after reviewing anatomical landmarks.

REFERENCES

Auroy Y, Benhamou D, Barques L, et al: Major complications of regional anesthesia in France: the SOS Regional Anesthesia Hotline Service. *Anesthesiology* 2002;97:1274–1280.

Benumof JL: Permanent loss of cervical spinal cord function associated with interscalene block performed under general anesthesia. *Anesthesiology* 2000;93:1541–1544.

Fanelli G, Casati A, Garancini P, Torri G, and the Study Group on Regional Anesthesia: Nerve stimulator and multiple injection technique for upper and lower limb blockade: failure rate, patient acceptance, and neurologic complications. *Anesth Analg* 1999;88:847–852.

Franco CD, Domasevich V, Vorono G, et al: The supraclavicular block with stimulator: to decrease or not to decrease, that is the question. *Anesth Analg* 2004;98:1167–1171.

Hadzic A, Vloka J, Hadzic, et al: Nerve stimulators used for peripheral nerve blocks vary in their electrical characteristics. *Anesthesiology* 2003;98:969–974.

Mulroy MF, Mitchell B: Unsolicited paresthesias with nerve stimulator: case reports of four patients. *Anesth Analg* 2002;95:762–763.

Sukhani R, Nader A, Candido KD: Nerve stimulator evoked motor response predicts the latency and success of single-injection sciatic block. *Anesth Analg* 2004;99:584–588.

Urmey WF, Stanton J: Inability to consistently elicit a motor response following sensory paresthesia during interscalene block administration. *Anesthesiology* 2002;96:552–554.

Peripheral Nerve Blocks

SERGIO ALVARADO

Peripheral nerve blocks have been used for many years to treat acute and chronic pain. The goal of regional analgesia is to provide prolonged pain relief to a specific portion of the body, thus limiting systemic administration of analgesics with their potential side effects. They can be useful diagnostically as well. When combined with modalities such as continuous nerve block catheters, cryoablation, and now pulsed radiofrequency, long-lasting relief can be obtained. This chapter focuses on a brief overview of commonly used blocks for chronic pain.

A. Techniques usually incorporate easily identifiable surface landmarks and take advantage of the most superficial locations of nerves to facilitate needle placement and limit complications. The advent of nerve stimulator techniques has increased the ease of performing these blocks as well as the reliability and safety of the procedures. Development of portable ultrasound may aid in actually visualizing the nerve or adjacent vascular structures, which should also increase safety and facilitate performance. Pain syndromes that are amenable to diagnosis and treatment via peripheral nerve blocks include peripheral neuralgias such as greater occipital, ilioinguinal, and iliohypogastric, and meralgia paresthetica. Facial pain and headache can be treated by blockade of the various branches of the trigeminal nerve. Shoulder and hip joint pain may benefit from blockade of articular branches of peripheral nerves as in suprascapular nerve block for shoulder pain and in blocking of branches of the femoral and obturator nerves for hip pain. Intercostal nerve blocks are useful in the treatment of chest wall pain. Various local anesthetics can be used. Corticosteroids are often included in the injectate although there is no evidence substantiating routine use. Liposomal formulations of local anesthetics are in development and would prolong the effect of single injection techniques.

B. Continuous peripheral nerve infusion can be useful in the treatment of chronic regional pain syndrome (CRPS) and phantom limb pain. Probably the most common site of continuous regional analgesia for chronic pain is the brachial plexus. Reliable analgesia can be obtained for the entire upper extremity via a single site of injection. Interscalene, subclavian perivascular, infraclavicular, and axillary approaches have been described, with choice of technique usually based on the experience and familiarity of the operator. Intensive rehabilitation can be pursued during the period of analgesia if desired. Long-acting local anesthetics are usually used, with bupivacaine and ropivacaine being the most common. Lower extremity plexus blocks including anterior (femoral nerve) and posterior lumbar plexus blocks, and sciatic nerve blocks can also be used as well for CRPS and phantom pain. Technically, lower extremity blockade has usually been difficult and unreliable. With the recent development of stimulating catheters, that may be changing. Strict aseptic technique should be adhered to during block administration.

C. Cryoablation is discussed in detail elsewhere in the book. When used for prolonged blockade of peripheral nerves, it can provide excellent analgesia with the potential for pursuing aggressive physical therapy. There may be significant numbness in the affected area.

D. Pulsed RF is also discussed in more detail in Chapter 117, p. 314. Its development has created a new option for providing long-term analgesia in the distribution of a peripheral nerve without destroying tissue or requiring equipment for continuous infusion.

REFERENCES

Hahn MB, Mcquillan PM, Sheplock GJ (eds): *Regional Anesthesia: An atlas of Anatomy and Techniques.* St. Louis, Mosby, 1996.

Raj PP: Nerve blocks: continuous regional analgesia. In: Raj PP (ed) *Practical Management of Pain,* 3rd ed. St. Louis, Mosby, 2000, pp. 710–720.

Saberski L, Fitzgerald J, Ahmad M: Cryoneurolysis and radiofrequency lesioning. In: Raj PP (ed) *Practical Management of Pain,* 3rd ed. St. Louis, Mosby, 2000, pp. 753–767.

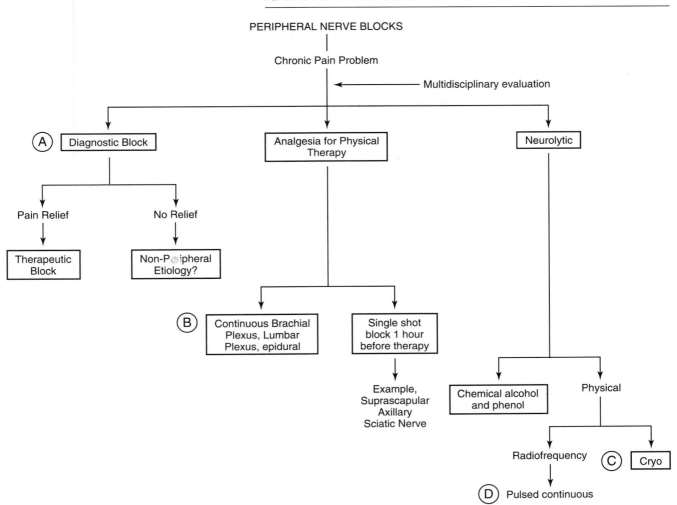

PERIPHERAL NERVE BLOCKS

Pediatric Extremity Blocks

LYNDA WELLS

Extremity blocks in pediatric patients are effective and extremely safe. In a study by Giaufre et al. (1996), the incidence of morbidity associated with peripheral nerve blocks in pediatric patients undergoing surgical procedures was 0 in 9396 cases. The indications, contraindications, advantages, disadvantages, and types of extremity block that can be performed in pediatric patients are identical to those used in adults. However, there are several differences in the clinical approach to performing extremity blocks in children that must be considered.

It is generally agreed that peripheral and plexus nerve block techniques should be learned and perfected in adult patients. Only practitioners who are facile in performing these blocks in adults should perform them in children. Unlike in adult practice, nerve blocks in children are usually performed under general anesthesia, and techniques that rely on eliciting parasthesia are contraindicated. Consequently, use of a peripheral nerve stimulator is mandatory except when performing a fascia iliaca block. When using a peripheral nerve stimulator, the negative electrode (cathode) should be connected to an insulated, short, beveled needle. Short, beveled needles allow easier appreciation of changes in tissue resistance and more distinct fascial "pops" in children whose fascial planes are thinner. Needles of an appropriate length should be used, especially in infants and small children when short needles are stiffer and easier to control. The positive electrode (anode) should be connected to the reference electrode. If a motor response is elicited at a current between 0.5 and 0.3 mA, the needle tip is adjacent to the nerve. If motor activity persists at currents less than 0.15 mA, it may indicate that the needle tip is within the nerve and should be withdrawn before injection. Appropriately sized indwelling catheters can be placed to allow continuous infusion of drugs for prolonged analgesia.

In specific circumstances, extremity blocks are performed in awake children. These situations include surgical blocks in older children in whom regional anesthesia without general anesthesia is considered preferable (e.g., malignant hyperthermia) and after trauma when concomitant injuries relatively contraindicate the use of sedation or anesthesia. "Older children" are more than 8 years of age: abstract cognition is not developed until this age. The maturity and personality of the child are also of importance. Extremity blocks in trauma victims are usually performed to relieve pain from fractures (e.g., femoral nerve block for a fractured femoral shaft, parascalene brachial plexus block for injuries below the elbow, anterior/lateral approaches to the sciatic nerve for injuries below the knee, and surgical procedures). All patients should have intravenous access and cardiorespiratory monitoring established before the block is performed. Whenever practicable, the preemptive use of a topical anesthetic preparation (e.g., EMLA cream) is recommended to reduce the discomfort of injections.

The pharmacokinetic characteristics of local anesthetic drugs change with age. Knowledge of maximum recommended doses and volumes, protein binding, metabolism, and duration of action at various ages is required and is especially important when treating neonates and infants. The most frequently encountered complication of extremity neural blockade is accidental intravascular injection, or rapid systemic absorption, of local anesthetic drugs leading to cardiovascular and neurologic toxicity. The following precautions help minimize this risk.

- Never exceed the maximum recommended dose.
- Aspirate before, and at frequent intervals during, injection.
- Inject the local anesthetic slowly.
- Continuously monitor the electrocardiogram and watch for changes in T wave morphology, heart rate, or QRS morphology.

Epinephrine in the local anesthetic solution does not reliably cause tachycardia on intravascular injection in infants and children who are anesthetized with volatile anesthetic drugs. Epinephrine-containing local anesthetic solutions should not be injected adjacent to end-arteries (e.g., digital blocks). The benefit of adding clonidine or other adjunctive drugs to local anesthetic solutions for extremity neural blockade has not been established.

REFERENCES

Dalens B (ed): *Regional Anesthesia in Infants, Children and Adolescents.* Baltimore, Williams & Wilkins, 1995.

Giaufre E, Dalens B, Gombert A: Epidemiology and morbidity of regional anesthesia in children: a one-year prospective survey of the French-Language Society of Pediatric Anesthesiologists. *Anesth Analg* 1996;83:904–912.

Peutrell JM, Mather SJ: *Regional Anaesthesia in Babies and Children.* New York, Oxford University Press, 1997.

PEDIATRIC EXTREMITY BLOCKS

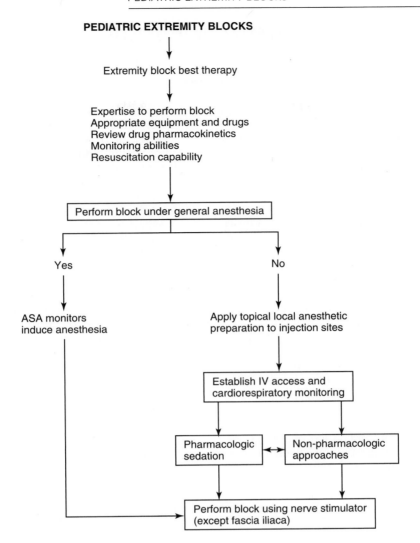

Extremity block best therapy

Expertise to perform block
Appropriate equipment and drugs
Review drug pharmacokinetics
Monitoring abilities
Resuscitation capability

Perform block under general anesthesia

Yes

No

ASA monitors
induce anesthesia

Apply topical local anesthetic
preparation to injection sites

Establish IV access and
cardiorespiratory monitoring

Pharmacologic
sedation

Non-pharmacologic
approaches

Perform block using nerve stimulator
(except fascia iliaca)

Epidural Block

DALE SOLOMON AND SOMAYAJI RAMAMURTHY

The epidural space is a space potentially filled with fat, lymphatics, and vascular structures located between the ligamentum flavum and vertebral laminae posteriorly and dura mater anteriorly. It extends from the foramen magnum to the sacral hiatus and can be entered with the needle anywhere along the length of its course. Drugs deposited in the space are taken up by adipose tissue and blood vessels so that significant systemic absorption occurs, but a portion of the drug diffuses through the dura mater or to the adjacent nerve roots to affect neural transmission.

A. Epidural blockade can modulate the pain of both acute and chronic conditions of the neck, extremities, and torso. Candidates for the procedure should have no systemic infection, coagulopathy, or local inflammation near the proposed site of injection. The patient should have stable neurologic function and should consent to the procedure. Patients with a low circulating blood volume have an exaggerated hypotensive response when a sympathectomy is caused by the local anesthetic block. The epidural space may be difficult to locate in areas of previous spinal surgery.

B. Place epidurally administered drugs as close as possible to the nerve root transmitting the pain impulses. For example, the thoracic epidural space may be entered for upper abdominal pain, the lumbar region for lower extremity pain, and caudal epidural space for pelvic pain. Use a midline or a paramedian approach in the lumbar region, but a paramedian approach in the midthoracic region of the spine because of the severe caudad angulations of the spinous processes.

C. Any drug injected into the epidural space should have a record of safety when used in the epidural space and be preservative free. Local anesthetics, opioids, and various other drugs have been placed into the epidural space to modulate the pain. Administer these drugs by intermittent bolus or by continuous infusion. Local anesthetics provide the most intense analgesia but impair sympathetic nerve activity and can impair motor function. Opioids preserve the motor and sympathetic nerve function but may cause respiratory depression, itching, urinary retention, and nausea and vomiting. The combination of low concentration of local anesthetic and opioid solutions has provided excellent analgesia with few side effects.

D. The dose and the volume of solution to be injected depends on (1) clinical aspects of the patient, (2) the distance from the site of injection to the pertinent nerve roots, (3) the region of the spine being entered, and (4) the physicochemical properties of the drug being administered. For example, 20 to 30 ml of local anesthetic solution may be required to reach the T4 dermatome from the lumbar region, but 5 ml of the same solution in the thoracic lesion may spread over several dermatomal levels. Three to five milligrams of

morphine in the lumbar region may be adequate for lower extremity pain, whereas 5 to 10 mg is needed to alleviate thoracic pain when injected from the same region of the spine.

E. Because of the risk of complications, resuscitation equipment and IV access must be present before proceeding with an epidural blockade. Scrub the skin over the spine with a disinfectant while the patient is sitting or in the lateral decubitus position. Obtain cutaneous and subcutaneous analgesia with local anesthetic, and pass an epidural needle through the ligamentum flavum. Advance the needle slowly until the epidural space is identified by the loss of resistance or hanging drop technique. After a negative aspiration for cerebrospinal fluid and blood, inject an appropriate solution, usually 3 ml of 2% lidocaine with 1:200,000 epinephrine, through the needle to detect IV or subarachnoid placement of the needle. Check vital signs every 5 minutes. For short surgical procedures inject the remainder of local anesthetic solution through the needle, and then withdraw it. For longer procedures and for short- and long-term pain management thread a catheter through the needle into the epidural space and secure it to the skin in a sterile fashion. For long-term use, the catheter can be tunneled subcutaneously away from the site of insertion.

F. Complications of epidural blockade local anesthetics include (1) hypotension caused by sympathetic blockade, (2) local anesthetic toxicity due to intravascular injection or uptake from the epidural space, and (3) the paralysis and apnea caused by high epidural, subarachnoid, or subdural injection. Epidurally administered opioids can cause respiratory depression, pruritus, nausea and vomiting, and urinary retention. Perform frequent inspection and redressing of long-term catheters to avoid infection. Epidural hematomas should be suspected with increasing back pain and progressive neurologic deficits. Accidental dural puncture may result in postdural puncture headache.

REFERENCES

Bromage PR: *Epidural Analgesia*. Philadelphia: WB Saunders, 1978, p. 8.

Cousins MJ, Mather LE: Intrathecal and epidural administration of opioids. *Anesthesiology* 1984;61:276.

Eisenach JC: Pain relief in obstetrics. In: Raj PP (ed) *Practical Management of Pain*. St. Louis, Mosby-Year Book, 1992, p. 391.

Elliott RD: Continuous infusion epidural analgesia for obstetrics: bupivacaine versus bupivacaine-fentanyl mixture. *Can J Anaesth* 1991;38:303.

Loeser JD, Cousins MJ: Contemporary pain management. *Med J Aust* 1990;153:208.

Mulroy MF: *Regional Anesthesia*. Boston: Little, Brown, 1989, p. 93.

Raj SP, Pai U: Techniques of nerve blocking. Conduction blocks. In: Raj P (ed) *Handbook of Regional Anesthesia*. New York: Churchill Livingstone, 1985, p. 237.

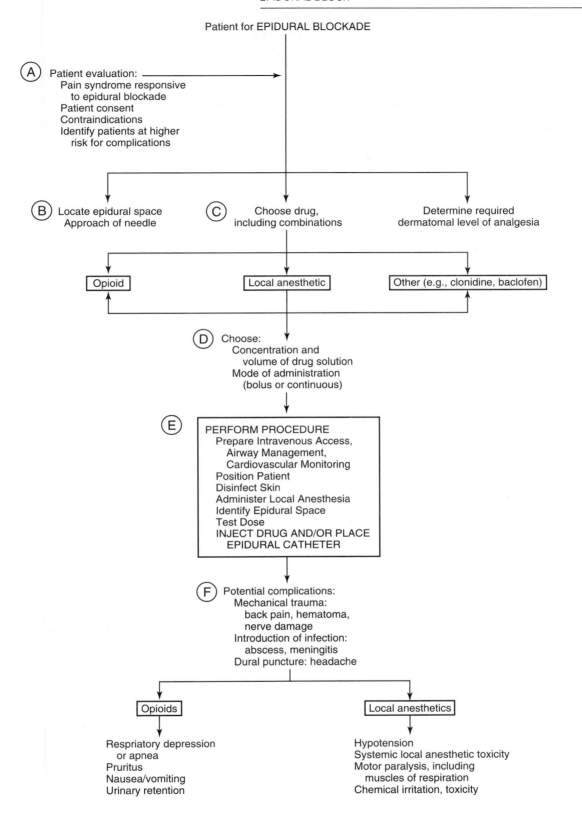

Patient for EPIDURAL BLOCKADE

(A) Patient evaluation:
    Pain syndrome responsive
        to epidural blockade
    Patient consent
    Contraindications
    Identify patients at higher
        risk for complications

(B) Locate epidural space
    Approach of needle

(C) Choose drug,
    including combinations

Determine required
dermatomal level of analgesia

Opioid

Local anesthetic

Other (e.g., clonidine, baclofen)

(D) Choose:
    Concentration and
        volume of drug solution
    Mode of administration
        (bolus or continuous)

(E) PERFORM PROCEDURE
    Prepare Intravenous Access,
        Airway Management,
        Cardiovascular Monitoring
    Position Patient
    Disinfect Skin
    Administer Local Anesthesia
    Identify Epidural Space
    Test Dose
    INJECT DRUG AND/OR PLACE
        EPIDURAL CATHETER

(F) Potential complications:
    Mechanical trauma:
        back pain, hematoma,
        nerve damage
    Introduction of infection:
        abscess, meningitis
    Dural puncture: headache

Opioids

Respriatory depression
    or apnea
Pruritus
Nausea/vomiting
Urinary retention

Local anesthetics

Hypotension
Systemic local anesthetic toxicity
Motor paralysis, including
    muscles of respiration
Chemical irritation, toxicity

Subarachnoid Block

DALE SOLOMON AND SOMAYAJI RAMAMURTHY

The subarachnoid space is contiguous with the intracranial cerebrospinal fluid (CSF) pathways and ends at the S2 spinal level in adults. Drugs injected into the CSF of the spine have a rapid action on exposed nerve membranes of the spinal cord and nerve roots. Subarachnoid blocks (SABs) are used to treat various acute and chronic pain syndromes, for diagnostic purposes, and to treat muscular spasms associated with cerebral, motor, or spinal cord dysfunction.

A. Candidates for SAB should consent to the procedure and have stable neurologic function, normal clotting function, no evidence of systemic sepsis, and no inflammation or infection over the proposed site of injection. Hypovolemic patients have an exaggerated hypotensive response to the sympathectomy caused by local anesthetics. Because of the risk of downward herniation of the brain, the dura must not be punctured when CSF pressure is elevated intracranially.

B. The subarachnoid space can be entered with a needle anywhere along its path, but to prevent injury to the spinal cord a site of entrance caudad to the conus medullaris (L1–2 in adults L2–3 in infants) is normally chosen. In the lumbar area, use either a midline or a paramedian approach to access the subarachnoid space through the interlaminar foramen. Because the spinous processes run nearly perpendicular to the long axis of the spine in this region, a spinal needle placed into the interspinous ligament is directed perpendicularly. Alternatively, the needle may be directed toward the midline from a position 1 cm lateral to the midline.

C. The choice and quantity of drug injected into the subarachnoid space are based on patient characteristics, the desired goal of the blockade, and the desired duration of the blockade. Any drug chosen should have a record of safety in the CSF and be preservative free. For short surgical procedures use of lidocaine has significantly decreased because of the high incidence of transient nerve root irritation syndrome. Preservative-free chloroprocaine is a good substitute. For longer procedures, use either tetracaine or bupivacaine. Vasoconstrictors (usually epinephrine, 1:200,000) can intensify the analgesia and prolong the blockade of most local anesthetics. The local anesthetic can be diluted with water, saline, or dextrose to make the specific gravity of the final solution less, equal to, or greater than the specific gravity of CSF. In the case of hypobaric or hyperbaric solutions, some degree of control of the spread of the local anesthetic in the CSF can be attained by patient positioning. For isobaric solutions, the spread of the blockade is governed primarily by the number of milligrams of local anesthetic injected, rather than the volume.

D. The required dermatomal level of any blockade depends on the level of the spinal cord at which the afferent pain impulses insert. For example, a blockade of somatic pain afferents may be effected by blockade of lower thoracic dermatomes during intraabdominal surgery, but visceral afferents passing through the celiac plexus and traveling along with the fibers of the sympathetic chain require a much higher level of blockade. Neurolytic agents can be placed into the subarachnoid space and directed toward the dorsal root ganglia while preserving motor fibers by using hypobaric or hyperbaric solutions.

E. Airway management devices must be at the bedside and there must be IV access before an SAB is instituted. Scrub the skin overlying the proposed site of entrance with disinfectant solution while the patient is in a sitting, lateral decubitus, or prone position. Obtain local anesthesia of the skin and subcutaneous area, and pass the needle toward the dura with the bevel oriented parallel to the long axis of the spine. As the dura is punctured, a distinct pop is often felt and CSF should return freely. Any blood cells should quickly clear, and there should be no paresthesias before or during injection. After an injection of local anesthetic, the patient may be turned immediately or left in the same position while the block is set up. Take vital signs every 5 minutes after injection of the local anesthetic, and follow the spread of anesthesia closely. For short surgical procedures, local anesthetics can be injected in a "one-shot" technique. For longer procedures and chronic pain therapy, pass a catheter through the spinal needle and leave it in the subarachnoid space for intermittent or continuous injections of local anesthetic or opiates. The catheter may also be tunneled subcutaneously.

F. Potential complications of SAB with local anesthetics include (1) backache in up to 40% of patients, (2) hypotension caused by sympathectomy, (3) postdural puncture headache, (4) nausea caused by unopposed vagal activity, (5) bradycardia from blockade of cardiac sympathetic fibers, (6) respiratory insufficiency due to hypotension or high motor blockade, (7) spinal cord or nerve root damage due to mechanical or chemical irritation, (8) chemical or bacterial meningitis, and (9) spinal and/or epidural hematoma and abscess. Subarachnoid opioids also cause the same complications as do epidural opioids.

REFERENCES

Albright AL, Cervi A, Singletary J: Intrathecal baclofen for spasticity in cerebral palsy. *JAMA* 1991;265:1418.

Bonnet F, Brisson VB, Francois Y, et al: Effects of oral and subarachnoid clonidine on spinal anesthesia with bupivacaine. *Reg Anesth* 1990;15:211.

Cousins JJ, Cherry DA, Gourlay GK: Acute and chronic pain: use of spinal opioids. In: Cousins MJ, Bridenbaugh PO (eds) *Neural Blockade in Clinical Anesthesia and Management of Pain*, 2nd ed. Philadelphia: JB Lippincott, 1988, p. 955.

Lee JA, Atkinson RS, Watt JM: *Lumbar Puncture and Spinal Analgesia: Intraduaral and Extradural.* Edinburgh: Churchill Livingstone, 1985, p. 60.

Mulroy MF: *Regional Anesthesia.* Boston: Little, Brown, 1989, p. 86.
Stienstra R, Greene NM: Factors affecting the subarachnoid spread of local anesthetic solutions. *Reg Anesth* 1991;16:1.

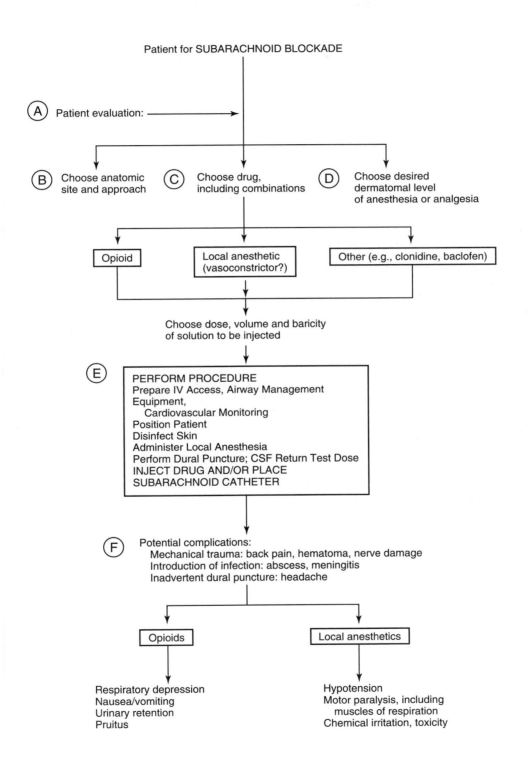

Patient for SUBARACHNOID BLOCKADE

(A) Patient evaluation:

(B) Choose anatomic site and approach

(C) Choose drug, including combinations

(D) Choose desired dermatomal level of anesthesia or analgesia

Opioid

Local anesthetic (vasoconstrictor?)

Other (e.g., clonidine, baclofen)

Choose dose, volume and baricity of solution to be injected

(E) PERFORM PROCEDURE
Prepare IV Access, Airway Management Equipment,
    Cardiovascular Monitoring
Position Patient
Disinfect Skin
Administer Local Anesthesia
Perform Dural Puncture; CSF Return Test Dose
INJECT DRUG AND/OR PLACE
SUBARACHNOID CATHETER

(F) Potential complications:
    Mechanical trauma: back pain, hematoma, nerve damage
    Introduction of infection: abscess, meningitis
    Inadvertent dural puncture: headache

Opioids

Local anesthetics

Respiratory depression
Nausea/vomiting
Urinary retention
Pruitus

Hypotension
Motor paralysis, including
    muscles of respiration
Chemical irritation, toxicity

Cranial Nerve Block

SOMAYAJI RAMAMURTHY

Cranial nerve blocks are utilized in the diagnosis and management of head and neck pain. The choice of the nerve block depends on the location and the distribution of the pain.

Dermatomal distribution. Most of the face is supplied by the divisions of the trigeminal nerve. Skin over the lower part of the mandible and the lower part of the pinna of the ear is supplied by the branches of C2 (greater articular nerve). The posterior part of the top of the head is supplied by greater and lesser occipital nerves that arise from C2. The anterior two thirds of the tongue is supplied by the lingual branch of the mandibular nerve. The posterior one third of the tongue is supplied by the branches of the glossopharyngeal nerve. The third, fourth, and sixth cranial nerves supply the muscles of the eye. The third cranial nerve carries sympathetic and parasympathetic fibers. These nerves are blocked doing the retrobulbar block performed for ophthalmic surgery. The vagus and the cranial portion of the accessory nerve together innervate the mucosa and the muscles of the pharynx and the larynx. The spinal portion of the accessory nerve innervates the sternocleidomastoid and the trapezius muscles. Block of this nerve is useful during neck and shoulder surgery and in the management of cervical dystonia.

A. *Trigeminal block.* The Gasserian ganglion is blocked with local anesthetic, steroids, and glycerol and radiofrequency techniques to manage the pain secondary to trigeminal neuralgia, usually under fluoroscopic guidance. The terminal branches such as supraorbital, supratrochlear, infraorbital, and mental branches are blocked when the pain is very localized in their distribution. The auriculotemporal nerve is blocked to relieve the pain originating from the temporomandibular joint. The mandibular and the maxillary divisions can be blocked percutaneously through the coronoid notch. These nerves also can be blocked transorally.

B. *Facial nerve block.* This nerve can be blocked as it exits from the stylomastoid foramen. A needle is advanced along the anterior surface of the mastoid process connected to a nerve stimulator until contraction of the facial muscles is noted. Two to three milliliters of local anesthetic will produce a block. This nerve block is useful in patients who have hemifacial spasms.

C. *Sphenopalatine ganglion block.* This ganglion can be blocked in three different ways. The most common method is to block it through the nose using local anesthetic–soaked Q-tips® through the nose and placing the Q-tips in contact with the nasopharyngeal wall just posterior to the middle turbinate. Percutaneously the ganglion can be blocked through the coronoid notch and by directing the needle just anterior to the lateral pterygoid plate into the pterygomaxillary fissure. Transorally the needle is placed through the greater palatine foramen and advancing that needle into the pterygomaxillary fossa.

D. *Glossopharyngeal nerve.* The 11th cranial nerve can be blocked transorally at the base of the posterior tonsillar pillar. Percutaneously the nerve can be blocked by advancing a needle just anterior to the mastoid process and redirecting the needle posteriorly after contacting the styloid process. The needle tip is very close to the carotid artery and the jugular vein.

   The vagus nerve is also blocked. This block is useful in the diagnosis of glossopharyngeal neuralgia.

E. *Spinal accessory nerve.* This nerve is blocked by injecting 5 ml of local anesthetic into the proximal portion of the sternocleidomastoid muscle.

Precautions and complications. The usual precautions necessary for any local anesthetic injection are taken. Even the injection of a very small quantity of local anesthetic agent into a branch of the facial artery can produce convulsion. The injections in the neck weakening the muscles can produce dizziness and lack of balance.

REFERENCE

Rosenberg M, Phero JC: Regional anesthesia and invasive techniques to manage head and neck pain. *Otolaryngol Clin North Am* 2003;36:1201–1219.

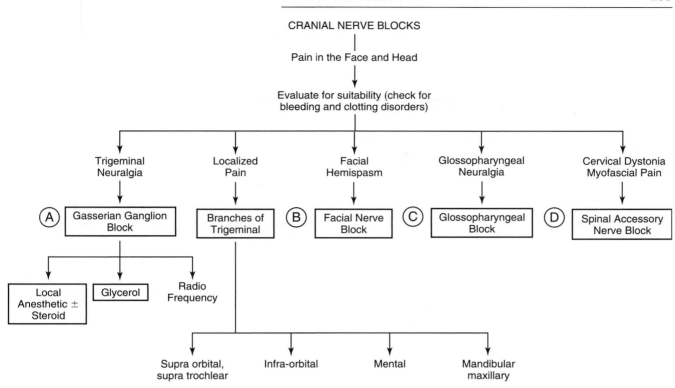

Sympathetic Blocks

EULECHE ALANMANOU

Substantial controversies still surround pain-relieving procedures that target the sympathetic nervous system. It is believed that sympathetic afferents may depolarize nociceptive afferent fibers at the site of nerve injury. It is also suggested that the cell bodies of sensory neurons in the dorsal root ganglion come under the closer influence of sympathetic axons following nerve injury, so sympathetic activity may be capable of initiating or maintaining activity in sensory fibers.

A. The list of indications for sympathetic nerve block is long, and much of the evidence does not include randomized clinical trials. The decision to block a specific site depends on the painful body part. The physician should be prepared to deal with potential side effects and complications. The patient should sign an informed consent that details the risks of the procedure.

B. Before the block is performed, a pain measurement (i.e., Visual Analogue Scale), any motor or sensory deficit, and a temperature over the affected area are compared to those on the contralateral site and documented.

C. Once a nerve block is performed, it is essential to confirm that the targeted nerve has been reached. It is also useful to know if an undesired block has occurred, such as blockade of an adjacent nerve. The postblock examination also includes assessment of temperature (a change of at least 1.5°C), sweating, and the sympathogalvanic response. Any sensory or motor change as well as a new pain measurement should be documented. The precision of sympathetic nerve blocks can be enhanced during their performance by techniques such as fluoroscopy, sonography, or computed tomography guidance.

D. Sympathetic denervation produces sudomotor, vasomotor, and ocular (stellate ganglion) changes. It leads to vasodilation, except in the trunk where vasoconstriction follows a segmental sympathetic block. In practice, only pain relief of more than 50% should lead to a repeat block. As for any block, a result should be interpreted cautiously after a sympathetic block. It is suggested that one should avoid the circular logic of defining sympathetically maintained pain as a condition relieved by sympathetic block, and a block is deemed successful if it relieves a pain that was assumed to be sympathetically maintained.

REFERENCES

Buckley FP: Regional anesthesia with local anesthetic. In: Loeser JD (ed) *Bonica's Management of Pain*, 3rd ed. Philadelphia, Lippincott Williams & Wilkins, 2000.

Hogan QH, Abram SE: Neural blockade for diagnosis and prognosis: a review. *Anesthesiology* 1997;86:216–241.

Justins D, Siemaszko O: Rational use of neural blockade for the management of chronic pain. In: Giamberardino MA (ed) *Pain 2002—An Updated Review: Refresher Course Syllabus*. Seattle, IASP Press, 2002.

Raja SN: Nerve blocks in the evaluation of chronic pain: a plea for caution in their use and interpretation. *Anesthesiology* 1997;86:4–6.

Ramamurthy S, Winnie AP: Regional anesthetic techniques for pain relief. *Semin Anesth* 1985;4:237.

SYMPATHETIC NERVE BLOCK

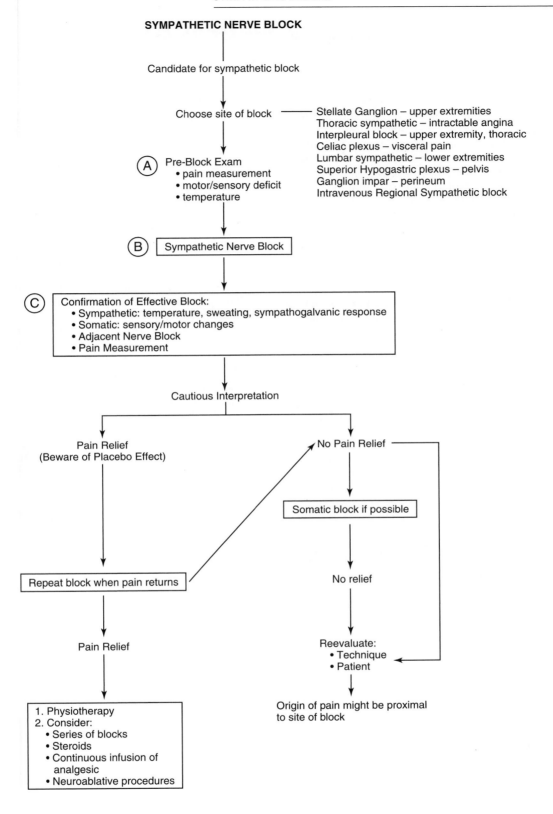

Candidate for sympathetic block

Choose site of block — Stellate Ganglion – upper extremities
Thoracic sympathetic – intractable angina
Interpleural block – upper extremity, thoracic
Celiac plexus – visceral pain
Lumbar sympathetic – lower extremities
Superior Hypogastric plexus – pelvis
Ganglion impar – perineum
Intravenous Regional Sympathetic block

(A) Pre-Block Exam
• pain measurement
• motor/sensory deficit
• temperature

(B) Sympathetic Nerve Block

(C) Confirmation of Effective Block:
• Sympathetic: temperature, sweating, sympathogalvanic response
• Somatic: sensory/motor changes
• Adjacent Nerve Block
• Pain Measurement

Cautious Interpretation

Pain Relief
(Beware of Placebo Effect)

No Pain Relief

Somatic block if possible

Repeat block when pain returns

No relief

Pain Relief

Reevaluate:
• Technique
• Patient

1. Physiotherapy
2. Consider:
  • Series of blocks
  • Steroids
  • Continuous infusion of
    analgesic
  • Neuroablative procedures

Origin of pain might be proximal
to site of block

Continuous Neural Block

SOMAYAJI RAMAMURTHY

The technology and the safety of the equipment used for continuous block have significantly improved over the last decade. Use of a nerve stimulator, availability of insulated Touhy needles, use of stimulating catheters, and fluoroscopic guidance have improved the accuracy of placement. It is important to make sure that the patient does not have any bleeding or clotting problems due either to a disease process or to pharmacotherapy. The wound site should be inspected carefully to recognize any signs of infection. Some clinicians use prophylactic antibiotics.

Various models of convenient, portable infusion pumps are available including battery-operated models and constant-flow balloon-type infusers.

A. *Indications.* When a local anesthetic block provides only a short-term but good quality pain relief, placing a catheter and providing longer term analgesia may be very useful for longer interruption of the pain cycle and also to provide analgesia for physical therapy. Continuous techniques are very commonly utilized to provide postoperative analgesia. These techniques are also utilized for performing epidural and intrathecal trials with opioids, local anesthetic, clonidine, and baclofen for spasticity.

B. *Brachial plexus block.* Continuous interscalene, infraclavicular, or axillary techniques provide excellent analgesia for upper extremity pain. These techniques are commonly utilized to provide prolonged postoperative analgesia. Patients who have chronic regional pain syndrome benefit significantly when the pain cycle is interrupted and analgesia is provided for physical therapy. After the initial block, 6 to 8 ml/hour of local anesthetic is usually sufficient to maintain good analgesia.

C. *Epidural block.* Continuous epidural block is the most common technique used for the management of lower extremity, abdominal and thoracic pain in the postoperative period. Thoracic epidural catheters are useful for management of thoracic and abdominal pain whereas lumbar catheters are useful for the management of lower extremity pain. With the catheter placed at the proper level, 5 to 8 ml/hour of local anesthetic with an opioid provides excellent analgesia over a long period, including for physical therapy. The patient should be monitored for complications such as respiratory depression, muscle weakness, pressure sores secondary to sensory loss, hypotension due to sympathetic block, urinary retention, and pruritus. For hygienic reasons, the sacral epidural technique is not commonly utilized.

D. *Peripheral nerve blocks.* The continuous block of the femoral and/or sciatic nerves or lumbar plexus is commonly utilized for the management of lower extremity pain. The sciatic nerve catheter can be placed utilizing parasacral, lateral, and popliteal approaches. The femoral and lateral femoral cutaneous nerves are blocked using either three-in-one block or fascia iliaca approach. An infusion of a weak local anesthetic 6 to 10 ml/hour is commonly used. Continuous intercostal, paravertebral, and interpleural blocks are useful to provide analgesia over the chest and the abdominal wall.

E. *Spinal (subarachnoid).* A continuous spinal (subarachnoid) catheter technique is most commonly utilized for intrathecal trial with opioids or baclofen before considering the patient for permanent placement of an intrathecal infusion system. An appropriate dose of the opioid together with 3 to 5 mg of ropivacaine or bupivacaine over a 24-hour period is commonly utilized. A continuous trial with opioids or baclofen over 3 to 4 days seems to provide much better information than single-shot spinal opioid or baclofen.

REFERENCES

Cousins MJ, Bridenbaugh PO: *Neural Blockade in Clinical Anesthesia and Management of Pain*, 3rd ed. New York, Lippincott-Raven, 1998.

Enneking EK, Chan V, Greger J, et al: Lower-extremity peripheral nerve blockade: essentials of our current understanding. *Reg Anesth Pain Med* 2005;30:4–35.

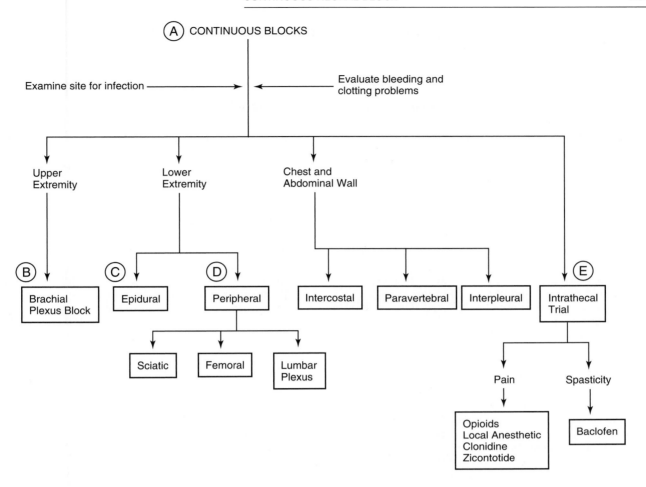

Intravenous Regional Block

SOMAYAJI RAMAMURTHY

A. This technique is commonly used for providing analgesia for short surgical procedures of the extremities. Intravenous regional anesthesia (IVR) is also utilized in the management of chronic regional pain syndrome. Technically, IVR is very easy to perform. Unlike other regional blocks, IVR can even be performed in patients who have bleeding and clotting disorders. Bilateral procedures can be done if needed. The popularity of the technique has significantly decreased because of the lack of availability of drugs such as guanethidine, bretylium, and so forth and the lack of clear evidence of a high level of efficacy. IVR is still useful to provide short-term analgesia to facilitate physical therapy.

B. The equipment is thoroughly checked. The availability of appropriate resuscitation equipment and drugs to treat local anesthetic toxicity is confirmed.

C. *Technique.* A small-gauge (22- or 24-) plastic intravenous cannula is placed in the involved extremity. A double-cuff tourniquet is applied over the proximal part of the extremity. The pressure required to obliterate the distal arterial pulse is noted, utilizing both cuffs of the tourniquet individually. The extremity is thoroughly exsanguinated using an Esmarch type of bandage. This can be a very painful procedure and may require sedation and analgesia. The proximal tourniquet is inflated and the absence of distal arterial pulse is confirmed. The Esmarch bandage is unwrapped. The mixture (30 ml for upper extremity and 50 ml for the lower extremity) containing 3 mg/kg of 0.5% lidocaine mixed with guanethidine (25 to 50 mg) or bretylium 1.5 mg/kg is injected very slowly into the IV cannula. After the onset of analgesia the joints of the extremity can be mobilized to improve the range of motion. The tourniquet is deflated intermittently, that is, 15 seconds of deflation followed by 30 seconds of reinflation, repeated for three cycles. This protocol reduces the peak blood level of local anesthetic drugs in the systemic circulation, thereby decreasing the incidence of systemic toxicity of the local anesthetic agents. If the patient experiences tourniquet discomfort before 20 minutes the distal tourniquet can be inflated over the anesthetized area, thereby increasing the tourniquet tolerance. The procedure is repeated twice a week for 2 weeks and the patient's improvement in pain level and function is reassessed.

REFERENCES

Glynn CJ, Basedow RW, Walsh JA: Pain relief following post-ganglionic sympathetic blockade with i.v. guanethidine. *Br J Anaesth* 1981;53:1297–1302.

Holmes CMK: Intravenous regional analgesia. A useful method of producing analgesia of the limbs. *Lancet* 1963;1:245–247.

Ramamurthy S, Hoffman J: Intravenous regional guanethidine. *Anesth Analg* 1995;81:718–723.

INTRAVENOUS REGIONAL BLOCK

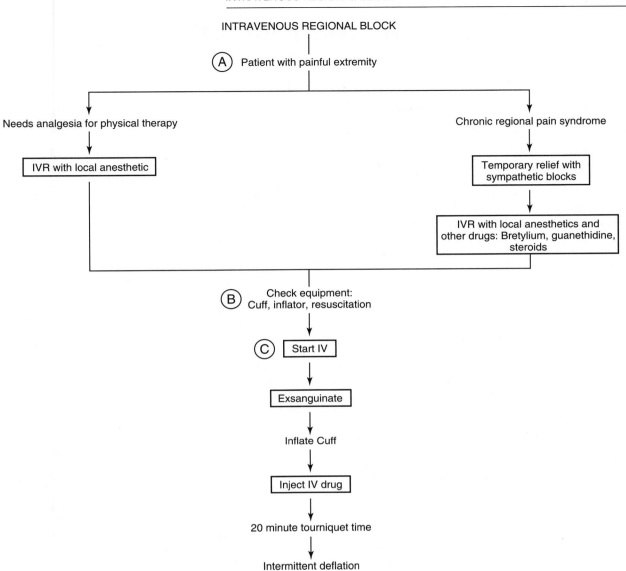

Steroid Joint Injections

LEY L. TAYLOR-JONES AND EULECHE ALANMANOU

Corticosteroids have glucocorticoid, antiinflammatory, and mineralocorticoid activity. Steroids also produce immunosuppressive effects in humans. The antiinflammatory effects of steroids are produced by the inhibition of prostaglandin synthesis, collagenase formation, and granulation tissue formation.

Corticosteroid joint injections are used to treat inflammatory processes. These injections may help determine the source of pain as articular or extraarticular. When oral medications, including nonsteroidal antiinflammatory drugs (NSAIDs), have failed, or are contraindicated, intraarticular injections may provide rapid pain relief and facilitate the utilization of appropriate physical therapy when indicated. Patients may also experience pain relief from other inflamed joints for a brief time.

The clinician performing the injection should have a thorough knowledge of the pharmacology of steroids and detailed knowledge of the anatomic basis of the procedure. Aseptic techniques should be respected at all times.

Contraindications to intraarticular joint injections include overlying soft tissue infection, bacteremia, articular instability, septic arthritis, avascular necrosis, osteonecrosis, neurotrophic joints, anatomic inaccessibility, and patient refusal. Steroid injection in the Charcot joint provides short-term relief only. A surgical prosthetic joint is more prone to infection than a normal joint and therefore is a contraindication for steroid injection.

Before an injection is started, the appropriate anatomic landmarks should be identified. A joint injection is done from the extensor surface where the synovium is closest to the skin. This minimizes the chance of injecting materials into arteries, veins, and nerves. To decrease the risk of a septic joint, sterile preparation and draping are mandatory, and the physician must wear sterile gloves, observe strict aseptic techniques, and use single-use vials. A skin wheal may be raised with 1% to 2% lidocaine. A 4 cm long 22- to 25-gauge needle is inserted through the skin and into the joint cavity. Aspiration is necessary to avoid intravascular injection. Aspiration of synovial fluid confirms the position of the needle, although one may not always obtain fluid, as tissue may be resting against the bevel of the needle. The aspirated fluid should be checked for inflammatory components unless the fluid is clear and straw-colored. If an infection is suspected, the steroid joint injection is delayed until infection is ruled out. The injection should be resistance-free, and once the medication is in place the needle should be flushed with normal saline or local anesthetic.

Several corticosteroid agents are suitable for joint injections. Potency, onset, duration of action, and side effects should be considered before injection. Table 1 provides guidelines only. The antiinflammatory potency is relative to the potency of hydrocortisone and the dose depends on the size of the joint to be injected.

Complications associated with steroid injection into a joint include infection and postinjection inflammation. The infection rate is reported to be extremely low (0.005%) if strict aseptic technique is used. Postinjection inflammation typically lasts 4 to 12 hours and is treated with NSAIDs and ice. If the postinjection pain lasts longer than 1 day, the patient should be reevaluated for infection. Tissue atrophy is a significant concern when injecting a steroid into joints. This can occur when the steroid leaks out of the joint or if the injection is too shallow or outside the joint. Repeated injections into the same joint can result in calcification and subsequent rupture of the ligaments. Trauma to the articular cartilage is also a concern. Weight-bearing joints should not be given injections more frequently than every 3 to 4 months to minimize damage to the ligaments and cartilage. A large joint should be given an injection only three or four times per year or a maximum of 10 times total. A small joint should only be injected two or three times per year or a maximum of four times total. Other systemic effects include increased blood glucose, hormonal suppression, fluid and electrolyte disturbances, gastrointestinal problems, dermatologic complications, and metabolic reactions. More discussion about steroids in Chapter 90, p. 248.

REFERENCES

Delisa J, Gans MB: Injection procedures. In: Delisa JA, Gans BM (eds) *Rehabilitation Medicine: Principles and Practice*, 3rd ed. Philadelphia, Lippincott Williams & Wilkins, 1998, p 553.

Hardman JG, Limbird LE (eds): ACTH: adrenocortical steroids and their synthetic analogs. In: *Goodman & Gilman's The Pharmacological Basis of Therapeutics*, 9th ed. New York, McGraw-Hill, 1996, p 1466.

Newman RJ, Kumar N: Complications of intra- and peri-articular steroid injections. *Br J Gen Pract* 1999;49:465.

Robinson DR: Prostaglandins and the mechanism of action of anti-inflammatory drugs. *Am J Med* 1983;75:26.

TABLE 1
Characteristics of Corticosteroids

Characteristic	Methylprednisolone (Depo-Medrol)	Hydrocortisone (cortisol)	Prednisolone (Hydeltra)	Triamcinolone (Aristospan)	Betamethasone (Celestone)
Antiinflammatory potency	5	1	4	5	25
Salt retention property	0	2+	1+	0	0
Onset	Slow	Fast	Fast	Moderate	Fast
Duration of action	Intermediate	Short	Intermediate	Intermediate	Long
Plasma half-life (min)	180	90	200	300	300
Concentration (mg/mL)	40–80	50	20	20	6
Usual dose (mg)	10–40	25–100	10–40	5–20	1.5–6.0

0: no salt retention.

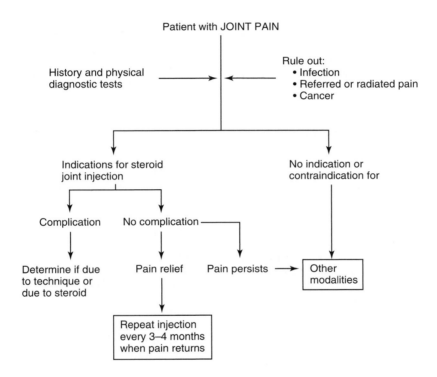

Epidural Steroid Injections

NIKESH BATRA

Epidural steroid injection (ESI) is perhaps one of the most commonly used weapons in the pain specialists' armamentarium. It has been used for back pain caused by annulus tear, chronic lumbar degenerative disc disease, herniated nucleus pulposus without neurologic deficits, and herniated nucleus pulposus with nerve root irritation or compression as well as pain caused by degenerative joint disease, spondylosis, scoliosis, spondylolisthesis, post-laminectomy syndrome, and spinal stenosis. It has also been used for postherpetic neuralgia.

A. Response to ESIs is predicted by nerve root irritation, recent onset of symptoms, and absence of psychological overlay. A favorable response is seen in patients with advanced educational background, primary diagnosis of radiculopathy, and pain of less than 6 months' duration. Factors associated with treatment failure include constant pain, frequent sleep disruption, and being unemployed owing to pain.

The rationale for epidural steroids focuses on the strong anti-inflammatory actions of the corticosteroids. Nerve root edema is seen in patients with herniated discs. Herniated discs have been found to contain high levels of the enzyme phospholipase A_2, which liberates arachidonic acid from cell membranes. Leakage of this enzyme may cause chemical irritation of nerve roots. Steroids interfere with the inflammatory process by inducing synthesis of a phospholipase A_2 inhibitor. Furthermore, administration of epidural solutions clears or dilutes the chemical irritants. Steroids also exert their effects by other modes, including membrane stabilization, inhibition of neural peptide synthesis or action, suppression of ongoing neuronal discharge, and suppression of the sensitization of dorsal horn neurons.

The most common steroids used in the epidural space include methylprednisolone acetate 80 mg or triamcinolone diacetate 50 mg. Usually a total volume of 6 to 10 ml is adequate for lumbar epidural administration, whereas 4 to 6 ml is used for the cervical region. Larger volumes 15 to 30 ml are required for administration through the caudal space. In contrast, only 0.5 to 2 ml is used for transforaminal injections.

The objective of epidural steroid injection is to deliver corticosteroid close to the site of pathology, presumably onto an inflamed nerve root. Caudal and interlaminar epidural injections are affected by the presence or absence of epidural ligaments or scarring, which may prevent migration of the posteriorly administered injectate to the anterior epidural space. For optimum results, the corticosteroid should reach the ventral epidural space in front of the dural sac and behind the disc. The transforaminal approach shows good ventral flow, whereas the interlaminar method predominantly shows dorsal flow, which is far removed from the usual site of inflammation.

B. The response of the patient is the most important factor determining the number or frequency of the epidural steroid injections. It is preferable to wait at least 2 weeks between injections. If the patient has an excellent response, the epidural steroid injection can be repeated on an as-needed basis if the pain returns.

C. If the patient has minimal relief with the interlaminar epidural injection, one transforaminal, site-specific, epidural steroid injection should be tried. During the initial stabilization phase, if the patient has good relief after 1 to 2 weeks and the pain comes back although not as severe as before, a second epidural injection becomes necessary. The need for a third injection is based on the response to the second. During the maintenance phase, the epidural steroid injection can be repeated every 3 months (maximum 3 times per year) only if the patient gets at least 50% relief for at least 6 weeks.

Disadvantages of the caudal approach include injection of a substantial volume of fluid, thereby diluting the injected corticosteroid, and unrecognized placement of the needle outside the epidural space or inside a blood vessel. The interlaminar approach also carries the disadvantages of diluting the injectate, extraepidural or intravascular placement of the needle, preferential cranial flow of the solution and preferential posterior flow of the solution, technical difficulties in postsurgical patients, dural puncture, and trauma to the spinal cord. The transforaminal epidural injections carry the potential complications of intraneural injection, neural trauma, intravascular injection, and spinal cord trauma. Other complications of epidural steroid administration include inadvertent intrathecal steroid injection causing aseptic meningitis, adhesive arachnoiditis, pachymeningitis, or conus medullaris syndrome, although clinicians have used intrathecal steroids without problems in the past. Epidural steroids affect the hypothalamus-pituitary-adrenal axis, resulting in depression of the plasma cortisol levels for up to 3 to 5 weeks. They can also cause iatrogenic Cushing's syndrome, congestive heart failure secondary to fluid retention, and changes in blood glucose levels in susceptible individuals.

REFERENCES

Atluri SL: Interlaminar epidural use of steroids. In: Manchikanti L, Slipman CW, Fellows B (eds): *Interventional Pain Management: Low Back Pain—Diagnosis and Treatment*. Paducah, KY, American Society of Interventional Pain Physicians, 2002.

Benzon HT: Epidural steroids. In: Raj PP (ed) *Pain Medicine: A Comprehensive Review*. St. Louis, Mosby, 1996.

Manchikanti L, Saini B, Singh V: Transforaminal epidural use of steroids. In: Manchikanti L, Slipman CW, Fellows B (eds) *Interventional Pain Management: Low Back Pain—Diagnosis and Treatment*. Paducah, KY, American Society of Interventional Pain Physicians, 2002.

Manchikanti L, Singh V: Caudal epidural use of steroids. In: Manchikanti L, Slipman CW, Fellows B (eds) *Interventional Pain Management:*

Low Back Pain—Diagnosis and Treatment. Paducah, KY, American Society of Interventional Pain Physicians, 2002.

Molloy R, Benzon H: Injection of epidural steroids. In: Benzon H, Raja SN, Borsook D, et al (eds) *Essentials of Pain Medicine and Regional Anesthesia*. New York, Churchill Livingstone, 1999.

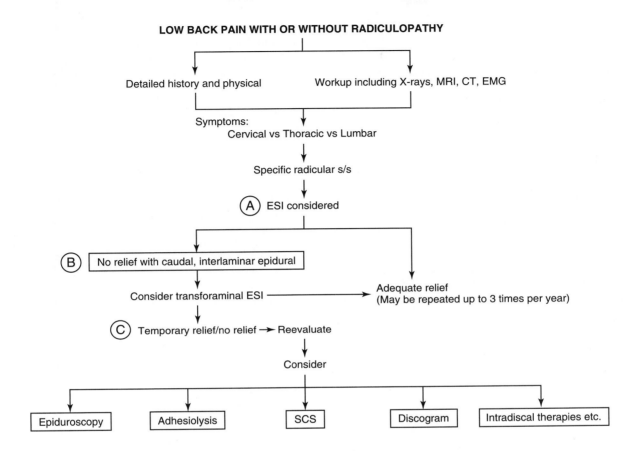

Radiographic Contrast Media

EULECHE ALANMANOU

Contrast agents have become useful for many pain management procedures requiring fluoroscopic assistance. They help visualize the needle tip, the spread of the substance injected, and the target structures. Radiographic contrast media are iodinated. Two types of contrast agent are commonly used. The ionic contrast agents have high osmolarity and include Renografim (diatrizoate) and Conray (iothalamate). The non-ionic agents have low osmolarity and include Isovue (iopamidol) and Omnipaque (iohexol).

A. In general, ionic contrast agents are neurotoxic and therefore not recommended for myelography, epidurography, or any other procedures in which dural puncture is likely (e.g., epidural injection, facet joint injection, selective nerve blocks, discography). Non-ionic agents are approved for those procedures and for intrathecal use. Non-ionic contrast agents are more expensive.

B. Adverse reactions to contrast media include nausea, vomiting, pruritus, dyspnea, bronchospasm, anaphylactic reaction, and cardiac arrest. The incidence of these reactions is increased in individuals with known sensitivities (asthma, multiple food and drug allergies, prior reaction to contrast media). Contrast agents should be used with caution in patients with poor renal function and paraproteinemias.

C. Patients at risk for allergic reactions to contrast agents should receive prophylactic treatment including steroids or H_1- and H_2-blockers (or both) before the exposure. In any case, the pain practitioner and his or her staff should be knowledgeable about resuscitation and prepared to manage adverse reactions that occur during pain management procedures.

REFERENCES

Curry NS, Schabel SI, Reiheld CT, et al: Fatal reactions to intravenous non-ionic contrast material. *Radiology* 1991;178:361.

Cusmano J: Premedication regimen eases contrast reaction. *Diagn Imaging* 1992;181–182, 185–186.

Greenberger PA, Patterson R: The prevention of immediate generalized repeated reactions to radiocontrast media in high-risk patients. *J Allergy Clin Immunol* 1991;87:867–872.

Lawrence V, Matthai W, Hartmaier S: Comparative safety of high-osmolality and low-osmolality radiographic contrast agents: report of multidisciplinary working group. *Invest Radiol* 1992;27:2–18.

RADIOGRAPHIC USES OF CONTRAST MEDIA

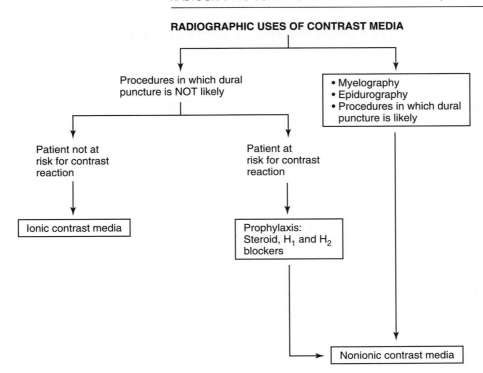

Intradiscal Therapies

OCTAVIO CALVILLO AND IOANNIS SHARIBAS

This chapter deals predominantly with intradiscal treatment of internal disc disruption (IDD). Identification of the precise etiology of back pain can be elusive, but it is fundamental for a successful outcome. Provocative discography followed by computed tomography (CT) provides the necessary information for accurately diagnosing low back pain due to IDD. Interbody fusion as a treatment for IDD is clearly indicated in some patients, although it can result in more complex pain and failed back syndrome with its attendant prolonged suffering.

Minimally invasive percutaneous intradiscal procedures have emerged as alternatives for patients with discographic evidence of IDD. This chapter discusses predominantly intradiscal electrothermal annuloplasty (IDET) and nucleoplasty.

INTRADISCAL ELECTROTHERMAL ANNULOPLASTY

IDET INCLUSION CRITERIA

1. Chronic pain persisting even after intensive conservative treatment
2. Discographic evidence of concordant pain
3. Annular fissures demonstrated on a CT scan
4. Single-level disease
5. Sometimes even in the presence of contained disc herniations

IDET EXCLUSION CRITERIA

1. Intervertebral disc herniation with radiculopathy
2. Disc height decreased 50%
3. Spinal stenosis
4. Prior discectomy
5. Spinal deformities
6. Coagulopathies

The IDET procedure utilizes an intradiscal catheter designed to achieve precise navigation and placement in the disc. The procedure is performed under monitored anesthesia and fluoroscopic guidance. The catheter delivers intradiscal thermal energy. The mechanism of analgesia is not entirely clear, although there is evidence that the collagen fibers in the annulus undergo structural changes so annular fissures can heal, thereby reducing pain. The possibility that the procedure is neurolytic on intradiscal nociceptive fibers can be reasonably entertained. IDET can reduce nuclear volume, so the procedure might be indicated for small, contained disc herniations. It is not recommended that more than two levels at one time be treated. Physical therapy is started 8 to 12 weeks after the procedure. Return to work is determined on an individual basis depending on the degree of analgesia attained. Signs of improvement usually occur 6 to 12 weeks after the procedure.

In a 16-month follow-up, case-controlled study, Saal and Saal (2000) reported a success rate approaching 60%.

NUCLEOPLASTY

Nucleoplasty utilizes a percutaneous approach to remove disc material. It is accomplished via a bipolar radiofrequency device that features coblation technology to ablate tissue alternating with thermal energy for coagulation. There is some evidence that nucleoplasty can relieve the pain associated with IDD, and the response is almost immediate compared to that seen with IDET. The mechanism of analgesia remains unknown, but it may be related to intradiscal neurolysis. Because removing disc tissue decompresses the annulus, the procedure is indicated in patients with contained disc herniations and radiculopathy. The inclusion and exclusion criteria for nucleoplasty are similar to those for IDET.

OTHER PROCEDURES

Percutaneous radiofrequency annular neurolysis pain has been reported to be efficacious in patients with discogenic pain. No long-term studies are available to determine its role in treating low back pain. However it might eventually become part of the armamentarium in the management of discogenic back pain.

LASER-ASSISTED SPINAL ENDOSCOPY

Percutaneous laser discectomy has been used extensively in the treatment of intervertebral disk herniation with concordant radiculopathy (Sherk 1993). The patient should exhaust all conservative options prior to considering laser-assisted spinal endoscopy (LASE). Inasmuch as it might be indicated for the treatment of IDD, it has been used predominantly to treat contained symptomatic intervertebral disc herniations and leg pain; back pain sometimes diminishes as well. In well selected patients, the results are comparable to those seen after open discectomy but without the attendant morbidity. The procedure is performed under monitored anesthesia care on an outpatient basis. The recovery phase is short. There is evidence that a significant amount of disc material can be ablated with LASE, thus explaining its mechanism of action.

REFERENCES

Saal JA, Saal JS: Intradiscal electrothermal treatment for chronic discogenic low back pain. *Spine* 2000;25:2622–2627.
Sherk HH: Lasers in orthopedic surgery, laser diskektomy. *Orthopedics* 1993;16:573–576.

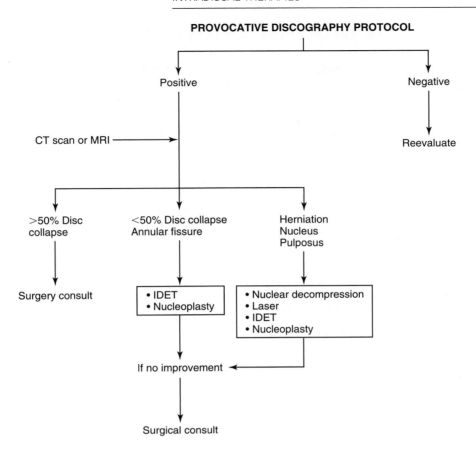

Epidural Endoscopy

MARCOS A. ZUAZU

Epidural endoscopy, epiduroscopy for short, has been utilized in the diagnosis and treatment of spinal conditions for many years. Its history dates to the work of Stern in 1936. In 1937, J. Lawrence Pool started performing diagnostic myeloscopy in patients and by 1942 he was reporting 400 cases that he had performed. With the advent of fiberoptic endoscopic technology, the diameter of flexible commercially available fiberscopes was reduced to a 0.8 to 1.0 mm OD (outer diameter), and therefore became suitable for percutaneous insertion through flexible introducer sheaths.

A. *Technical aspects.* Epiduroscopy is usually performed with the patient in the prone position using the caudal approach via the sacral hiatus. A guidewire placed through an epidural needle facilitates the insertion of a flexible and maneuverable sheath containing separate channels for the endoscope itself and for irrigation and injection of solutions. During endoscopy the epidural space can be visualized only if it is distended by repeated injections of saline flushing solution. Fluoroscopic control for localization of endoscope location is fundamental to the technique, and contrast dye is used to guide the operator and to evaluate regional pathology. The presence of a dorsomedial band (plica medialis dorsalis) has been reported in some studies. Injections of medications is routinely used in the procedure. For safety and patient feedback during the procedure, the procedure should not be performed under general anesthesia and only appropriate light sedation is employed for patient comfort.

Rigorous control of total volume of irrigation solutions (used during the procedure to distend the epidural space and provide good visualization) is essential to prevent complications due to overdistension of the lumbar epidural space, with resultant excessive increases in intraspinal pressures. The volume limits advocated by most clinicians is 100 ml. Cases of macular hemorrhage and visual impairment following the procedure have been reported. Other complications are epidural abscess, dural puncture, and prolonged headaches. As a safety measure, a time limit of 30 minutes has been proposed by some authors for the endoscopic time itself to aid in prevention of post-procedure problems. Many practitioners use prophylactic antibiotics prior to the endoscopy.

B. *Indications and patient selection.* Scarce literature is available to help in the evaluation of the benefits of epidural endoscopy in the management of patients with chronic pain. There are several indications for the use of epidural endoscopy. The most common is the diagnostic examination of the epidural space in patients with chronic radicular pain without evidence of disc injury. Visualization of inflammatory changes in the nerve roots corresponding to the patient's symptoms can be useful in establishing mechanical compression as the basis for the patients complaints.

Epidural endoscopy can be useful in the evaluation and lysis of epidural adhesions in patients not responsive to conventional treatments, and in patients suspected of scar entrapment of painful nerve roots as suggested by gadolinium-enhanced magnetic resonance imaging (MRI). It is also useful in the treatment of the "failed back surgery syndrome." Epidural endoscopy allows mechanical lysis of the adhesions that entrap the corresponding symptomatic root, by gentle manipulation of the fiberscope and the injection of "targeted" medications at the site of pathologic findings. Injections of corticosteroids, hyaluronidase, clonidine, hypertonic saline, and opiates have been described in the literature. The reason given for resorting to this injection treatment is the failure of the classic epidural steroid injection techniques to reach the pathologic areas because of the presence of fibrous scar tissue or adhesions. Targeted injections after adhesiolysis, then, become a viable mode of administration, overcoming disadvantages of previous epidural administrations.

C. *Efficacy and results.* Despite widespread practice of epiduroscopy, there is a shortage of controlled studies of its benefits. A recent small series from the Netherlands by Geurts et al. offers a prospective study with good results. No randomized, controlled studies are available and the literature mainly offers case and series reports from various symposia. Lysis of epidural adhesions by mechanical means (wire spiral catheters) is largely based on the work of Racz and others. Further studies are needed to evaluate the benefit of epidural endoscopy, as well as patient selection criteria, to fully understand the indications of this treatment.

Epidural endoscopy offers a sensible approach to treat a group of patients in which other options are more aggressive and require either a repeat surgical procedure or the use of implantable devices for pain control.

REFERENCES

Geurts JW, Kallewaard JW, Richardson J, Groen GJ: Targeted methylprednisolone acetate/hyaluronidase/clonidine injection after diagnostic epiduroscopy for chronic sciatica: A prospective, 1 year follow up study. *Reg Anesth Pain Med* 2002;27:343–352.

Pool JL: Myeloscopy: Intraspinal endoscopy. *Surgery* 1942;11:169–182.

Raj PP, Lou L, Erdine S, Staats PS: Epiduroscopy. In: Raj PP, Lou L, Erdine S, et al (eds) *Radiographic Imaging for Regional Anesthesia and Pain Management*: Philadelphia, Churchill Livingstone, 2003, pp. 272–281.

Saberski LR: Spinal endoscopy: Current concepts. In Waldman SD (ed) *Interventional Pain Management*, 2nd ed. Philadelphia, WB Saunders, 2001, pp. 143–161.

Stern EL: The Spinascope: A new instrument for visualizing the spinal canal and its contents. *Med Rec* (NY) 1936;143: 31–32.

EPIDURAL ENDOSCOPY

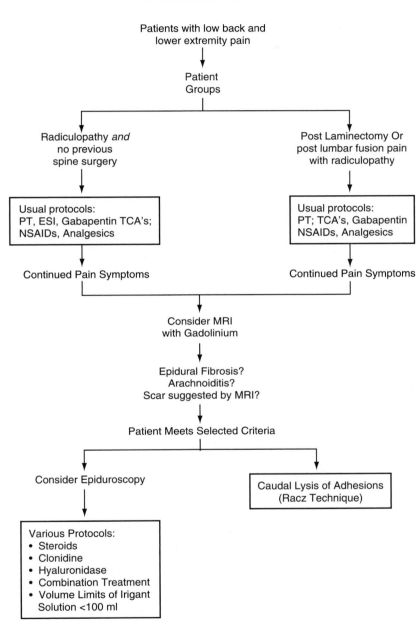

Intravertebral Analgesics

SERGIO ALVARADO

Instillation of analgesic agents into the subarachnoid and epidural spaces provides an effective therapeutic option for management of acute and chronic pain. In the setting of chronic pain, neuraxial analgesics can provide diagnostic information, but more commonly they are a tool for treatment of pain refractory to more conservative therapies. Cocaine was probably the first agent used, with Augustus Bier reporting surgical anesthesia in 1899 via subarachnoid block (SAB), and James Leonard Corning reporting on treatment of "spinal weakness and seminal incontinence" with cocaine injected "spinally" in 1885. Although Corning did not describe or accurately document needle insertion epidurally, it is felt that based on onset and duration of analgesia, the local anesthetic was placed in the epidural space. Opioid receptors were first discovered by Goldstein in 1970, isolated in neural tissue in 1973, discovered in the brain in 1974, and reported in the spinal cord in 1976. Administration of opioids intraspinally has since evolved and is now commonly used for various types of acute and chronic pain states.

Intrathecal infusion of baclofen has emerged as an effective therapy for refractory spasticity and the pain associated with it.

A. Local anesthetics were the original analgesics used for intravertebral injection. The most commonly used intraspinal local anesthetic today is bupivacaine. Because of its cardiotoxicity and rapid progression from central nervous system (CNS) effects to cardiac effects, newer analogs with less potential for cardiac effects have gained increasing popularity. Improved safety profiles are claimed for mepivacaine, ropivacaine, and levobupivacaine. Of the newer agents, ropivacaine is most commonly used in the chronic pain setting. None of the local anesthetics are FDA approved for chronic intraspinal infusion, and often must be compounded to provide a higher concentration than is commercially available in order to prolong intervals between refilling of the infusion device. The maximum concentration varies by pharmacy, with the dose of bupivacaine ranging from 15 to 40 mg/ml. Ropivacaine is more soluble. Side effects include sensory or motor changes at the level of administration, as well as sedation, hypotension, and bradycardia. Gradual upward titration can decrease the incidence of these effects. As expected, epidural administration requires larger volumes.

B. Opioids have become a mainstay of intravertebral analgesia. They appear to be better suited to treatment of nociceptive pain, which is mediated by nociceptors throughout the body, often described as dull, aching, sharp, throbbing, and commonly due to trauma, as well as tissue injury resulting from cancer and surgery. Opioids are much less effective for neuropathic pain, which is often described as tingling, burning, shooting, and due to damage to the peripheral or central nervous system. The classic opioid used for intraspinal therapy is morphine, which is the only one approved by the FDA for this purpose. Hydromorphone, fentanyl, sufentanil, meperidine, and methadone have also been used. Onset of action, duration, metabolism, and CNS side effects are all a function of a particular opioid's lipid solubility. Morphine and hydromorphone have a low lipid solubility, resulting in slower onset, prolonged duration, and greater extent of spread. They also have a greater risk of CNS side effects such as sedation, nausea and vomiting, and respiratory depression. Fentanyl and sufentanil are highly lipophilic, resulting in a decreased extent of spread and requiring placement of the catheter tip as close as possible to the spinal level associated with the patient's pain. Methadone and meperidine do not appear to offer any advantages, with meperidine suspected of causing damage to infusion devices. Effective doses are highly individualized, with higher doses required for neuropathic pain. Older patients often need lower doses than younger patients. Converting systemic opioid to intraspinal doses involves multiplying the daily oral morphine equivalent by 0.33 for epidural use and by 0.033 for intrathecal. Known side effects include those mentioned earlier as well as generalized pruritus, constipation, sedation, and confusion. Other complications include paranoia, hyperalgesia/myoclonus syndrome, vestibular disturbances, and herpes reactivation. Switching opioids may overcome these problems; however, an attempt should be made to treat the effects pharmacologically first. High opioid concentrations are thought to play a role in the formation of catheter-tip granulomas; however, it appears from animal studies that morphine is more likely than hydromorphone to be involved in granuloma formation.

C. Clonidine is a centrally acting alpha-2 adrenergic agonist that has been shown to be effective for intraspinal use in both nociceptive and neuropathic pain. It appears to act postsynaptically on nociceptive neurons to inhibit release of substance P. It is approved for medium-term epidural use in cancer pain and is commercially available as a 100 µg/ml formulation, although it is used extensively in intrathecal infusion devices for various pain syndromes. It has been well studied for safety and animal studies have not shown any toxicity. Side effects include hypotension, bradycardia, and sedation. Hypotension appears to be less common at higher doses. Tizanidine and dexmedetomidine are related alpha-adrenergic agonists that are being studied for intraspinal use.

INTRAVERTEBRAL ANALGESICS

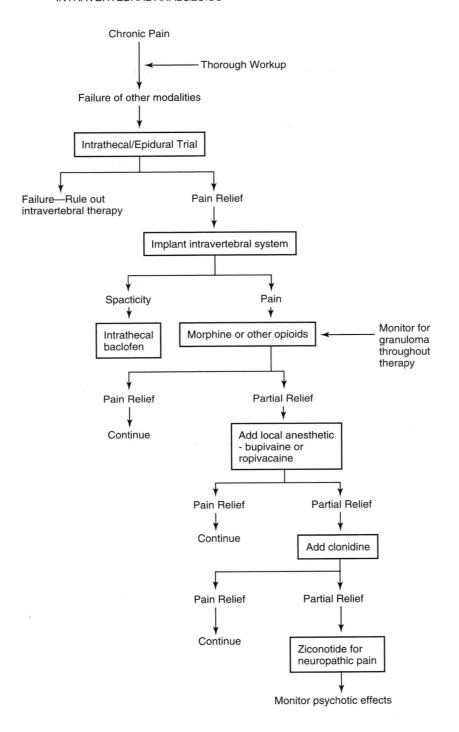

D. Midazolam has gained recent attention as a possible intraspinal analgesic via its GABAergic mechanism. Much controversy was generated over human studies performed prior to adequate toxicity studies; however, results of both were published simultaneously. The human studies involved analgesia for obstetrics and may lead to chronic pain studies.

E. Ketamine is an *N*-methyl-D-aspartate (NMDA) antagonist and has been studied for intrathecal use where it may have a role in the treatment of neuropathic pain and as an adjunct to prevent opioid tolerance. It is commercially available outside the United States as a preservative-free formulation of solely the (S)-enantiomer, which is thought to be less likely to produce adverse psychiatric effects. Some compounding pharmacies will manufacture a preservative-free formulation, although it is not approved in the United States for intraspinal use.

F. Early studies have been initiated with the non-steroidal antiinflammatory agent ketorolac for intrathecal use. Toxicity studies found no significant problems. The cyclooxygenase enzyme has been found to play a role in CNS pain signal processing.

G. Ziconotide, an N-type calcium channel blocker derived from a neurotoxin produced by the giant cone snail of the South Pacific and developed specifically for intrathecal use, recently gained FDA approval for use in Medtronic SynchroMed infusion systems. The development of psychotic adverse effects prompted further study and resulted in a revised dosing schedule with a lower dosing range than initially proposed.

H. Neurolytic agents such as phenol and alcohol are discussed in detail elsewhere in this book and have a role as intravertebral agents primarily in the management of cancer pain, but may also be used in refractory pain syndromes such as chronic regional pain syndrome (CRPS).

I. Baclofen is FDA approved for intrathecal use in managing spasticity, for which it has proven to be extremely effective. It is indicated for patients who do not respond to maximum doses of oral baclofen or who develop intolerable side effects. Its use as an analgesic is related to treatment of pain caused by the spasticity itself. Major side effects are usually a result of overdosage and include sedation, nausea respiratory depression, and weakness.

J. At the present time, intrathecal infusion of analgesics appears to be preferable to the epidural route, primarily because of the much smaller volume needed for intrathecal infusion, resulting in an overall easier system to manage than for epidural administration. The need for more frequent manipulation of the system may increase the risk of infection.

K. Intravertebral administration of analgesics represents a therapeutic option for refractory pain syndromes, especially the severe pain associated with cancer. If an implantable system is to be considered for drug administration, strict patient selection criteria should be adhered to including performance of an adequate trial of medication to prove efficacy. If non-FDA-approved agents are used and manufactured by a compounding pharmacy, documentation of strict stability and sterility testing, including bacterial and fungal analysis by an independent lab, should be obtained. Agents of different classes are often combined with opioid/local anesthetic/clonidine mixtures.

REFERENCES

Candido K, Stevens RA: Intrathecal neurolytic blocks for the relief of cancer pain. *Best Pract Res Clin Anesthesiol* 2003;17: 407–428.

Garber JE, Hassenbusch SJ: Spinal administration of nonopiate analgesics for pain management. In: Waldman SD (ed) *Interventional Pain Management,* 2nd ed. Philadelphia, WB Saunders, 2001, pp. 621–626.

Product information, Prialt. Elan Pharmaceuticals, 2005.

Rames ES: Intraspinal analgesia for nonmalignant pain. In: Waldman SD (ed) *Interventional Pain Management,* 2nd ed. Philadelphia, WB Saunders, 2001, pp. 609–618.

Rauck RL, Eisenach JC, Mitchell M, Curry G: Phase I safety assessment of intrathecal ketorolac in patients with chronic pain. *Anesthesiology* 2004;101:A965.

Tucker AP: Intrathecal midazolam II: combination with intrathecal fentanyl for labor pain. *Anesth Analg* 2004;98:1521–1527.

Complications of Neurolytic Blocks

SERGIO ALVARADO

Complications associated with neurolytic procedures can be severe and devastating to the patient. The risks and benefits of neurolysis should be discussed thoroughly with the patient before any procedure is performed and should be considered only after more conservative therapy has failed. Complications are directly related to the site of injection or intervention and injury at the site or to adjacent structures. A detailed description of all possible adverse effects is beyond the scope of this chapter.

A. Complications related to chemical agents are the result of their inherent properties and difficulty in controlling the extent of the lesion created with a liquid medium. One of the most common complaints with alcohol is a neuralgia. Recovery can be slow and ranges from weeks to months. Rarely hypesthesia or analgesia occurs, but is usually short lived. Problems that can occur with either phenol or alcohol include loss of motor function of extremities and loss of bowel and bladder function. These often are attributable to intrathecal injection in the lower lumbar spine and sacral areas. Genitofemoral neuralgia with severe groin pain can result from alcohol lumbar sympathetic block. Paraplegia can occur if injection of alcohol causes spasm of the artery of Adamkiewicz. Phenol has potential for systemic toxicity with central nervous system (CNS) depression and cardiovascular collapse; however, at commonly used clinical doses, these effects are extremely rare. If injected subcutaneously, phenol may produce local skin ulceration. As with any neurolytic technique, loss of sensory and motor function are potential side effects. Anesthesia dolorosa (constant severe deafferentation pain) can also occur. In the case of neurolytic Gasserian rhizotomy, cranial nerve deficits, corneal numbness, meningitis, dysesthesias, masticatory weakness, and keratitis may all occur and should be mentioned to the patient as possible complications.

B. Cryoablation is a reversible process with relatively minor complications including cold injury, skin discoloration, and numbness in the distribution of the treated nerve. As with any percutaneous procedure, complications may also be related to needle placement.

C. Complications associated with radiofrequency (RF) techniques are theoretically similar to chemical neurolysis; however, the purported advantage of RF is the ability to perform motor and sensory stimulation prior to lesioning, as well as control of the size of the lesion. Complications vary based on the site of lesioning, the technique of needle placement, and vulnerability of adjacent structures. Those directly related to neurolysis are similar to complications associated with chemical neurolysis, with neurologic deficits, deafferentation pain, and neuritis possible. One difference is the possibility of burns associated with the generator and improper grounding. In actuality, the incidence of complications is low, especially with the most common applications such as facet denervation. A recent 5-year retrospective analysis of complications after lumbar facet denervation using a standard traditional RF protocol found complications to be minor and rare, with an incidence of minor complications less than 1% per lesion site. Mild ataxia can occur after cervical facet denervation, is usually well tolerated, and is an acceptable side effect for many patients with chronic pain. In contrast, an analysis of ablative techniques for trigeminal neuralgia found sensory deficits more common with RF than glycerol rhizolysis or stereotactic radiosurgery, and they had a significant impact on quality of life, although data were heterogenous with protocols not standardized. The advent of pulsed RF technology may further enhance the safety of this technique. Some operators inject a small amount of corticosteroid at the site after lesioning to prevent neuritis, but its efficacy is theoretical and has not been proven.

The importance of discussing with patients the potential complications of neurolytic procedures cannot be stressed enough. Some patients with terminal illnesses and/or refractory pain may be willing to accept the adverse effects while others may not.

REFERENCES

Candido K, Stevens RA: Intrathecal neurolytic blocks for the relief of cancer pain. Best Pract Res Clin Anesthesiol 2003;17:407–428.

de Leon-Casasola OA, Ditonto E: Drugs commonly used for nerve blocking: Neurolytic agents. In: Raj PP (ed) *Practical Management of Pain*, 3rd ed. St. Louis, Mosby, 2000, pp. 575–578.

Kornick C, Kramarich SS, Lamer TJ, Todd Sitzman B: Complications of lumbar facet radiofrequency denervation. *Spine* 2004;29:1352–1354.

Lopez BC, Hamlyn PJ, Zakrewska JM: Systematic review of ablative neurosurgical techniques for the treatment of trigeminal neuralgia. *Neurosurgery* 2004;54:973–983.

Sluijter M: *Radiofrequency, Part I: Flivopress SA*. Switzerland, Meggan (LU), 2001.

COMPLICATIONS OF NEUROLYTIC BLOCKS

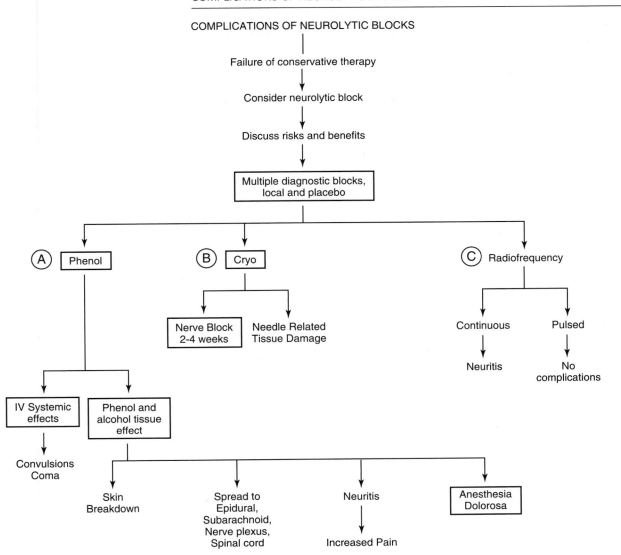

Cryoanalgesia

THOMAS A. EDELL

Cryoanalgesia, the relief of pain by application of cold, has been used for millennia. The presurgical use of cold for operative analgesia was described by Hippocrates, Avicenna of Persia, Severino of Naples, and Larré. During the 1920s Trendelenberg studied the destructive effects on nerves, noting prolonged loss of function and regeneration without scar or neuroma formation. The real advent of cryoanalgesia and cryoneurolysis in modern medicine began with the introduction of the first cryoprobe by Cooper in 1961. The potential for medical use was further enhanced when Amoils introduced the much smaller, more easily handled CO_2 cryoprobe in 1967. Only gas expansion (the Joule-Thompson effect with CO_2 or N_2O) cryomachines are used for pain control today. Important features of the cryomachine include a thermocouple at the tip to monitor temperature, a nerve stimulator at the tip allowing both motor and sensory stimulation for nerve localization, a flowmeter to monitor high-pressure gas flow, a pressure gauge to monitor cylinder contents, and freeze and defrost indicators.

The exact mechanism(s) of freeze injury is unknown. Theories include direct ice crystal destruction, hypertonicity, protein denaturation, critical reduction of cell volume, dehydration, cell membrane rupture, ischemia, and antibody formation. Ice crystal formation is the underlying process with any type of freeze injury. It involves removal of pure water from solution and the formation of crystals both intra- and extracellularly. The rate of crystal formation is one of the most important aspects of the degree of cell injury. A temperature of $-20°C$ must be reached in the tissues to result in uniform cell death. Therefore one can see that when using a gas expansion cryoprobe, which cools to $-70°C$ (using N_2O), the center of the ice ball must be within approximately 4 to 5 mm of the nerve for lethal application. The temperature reached at the probe tip, the probe size and geometry, and the surrounding structures (i.e., thermal conductivity and vascularity) determine the ultimate size of the ice ball. Cryolesioning produces a second-degree nerve injury according to Sunderland's classification; this is in contrast to third-, fourth-, and fifth-degree injuries caused by high-temperature radiofrequency, phenol, alcohol, and surgical resection. In contradistinction to the more severe nerve injuries, cryoneurolysis preserves the fibrous architecture, especially the endoneurium, allowing more organized regeneration without neuroma formation and a low incidence of neuritis. Freezing results in axonal disruption followed by wallerian degeneration of the axon distal to the lesion. Nerve regeneration follows and proceeds at a rate of approximately 1 to 3 mm/day. Whereas return of function depends in part on the distance of the lesion from the end-organ, functional measures can return to normal as early as 3 weeks. Pain relief can outlast the return of function by weeks.

Evans (1981) demonstrated that so long as the critical temperature of less than $-20°C$ was reached for 1 minute, there is no benefit to prolonging or repeating the freezing period for an exposed nerve. In practice, percutaneous applications, with less than ideal nerve localization, benefit from extending the duration of cryolesioning from 2 minutes to 4 minutes and repeating the freeze-thaw cycle two or three times; this measure may enlarge the ice ball up to 15% with the gas-expansion cryoprobe. The longer freeze time and repeat cycles are especially important when freezing nerves in close proximity to vascular structures (e.g., intercostal nerves), which act as heat sinks.

A. Lloyd et al. (1976) coined the term cryoanalgesia, which is the clinical application of cryotherapy for pain management. Cryoneurolysis is essentially a prolonged somatic block. It has been used for both acute (primarily postoperative) and chronic pain conditions. In this capacity, it is principally utilized for peripheral neurolysis. As all peripheral nerves regenerate following neurolysis, the most appropriate use of cryoanalgesia is in clinical settings where pain management is needed for weeks to months.

B. Cryoanalgesia for postsurgical pain allows use of the more effective open/surgical (direct vision) technique. The two most common uses for cryoanalgesia in postoperative pain management today are to establish an ilioinguinal nerve block for postherniorrhaphy pain or an intercostal nerve block for postthoracotomy pain. Of particular interest to clinicians dealing with pain is the fact that cryoneurolysis for postsurgical pain has never been shown to reduce the incidence of chronic postthoracotomy or postherniorrhaphy pain syndromes. Cryoneurolysis under direct vision results in more predictable pain relief than the percutaneous technique.

C. Although most peripheral nerves have been treated with cryoanalgesia, not all nerves appear to be amenable to this treatment. The following nerves are the most commonly subjected to cryoanalgesia during chronic pain management: neuromas, intercostal nerves, superficial primarily sensory nerves (e.g., ilioinguinal), and medial branches of the posterior primary rami of the spinal roots. The percutaneous technique requires use of a nerve stimulator (in addition to fluoroscopy for deep nerves) for localization. The cyroprobes (or angiocaths used for tissue penetration, if round-tipped probes used) are relatively large and result in significant intervening tissue trauma (for this reason, radiofrequency neurolysis has largely supplanted cryoneurolysis in most pain clinics).

D. As with any invasive procedure used for pain management, and with neurolysis in particular, patient selection and education are paramount to a successful outcome. Prior adequate pain relief with local anesthetic blockade is no guarantee that subsequent neurolysis will result in equally successful results. Patients must also be made aware of the difficulty of

316

foreseeing the actual duration of analgesia, especially with the percutaneous technique. They must understand that the analgesia is temporary (to facilitate other treatment modalities), that there is a possibility of increased pain (whether true or perceived) following regeneration, that full-thickness skin damage may occur (with superficial nerves), and that there are the usual risks of invasive procedures (including pneumothorax for intercostal neurolysis). See Table 1 for techniques.

REFERENCES

Evans PJD: Cryoanalgesia: the application of low temperatures to nerves to produce anaesthesia or analgesia. *Anaesthesia* 1981;36:1003–1013.

Kalichman MW, Myers RR: Behavioral and electrophysiological recovery following cryogenic nerve injury. *Exp Neurol* 1987;96:692–702.

Lloyd JW, Barnard JDW, Glynn CJ: Cryoanalgesia: a new approach to pain relief. *Lancet* 1976;2:932–934.

Sunderland S: A classification of peripheral nerve injuries producing loss of function. *Brain* 1951;74:491–516.

TABLE 1
Cryoneurolysis Techniques

Cryoneurolysis, open technique
1. Freeze at –60° to –70°C for 30–120 seconds (longer time is needed for intercostal neurolysis, if nerve is not separated from the vasculature).
2. A second freeze is not needed with a complete first freeze (if used, thaw the ice ball completely between freezes).
3. *Do not remove the ice ball from the tissue*: Wait until it is completely thawed.

Percutaneous cryoneurolysis
1. Freeze at –60° to –70°C for 2–4 minutes (the longer time for intercostal neurolysis).
2. Repeat 2–3 times, ensuring adequate thaw times between freezes.
3. *Do not remove the ice ball from the tissue*: Wait until it is completely thawed.

CRYOANALGESIA

(A) Patient selection: Appropriate nerve(s) serving areas of pain

(B) Acute, postoperative pain - anticipated (e.g. intercostal or ilioinguinal nerve)

    → Cryoneurolysis - open technique

    → No pain relief → Reassess differential diagnosis

(C) Chronic, intractable pain (e.g. neuromas, intercostal neuralgia, facet arthropathy)

    → Diagnostic blocks (± steroid)

    → Temporary pain relief → Percutaneous cryoneurolysis

    → Significant motor block or patient dislikes insensate state → Alternative treatment options

(D) Risks include infection, bleeding, adjacent tissue damage (including skin, vessels), no pain relief, less pain relief than local anesthetic blocks, unable to predict duration of pain relief, the possibility of increased pain following nerve regeneration, pneumothorax (intercostals), neuritis (but less than with other neurolytic techniques), neuroma (if ice ball removed or direct trauma during cryoprobe placement). If percutaneous cryoneurolysis inadequate, consider repeat cryoneurolysis under direct vision/surgical exposure; I will do this only when surgery already planned.

Radiofrequency Ablation

STUART W. HOUGH

Therapeutic neurolysis may be accomplished by chemical or thermal means. Modern radiofrequency (RF) generators and cannulas allow precision thermal lesion placement, minimizing damage to surrounding tissue. Various cannulas are available to produce different lesion sizes and shapes. Continuous temperature monitoring gives the operator additional control over lesion size. Built-in nerve stimulators ensure proximity to the target nerve and adequate distance from unintended neural targets. Impedance monitors detect electric circuit malfunctions and may signal close proximity to bone (high impedance) or blood vessels (low impedance).

Radiofrequency thermal ablation is well suited to small neural targets that can be identified by radiologic or functional (electrical stimulation) means (or both). Such targets include sympathetic and dorsal root ganglia, the gasserian ganglion, and medial branches of the posterior primary rami of spinal nerves (for zygapophyseal joint denervation). Larger nerves are not good candidates for ablation, as the resulting sensory and motor dysfunction could disable the patient.

Radiofrequency heat lesions are produced by exciting ions within a field of alternating electric current at 500,000 Hz. Because current density decreases rapidly with distance from the electrode tip, the volume of the lesion is limited. The determinants of lesion size are electrode size, tissue conductivity (water content), adjacent tissues (bone, blood vessels), and RF generator output. Heating tissue to 80°C for 60 seconds creates a maximal lesion. A clinical effect may also be possible, without heating the tissue significantly, using pulsed RF energy. The inactive period between pulses allows heat to dissipate, minimizing procedural discomfort and tissue injury and possibly reducing the likelihood of postoperative neuralgia. It is speculated that the high-energy field or current density can produce sustained interruption of pain transmission without affecting large-fiber function.

Prior to performing radioablation of a target nerve, the physician should be convinced that it is either generating or transmitting noxious stimuli. After selecting a potential target, a prognostic nerve block is performed. The physician should use nerve stimulation or radiologic reference points (or both) to identify the target, so a small volume of local anesthetic (less than 1 mL) can produce a complete block. This small volume approximates the size of an RF lesion and prevents spread of the anesthetic to adjacent nerves. If the patient responds favorably to the prognostic injection, he or she may be a candidate for RF ablation.

To maximize the predictive value of a positive prognostic nerve block, the physician may perform additional blocks with other local anesthetics. It is helpful to examine the patient before and after each block using provocative maneuvers that would ordinarily cause pain. The quality of the initial analgesic response should be documented. The patient then identifies an activity that normally produces the pain and keeps a record of activity and pain intensity for at least a day after each block. He or she should note the exact time of pain recurrence and the associated activity. Patients whose response durations are inconsistent with the agents injected may be placebo responders and should be reconsidered for neural ablation.

REFERENCES

Barnsley L, Lord S, Bogduk N: Comparative local anaesthetic blocks in the diagnosis of cervical zygapophysial joint pain. *Pain* 1993;55:99.

Lord SM, Barnsley L, Wallis BJ, et al: Percutaneous radio-frequency neurotomy for chronic cervical zygapophysial-joint pain. *N Engl J Med* 1996;335:1721.

Schwarzer AC, Aprill CN, Derby R, et al: The false-positive rate of uncontrolled diagnostic blocks of the lumbar zygapophysial joints. *Pain* 1994;58:195.

Sluijter ME, van Kleef M: Characteristics and mode of action of RF lesions. *Curr Rev Pain* 1998;2:143.

CANDIDATE FOR RADIOFREQUENCY LESION?

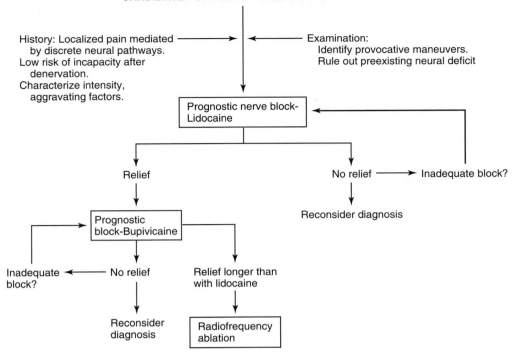

History: Localized pain mediated by discrete neural pathways. Low risk of incapacity after denervation. Characterize intensity, aggravating factors.

Examination: Identify provocative maneuvers. Rule out preexisting neural deficit

Prognostic nerve block-Lidocaine

Relief

No relief → Inadequate block?

Reconsider diagnosis

Prognostic block-Bupivicaine

Inadequate block? ← No relief

Relief longer than with lidocaine

Reconsider diagnosis

Radiofrequency ablation

Spinal Cord Stimulation

THOMAS A. EDELL

Electrical stimulation for pain control has a long and storied past: from the torpedo fish of Dioscorides to Franklinization. It was not until Melzack and Wall's gate control theory of pain in 1965 that the scientific application of electrical stimulation to the spinal cord began to emerge as a clinical reality. Since that time, advances in technology, materials, and our understanding of spinal cord physiology have resulted in myriad applications for spinal cord stimulation (SCS).

Spinal cord stimulation is a nondestructive, reversible, "augmentative" treatment for chronic pain. The exact mechanism of action of SCS in analgesia remains a mystery. Initially, it was thought that stimulation of the dorsal columns (stimulation of large sensory fibers "closing the gate") was responsible for pain control—hence dorsal column stimulation (DCS). It is now known that if DCS plays a role it is not the only mechanism. Other proposed mechanisms include sympathetic inhibition, spinothalamic tract inhibition, direct effect on spinal cord neuromodulators, and supraspinal effects. The cathode (negative pole) causes depolarization of the neuron, leading to an action potential that is propagated along the nerve. Close proximity of the anode to the cathode, as with all SCS multielectrode leads in use today, allows a narrow, targeted stimulation field. The success of SCS has continuously improved since its inception. In addition to the advances in technology, materials, and design, the most important aspect of improved outcome has been better patient selection.

A. Careful patient selection is of critical importance. Important negative predictors for SCS success include inadequately treated depression or other psychiatric disorders, nonorganic or questionable etiologies of pain, ongoing drug or alcohol abuse, and ongoing legal issues related to the painful condition. After establishing a pain diagnosis (demonstrable pathology) and the failure of appropriate treatment modalities, including injections, medications, and physical and psychological therapies, SCS may be considered a treatment option. Comprehensive patient education, concerning both the trial and implant phases, is paramount. This should be followed by an assessment by a mental health specialist to ensure an understanding of the SCS treatment objectives, appropriate expectations, and the absence of any significant psychological impairment.

B. Spinal cord stimulation seems to work best for two broad categories of pain: neuropathic and ischemic. (Nociceptive pain responds poorly if at all.) The most common use of SCS in the United States is for the treatment of radiculopathies following back or neck surgery; in Europe one of its most common uses is the treatment of ischemic pain due to vascular diseases, including inoperable angina. Other less common diseases have also proven amenable to treatment with SCS: chronic regional pain syndromes (especially sympathetically mediated components); some peripheral neuropathies, plexopathies, and nerve root avulsions; regionalized pain due to multiple sclerosis and spinal cord lesions. More recently, with the advent of simultaneous stimulation of dual, parallel leads, there has been some success in including the low back or neck, thereby reducing the pain in these areas due to failed back/neck syndromes. Finally, the same electrical stimulation systems are currently being used with some success in direct peripheral nerve or nerve root stimulation for such conditions as occipital neuralgia, ilioinguinal neuralgia, interstitial cystitis, sacral/perineal pain of various etiologies, and a host of other neuropathies.

C. The next step is a trial with SCS. (Note that although the transcutaneous electrical nerve stimulator was originally designed for a trial of SCS, it was never proven effective for this use.) The SCS trial is performed by placing stimulating leads into the epidural space (cervical level for upper extremity pain and low thoracic level for lower extremity pain), either percutaneously or surgically (where leads are anchored and tunneled in the operating room). Leads with four or eight electrode arrays may be used. Dual leads may be used in an attempt to treat bilateral or midline pain. *The patient must experience parasthesias in the areas of pain.* The patient is awake to ensure adequate, appropriate stimulation parasthesias. SCS uses electrical pulses. The electrical stimulating parameters of pulse width (10 to 500 ms) and frequency (5 to 1500 Hz; see below) are adjusted to fine-tune the stimulation pattern; the amplitude is adjusted to patient tolerance. The trial should last at least 3 days, preferably on an outpatient basis while the patient engages in his or her normal painful activities. If the patient declares that the pain is reduced significantly (e.g., 50% or more), with or without a reduction in medications, the trial is considered successful.

D. A permanent SCS system is implanted with the patient in the operating room. After trials with percutaneous leads, new leads are used; after surgical trials, the already tried electrode arrays are permanently implanted. Alternatively, laminotomy leads may be placed in lieu of catheter leads. They require greater surgical invasion but migrate less, may require lower amplitudes, and are "insulated" posteriorly. The leads are anchored and connected to extensions that are subcutaneously tunneled into the subcutaneous pocket containing the generator/receiver. The decision to utilize a totally implanted system—implanted pulse generators (IPGs) with internal battery—versus the radiofrequency (RF) system (receiver implanted, with external antenna and battery) should be based on the stimulation requirements during the trial along with patient preference. IPGs can stimulate up to eight electrodes, whereas one RF system can handle up to 16 contacts. The newer IPGs allow independent programming of multiple leads and utilization of two stimulating sets; the 16-electrode RF system allows multiple stimulation sets and much higher frequencies (up to 1500 Hz, compared with 130 Hz). The totally implanted system requires surgical replacement of the generator/battery every 3 to 5 years depending on the amplitudes and hours of use, whereas the RF system requires a second surgery only for removal (due to malfunction or loss of pain control). Following implantation, the stimulating electrodes, parameters, and limits are set. Automatic on/off cycling of the IPGs can be programmed to prolong battery life. The patient can turn the unit on and off and adjust the amplitude, frequency, and pulse width up to the preset limits. The patient should avoid activities (strenuous bending, twisting, lifting) that might cause lead migration until the leads become fibrosed in the epidural space within 4 to 8 weeks (some advocate soft collars or corsets as "reminders"). The patient should be warned that the stimulation intensity may change with different positions, even after the fibrosis is complete, and that they should not drive while the stimulator is turned on.

E. Loss of adequate stimulation, pain control, or both requires intervention. Leads can migrate or break. Reprogramming may restore adequate stimulation with migrated leads (some implanters use dual leads or eight-electrode leads for unilateral pain to enable greater reprogramming possibilities if leads migrate). If reprogramming is unsuccessful or the leads are nonfunctioning, new leads (possibly the laminotomy type with little or no migration) must be placed.

Extensions can break or generators/receivers can malfunction, requiring surgical replacement. "Tolerance" can also develop: Epidural fibrosis may cause insulation of the electrodes and loss of stimulation, or neural plasticity may result in loss of pain control despite continued appropriate stimulation parasthesias. For the latter, consider a trial "holiday" to see if adequate pain control can be restored. Otherwise removal of the system is warranted. These risks should be discussed with the patient *before* the trial and implantation.

REFERENCES

Barolat G: Current status of epidural spinal cord stimulation. *Neurosurg Q* 1995;5:98–124.

Burchiel KJ, Anderson VC, Wilson BJ, et al: Prognostic factors of spinal cord stimulation for chronic back and leg pain. *Neurosurgery* 1995;36:1101–1111.

DeJongste MJL: Spinal cord stimulation for ischemic heart disease. *Neurol Res* 2000;22:293–298.

Jacobs MJ, Jörning PJ, Joshi SR, et al: Epidural spinal cord electrical stimulation improves microvascular blood flow in severe limb ischemia. *Ann Surg* 1988;207:179–183.

Kumar K, Toth C, Nath RK, et al: Epidural spinal cord stimulation for treatment of chronic pain: some predictors of success; a 15-year experience. *Surg Neurol* 1998;50:110–127.

Melzack R, Wall PD: Pain mechanisms: a new theory. *Science* 1965;150:971–979.

North RB, Roark GL: Spinal cord stimulation for chronic pain. *Neurosurg Clin North Am* 1995;6:145–155.

North RB, Wetzel FT: Spinal cord stimulation for chronic pain of spinal origin: a valuable long-term solution. *Spine* 2002;27:2584–2591.

Oakley JC, Prager JP: Spinal cord stimulation: mechanisms of action. *Spine* 2002;27:2574–2583.

SPINAL CORD STIMULATION

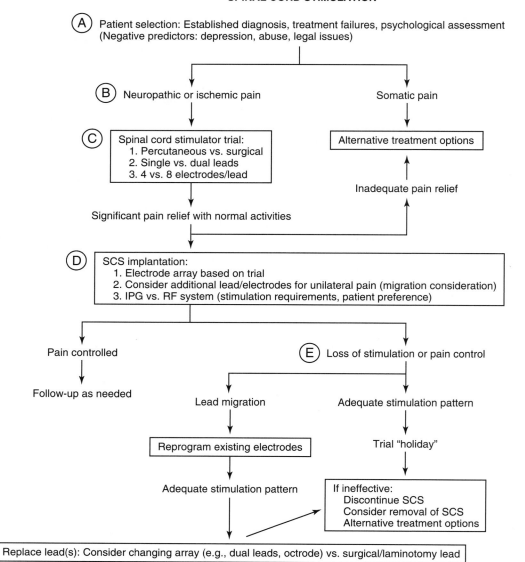

(A) Patient selection: Established diagnosis, treatment failures, psychological assessment
(Negative predictors: depression, abuse, legal issues)

(B) Neuropathic or ischemic pain

Somatic pain

(C) Spinal cord stimulator trial:
1. Percutaneous vs. surgical
2. Single vs. dual leads
3. 4 vs. 8 electrodes/lead

Alternative treatment options

Inadequate pain relief

Significant pain relief with normal activities

(D) SCS implantation:
1. Electrode array based on trial
2. Consider additional lead/electrodes for unilateral pain (migration consideration)
3. IPG vs. RF system (stimulation requirements, patient preference)

Pain controlled

(E) Loss of stimulation or pain control

Follow-up as needed

Lead migration

Adequate stimulation pattern

Reprogram existing electrodes

Trial "holiday"

Adequate stimulation pattern

If ineffective:
Discontinue SCS
Consider removal of SCS
Alternative treatment options

Replace lead(s): Consider changing array (e.g., dual leads, octrode) vs. surgical/laminotomy lead

Neurosurgical Procedures for Pain

SOMAYAJI RAMAMURTHY

Advances in pharmacologic techniques and neuraxial delivery systems have significantly decreased the need for ablative surgical procedures. Neurosurgical techniques can be valuable if used in highly selected patients.

A. A thorough history, physical examination and diagnostic work up are important in patient selection.

B. Multidisciplinary evaluation with special attention to psychological factors, drug seeking behavior, and secondary gain factors is important. Noninvasive modalities and nonsurgical approaches including physiotherapy, pharmacotherapy, nerve blocks, and psychological methods should be given an adequate trial before considering surgical approaches.

C. Patients with pain due to malignancy that is not controlled by pharmacotherapy including opioids, nonsteroidal antiinflammatory drugs (NSAIDs), antineuropathic medications, and neuraxial opioids should be considered for operative procedures. If the pain is localized, diagnostic nerve blocks are performed. If the pain is relieved by a somatic or a sympathetic nerve block, the blocks are repeated to be certain that the patient obtains pain relief consistently and is not a placebo responder. This also gives the patient an opportunity to evaluate the numbness, weakness, and other effects of interruption of neural pathways. Dorsal rhizotomy and sympathectomy in the lumbar and thoracic area can provide excellent pain relief. Patients who have diffuse pain may benefit from cordotomy, myelotomy, thalamotomy, or singulotomy. Patients with diffuse pain secondary to metastatic breast or prostate cancer have received excellent pain relief from hypophysectomy with the use of alcohol, cryo, or thermal lesions or an open surgical procedure.

D. Patients with trigeminal neuralgia unresponsive to pharmacotherapy or who have intolerable side effects are candidates for neurosurgical procedures. Glycerol rhizotomy and radiofrequency lesion are very effective. Despite the incidence of recurrence, these procedures seem to give excellent pain relief without significant sensory loss and motor function of the mandibular nerve. Microvascular decompression has a high success rate but involves posterior fossa exploration with a significant surgical risk.

E. Patients with pain from nonmalignant conditions may be considered for decompressive or ablative surgery or stimulation techniques depending on the type, extent, and location of the pain.

F. Patients who have compressive neuropathy such as carpal tunnel syndrome, ulnar and other nerve compression syndromes, or radicular or spinal cord compression from spinal stenosis may benefit from decompressive surgery.

G. Older patients who have pain from nonmalignant conditions are not good candidates for neuroablative surgery. There is a significant incidence of recurrence. Any impairment of function secondary to weakness or bladder/bowel incontinence can seriously impair the quality of life. Dysesthesias and anesthesia dolorosa can produce discomfort worse than that of the original pain. Patients with localized pain unresponsive to all other modalities may benefit from dorsal root rhizotomy or ganglionecteomy. This may spare the motor function. Sectioning more than five roots can result in loss of proprioception and motor incoordination. Patients with diffuse unilateral pain may benefit from cordotomy. Patients with significant respiratory impairment are not suitable candidates for this procedure. Percutaneous cordotomy is preferred to open cordotomy. Patients with deafferentation pain resulting from avulsed spinal roots, postherpetic neuralgia, and phantom pain may benefit from dorsal root entry zone lesions (DREZ).

H. When the pain is in a single nerve distribution, peripherally implanted nerve stimulators have provided effective pain relief. Spinal cord stimulation with epidurally placed electrodes with a trial followed by permanent implantation can control pain resulting from chronic regional pain syndrome and neuropathic pain. Deep brain stimulation may be used for patients who have more diffuse pain and pain of central origin.

REFERENCE

Hassenbusch SJ: Surgical techniques in pain management. In: Raj PP (ed). *Practical Management of Pain,* 3rd ed. St. Louis, Mosby, 2000, pp. 792–806.

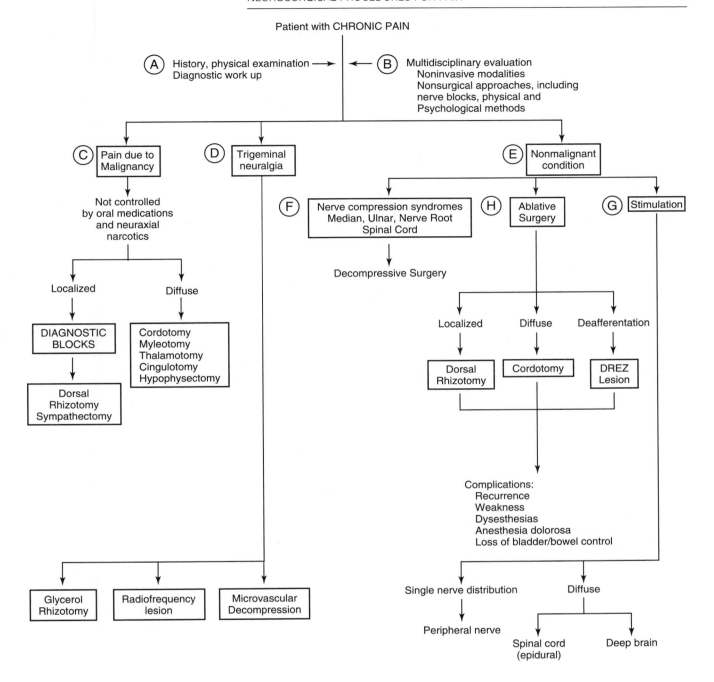

Patient with CHRONIC PAIN

(A) History, physical examination →   ← (B) Multidisciplinary evaluation
     Diagnostic work up   Noninvasive modalities
                                                  Nonsurgical approaches, including
                                                  nerve blocks, physical and
                                                  Psychological methods

(C) Pain due to   (D) Trigeminal   (E) Nonmalignant
     Malignancy   neuralgia   condition

Not controlled   (F) Nerve compression syndromes   (H) Ablative   (G) Stimulation
by oral medications   Median, Ulnar, Nerve Root   Surgery
and neuraxial   Spinal Cord
narcotics
                                            Decompressive Surgery

Localized   Diffuse   Localized   Diffuse   Deafferentation

DIAGNOSTIC   Cordotomy   Dorsal   Cordotomy   DREZ
BLOCKS   Myleotomy   Rhizotomy   Lesion
                Thalamotomy
Dorsal   Cingulotomy
Rhizotomy   Hypophysectomy
Sympathectomy

                                                         Complications:
                                                            Recurrence
                                                            Weakness
                                                            Dysesthesias
                                                            Anesthesia dolorosa
                                                            Loss of bladder/bowel control

Glycerol   Radiofrequency   Microvascular   Single nerve distribution   Diffuse
Rhizotomy   lesion   Decompression
                                                         Peripheral nerve   Spinal cord   Deep brain
                                                                                 (epidural)

Prosthetic Support

GORDON BOSKER AND ANDREW GITTER

Amputation-related pain can be caused by multiple factors including surgery and wound healing complications, tissue loading effects from prosthetic limbs, and peripheral and central neuropathic phenomena. The intensity and response of the individual amputee to these potential pain sources varies considerably and is influenced by past pain experiences, cultural conditioning, and psychological issues. Prosthetic appliances and support services play several roles in the management of amputation-related pain. Such roles include facilitating wound healing and pain control during the immediate postoperative period, restoring lost function, and managing persistent residual limb pain.

A. During the immediate postoperative period clinical management of the amputated limb focuses on successful wound healing, control of pain, and prevention of trauma and joint contractures. Pain control is enhanced when wound healing occurs rapidly. Prosthetic appliances and services are used to promote healing and reduce postoperative pain by controlling edema and protecting the limb from external trauma. This is accomplished through the use of removable elastic wraps, elastic stump socks, semirigid (Unna) dressings, or rigid plaster casting of the residual limb. With the rigid dressing, the residual limb is protected from external trauma during transfers and falls, and joint contractures are minimized. The immediate postoperative prosthesis, which consists of a rigid dressing with prosthetic components mounted, enables early evaluation and training in prosthetic limb use but must be closely monitored. Immediate postoperative prosthetic limb fitting is most appropriate for the upper limb amputee or nondysvascular lower limb amputee.

B. Fitting the amputee with a prosthetic limb enhances self-image, improves function, and can assist in managing amputation-related pain. The initial prosthetic limb given to the amputee is called the preparatory, or temporary, prosthesis. The preparatory prosthesis is simple in design and allows the amputee to continue the process of stump maturation and shrinkage, develop tolerance to weight-bearing, and participate in training and skill development regarding the functional use of the device. The definitive prosthetic limb is prescribed following stump maturation typically after 3 to 12 months of preparatory limb use. Appropriate use of specialized prosthetic components can optimize loading and shear forces on the residual limb and assist in eliminating specific pain problems. An example is the use of transverse and multiaxis adapters that allow mediolateral movement of the residual limb and socket while the foot stays stationary on the ground.

C. Phantom limb pain is a common occurrence following amputation. Effective treatment of this pain syndrome requires multiple strategies, and use of a prosthetic device is often helpful.

D. In contrast to phantom limb pain, residual limb pain is perceived as originating and predominantly affecting the residual portion of the limb. Persistent residual limb pain occurs in up to 70% of lower limb amputees, with about half reporting the pain as moderately to severely bothersome. Residual limb pain is commonly described as aching, sharp, throbbing, and hotly burning in character. The underlying causes of residual limb pain can be classified as intrinsic or extrinsic.

1. Intrinsic residual limb pain is caused by changes or complications in the underlying bony or soft tissues of the residual limb. The intrinsic causes of residual limb pain include neuromas, bony abnormalities, poor surgical technique, and underlying disease processes. Neuroma-related pain is characterized by paroxysmal radiating pain and paresthesias usually in the distribution of the affected nerve. This pain may be precipitated by direct compression due to manual palpation or socket pressure, percussion (Tinel's sign), or traction on an adherent scarred nerve. When prosthetic use exacerbates neuroma pain, the use of gel socks or liners, flexible sockets, or socket modification to relieve and off-load sensitive areas may be effective. Bony overgrowth and heterotopic bone formation can occur in any amputee but is most problematic in pediatric amputees. Excessive pressure over the abnormal bone leads to localized pain and tenderness, which can lead to the development of adventitial bursa or frank soft tissue ulceration. Initial management includes prosthetic socket modifications to relieve pressure, although surgical revision may be needed for lasting improvement. Poor surgical technique may contribute to a painful residual limb by compromising weight-bearing tolerance, and it may interfere with obtaining a comfortable socket fit. These potentially preventable problems include incorrect shaping and beveling of cut bone ends, inadequate stabilization of soft tissues through myoplasty or myodesis, or inadequate soft tissue padding. Osteomyelitis, tumor recurrence, and persistent limb ischemia may cause more generalized residual limb pain and require medical and surgical management.

2. Extrinsic residual limb pain is caused by a mismatch between the residual limb and the prosthesis because of poor socket fit or limb malalignment. Most contemporary prosthetic sockets are designed for total contact with modifications to the socket shape to load weight tolerance tissues preferentially. The initial good fit of a socket is inevitably compromised, as residual limb shape, volume, and muscle bulk

change with time. Typically, amputees add socks over the residual limb to accommodate these changes. An inadequate fit occurs when weight-bearing loads shift to tissues with poor pressure tolerance, creating pain when standing or walking. Malalignment of the components of a lower limb prosthesis can create abnormally high or prolonged loading forces in the residual limb. Sagittal plane alignment problems more frequently affect the distal tibia region, whereas frontal plane malalignment primarily affects loading forces along the fibula. Clinical manifestations of poor fit and excessive local tissue loading include persistent erythema following limb use, bursa development, proximal choking with distal edema formation, and skin breakdown. Replacing or changing the liner or using gel-impregnated socks can offer temporary improvement, but ultimately correction of the alignment problem or socket replacement is required.

REFERENCES

Ehde DM, Czerniecki JM, Smith DG, et al: Chronic pain sensations, phantom pain, residual limb pain, and other regional pain after lower limb amputation. *Arch Phys Med Rehabil* 2000; 81:1039–1044.

Gallagher P, Allen D, Maclachlan M: Phantom limb pain and residual limb pain following lower limb amputation: a descriptive analysis. *Disabil Rehabil* 2001;23:522–530.

Henrot P, Stines J, Walter F, et al: Imaging of the painful lower limb stump. *Radiographics* 2000;20:S219–S235.

Leonard JA, Meier RH: Upper and lower extremity prosthetics. In: DeLisa JA, Gans BM (eds) *Rehabilitation Medicine: Principles and Practice.* Philadelphia, Lippincott-Raven, 1998, p 669.

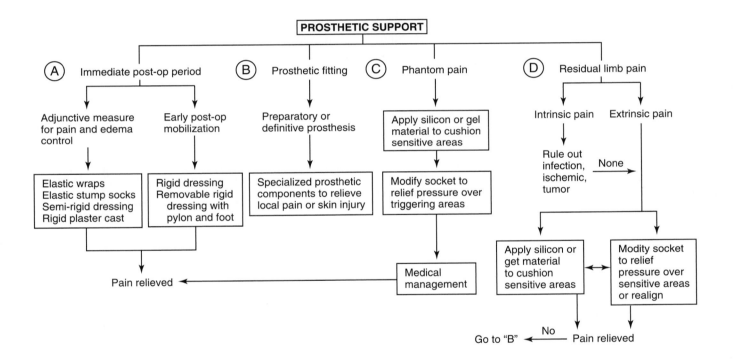

Psychological Interventions

LAWRENCE S. SCHOENFELD AND CATHERINE HOERSTER

The comprehensive evaluation of patients with pain results in identification of dysfunctional factors in four primary areas: cognition, affect, physical (somatic) well-being, and motivation. Each of these factors contributes to pain perception and can be modified through psychological interventions. To intervene successfully with chronic pain, it is vital first to conduct a comprehensive evaluation of the patient's pain history and current level of psychological functioning. Successful pain programs must then identify the dysfunctional components and initiate appropriate psychological intervention strategies to decrease pain perception and abnormal illness behavior. A multidisciplinary approach may maximize benefits to the pain patient.

A. Dysfunctional beliefs, attributions, and expectations often perpetuate pain behavior. Cognitive behavioral therapy (CBT) utilizes education, coping skills training, and behavioral rehearsal to help patients restructure their thoughts, behaviors, and emotions about pain and to change their overall perceptions of pain. Group therapy can also address these issues in a social context.

B. Depression, anxiety, and anger often magnify pain. Relaxation therapies, including biofeedback and hypnosis, serve as useful anxiolytic interventions. Antidepressant medication, exercise, and CBT can also have antidepressant, analgesic, and sleep-normalizing properties. Supportive psychotherapy may facilitate compliance with rehabilitation plans. Although not the treatment of choice for pain, psychodynamic psychotherapy may address the psychological issues such as sexual and physical abuse, anger, helplessness, and depression that may prolong or exacerbate pain issues.

C. Narcotic and anxiolytic drug abuse requires detoxification and appropriate psychological support. Myofacial pain and disuse can be reduced through operant behavior modification strategies, exercise, biofeedback, and psychotropic medication.

D. Primary and secondary gains through interpersonal manipulations, avoidance of responsibilities through pain behavior, or both require direct resolution if the patient is to improve. Job-related stress, social acceptance, sexual dysfunction, and marital difficulties may contribute significantly to pain and are addressed through behavior modification, supportive psychotherapy, marital or sex therapy, and vocational rehabilitation.

REFERENCES

Eimer BN, Freeman A: *Pain Management Psychotherapy: A Practical Guide.* New York, Wiley, 1998.

France R, Krishnau KRR (eds): *Chronic Pain.* Washington, DC, American Psychiatric Press, 1988.

Gatchel RJ, Turk DC (eds): *Psychological Approaches to Pain Management: A Practitioner's Guide.* New York, Guilford Press, 1996.

Miller L: Psychotherapeutic approaches to chronic pain. *Psychotherapy* 1993;30:115–124.

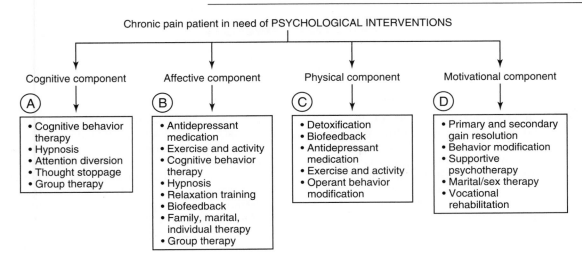

Chronic pain patient in need of PSYCHOLOGICAL INTERVENTIONS

Cognitive component

(A)

- Cognitive behavior therapy
- Hypnosis
- Attention diversion
- Thought stoppage
- Group therapy

Affective component

(B)

- Antidepressant medication
- Exercise and activity
- Cognitive behavior therapy
- Hypnosis
- Relaxation training
- Biofeedback
- Family, marital, individual therapy
- Group therapy

Physical component

(C)

- Detoxification
- Biofeedback
- Antidepressant medication
- Exercise and activity
- Operant behavior modification

Motivational component

(D)

- Primary and secondary gain resolution
- Behavior modification
- Supportive psychotherapy
- Marital/sex therapy
- Vocational rehabilitation

Biofeedback

SOMAYAJI RAMAMURTHY

Biofeedback is a technique that improves the ability of an individual to voluntarily control physiologic activities by providing information back to the individual. The most common feedback given is regarding muscle tension using surface electromyography (EMG) electrodes or the skin temperature using a thermistor. These noninvasive techniques are without any significant side effects. Biofeedback requires use of machines and computers, the cost of which has decreased significantly in recent years. After the initial evaluation the subsequent biofeedback therapy can be administered by a trained technician, thus reducing the cost.

The selection of candidates for biofeedback is typically preceded by an assessment process. In many cases, patients are selected for conservative treatment because more invasive approaches have failed or are deemed inappropriate. Psychological testing may be helpful in identifying patients with concentration difficulties, secondary to depression, which may limit their capacity to participate in self-regulatory approaches to treatment. Patients with elevated scores on the Minnesota Multiphasic Personality Inventory (MMPI), hypochondriasis, and hysteria scales have been shown to experience poorer outcomes, and younger patients sometimes may have more favorable outcomes than older individuals. Patients with previously untreated depression should usually be referred for treatment of the mood disturbance before biofeedback training. Hypochondriacal trends are not a definitive contraindication to biofeedback treatment, but may suggest a pattern of illness behavior or secondary gain that needs to be modified before a self-regulatory approach, such as biofeedback, has a reasonable chance for success.

Biofeedback has proven to be most effective in managing muscle tension headache with a success rate of 45% to 60%. Success rate is further increased to 70% to 75% when biofeedback is combined with progressive relaxation techniques. Vascular headache such as migraine is less responsive whereas cluster headache is least likely to benefit from biofeedback.

Biofeedback has been used for various other painful conditions with variable reported success. Musculoskeletal low back pain and temporomandibular joint syndrome (myofascial pain dysfunction syndrome) are two major categories of chronic pain that are likely to benefit significantly with biofeedback training. Thermal biofeedback has been successfully utilized in the treatment of Raynaud's disease. Pain secondary to constipation has been treated with biofeedback both in children and in adults. Children appear to prefer temperature feedback. Irritable bowel syndrome, intractable rectal pain, vulvar vestibulitis and dyspareunia, fibromyalgia, and chronic regional pain syndrome have also been treated with biofeedback with varying results.

After a thorough evaluation of the chronic pain patient, biofeedback combined with relaxation can be used as the primary therapeutic modality in patients with muscle tension headache with high likelihood of benefit. The ability of the patient to influence and control physiologic activity can be assessed and monitored by assessing the ability of the patient to influence the physiologic activity prior to biofeedback and after the training session. Ten to 15 treatment sessions may be necessary to achieve useful level of control of pain and discomfort.

REFERENCES

Arena JG, Blanchard EB: Biofeedback therapy for chronic pain disorders, pp. 1759–1767.

Blanchard EB, Ahles TA: Biofeedback therapy. In: Bonica JJ (ed) *The Management of Pain*, 2nd ed. Philadelphia, Lea and Febiger, 1990, p. 1722.

Keefe FJ: EMG assisted relaxation training in the management of chronic low back pain. *Am J Clin Biofeedback* 1981;4:3.

Wolf SL, Nacht M, Kelly JL: EMG biofeedback training during dynamic movement for low back pain patients. *Behav Ther* 1982; 13:395.

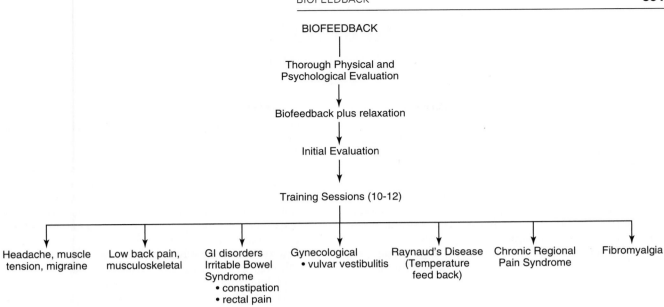

BIOFEEDBACK

Thorough Physical and
Psychological Evaluation

Biofeedback plus relaxation

Initial Evaluation

Training Sessions (10-12)

Headache, muscle
tension, migraine

Low back pain,
musculoskeletal

GI disorders
Irritable Bowel
Syndrome
• constipation
• rectal pain

Gynecological
• vulvar vestibulitis

Raynaud's Disease
(Temperature
feed back)

Chronic Regional
Pain Syndrome

Fibromyalgia

Hypnosis

LAWRENCE S. SCHOENFELD AND SUZETTE M. STOKS

Hypnosis is a pain-attenuating procedure that has been endorsed by the American Medical Association as an accepted treatment modality. It can be used effectively in both children and adults. Hypnosis does not cause significant side effects or a reduction in mental status. A recent meta-analysis indicated that hypnosis provided substantial pain relief for 75% of the populations studied. The mechanism by which hypnotic pain achieves relief remains unclear. For most patients with chronic pain, hypnosis serves as an adjunct to other interventions by enhancing the relaxation response and augmenting self-control strategies. Some patients can achieve total pain control through self-hypnosis.

A. Hypnosis requires the patient to engage in sustained or focused attention or concentration. When the ability to sustain focused attention is compromised, hypnosis provides little or no therapeutic value and may further frustrate the patient, diminishing motivation and compliance. An initial clinical evaluation should exclude patients with psychosis, organic brain syndrome, mental retardation, or severe depression. Patients with significant depression should undergo antidepressant treatment before a trial of hypnosis.

B. Patients are given a full explanation of hypnosis for pain control and then undergo a trial hypnotic induction to establish their susceptibility to hypnosis and to desensitize them to the procedure. Clinicians should also take into account that good therapeutic rapport can lead to increased suggestibility. Formal hypnotic susceptibility scales such as the Stanford Hypnotic Susceptibility Scale and the Hypnotic Induction Profile may be used but are not necessary. Both direct and indirect hypnotic induction techniques are useful for pain control.

C. Patients with low susceptibility to hypnosis may still find the technique useful for facilitating the relaxation response and as a strategy for attention diversion. These two factors provide the patient with perceived control over aspects of the pain.

D. Patients who demonstrate moderate to excellent ability to be hypnotized are able to modify the perception of pain to a significant degree. These patients undergo repeated induction and are provided with direct and indirect suggestions that facilitate dissociation, analgesia, and anesthesia. Pain perception can be moved to alternate locations in the body, and pain characteristics can be altered to increase tolerance. Life-enhancing attitudes to facilitate other treatment modalities may be suggested.

E. After an introduction to hypnosis, the patient may choose to use this procedure for pain management. An audio recording of the procedure can help the patient practice hypnosis daily. Often patients can use self-hypnosis after repeated tape-recorded inductions. Some patients can learn self-hypnosis for pain control after a single trial of hypnosis. Repeated follow-up can reinforce the use of hypnosis to facilitate compliance and to modify the pain experience.

REFERENCES

Barber J: Rapid induction analgesia: a clinical report. *Am J Clin Hypn* 1977;19:138.

Crasilneck HB, Hall JA: *Clinical Hypnosis: Principles and Applications.* Orlando, Grune & Stratton, 1985.

Eimer BN: Clinical applications of hypnosis for brief and efficient pain management psychotherapy. *Am J Clin Hypn* 2000;43:17.

Montgomery GH, DuHamel KN, Redd WH: A meta-analysis of hypnotically induced analgesia: how effective is hypnosis? *Int J Clin Exp Hypn* 2000;48:138.

Oullette EA: Pain management and medical hypnosis. *AAOS Instruct Course Lect* 2000;49:541.

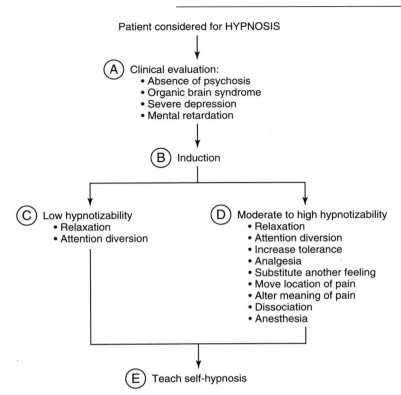

Patient considered for HYPNOSIS

(A) Clinical evaluation:
- Absence of psychosis
- Organic brain syndrome
- Severe depression
- Mental retardation

(B) Induction

(C) Low hypnotizability
- Relaxation
- Attention diversion

(D) Moderate to high hypnotizability
- Relaxation
- Attention diversion
- Increase tolerance
- Analgesia
- Substitute another feeling
- Move location of pain
- Alter meaning of pain
- Dissociation
- Anesthesia

(E) Teach self-hypnosis

Acupuncture

SOMAYAJI RAMAMURTHY

Acupuncture has its origin in ancient Chinese medicine and has been used to treat all types of the diseases. It is believed that energy *chi* flows through a complex system of meridians, and the imbalances in energy can be corrected by careful diagnosis and appropriate treatment by inserting needles in the acupuncture points located on these meridians. So far, scientific investigations have failed to demonstrate any anatomic or neurophysiologic evidence to support the claims of the classic acupuncture theories.

Despite innumerable animal and human studies, there is no consensus regarding the mechanisms, indications, number of treatments needed, number and location of needle placements, efficacy of acupuncture points versus nonacupuncture points, manual versus electrical stimulation, or evidence of long-term significant relief. Studies indicate that acupuncture, needling, or electrical stimulation of the trigger points are equally effective. There is a consensus that acupuncture is beneficial for headache and muscular back pain. Patients who believe in the effectiveness of acupuncture are more likely to benefit.

Acupuncture should be considered one of the modalities, not a complete system of treatment, for management of pain. Acupuncture should be considered only after a thorough workup of the patient's problem by a physician. Otherwise, an early diagnosis and treatment of serious illnesses can be missed. Knowledge of anatomy and sterile techniques is necessary for the administration of acupuncture.

ACUPUNCTURE PROCEDURE

Because of the lack of consensus, the following approach is utilized at our pain management center. Patients with bleeding and clotting disorders and patients with infection in the proposed area of needle insertion are excluded. Informed consent is obtained. The patient is placed in a horizontal position to avoid vasovagal reactions. The skin is cleansed with alcohol, and 28- to 30-gauge disposable needles that are 2 to 4 cm long are inserted into the classic myofascial trigger points. (We do not recommend the use of reusable needles.) Approximately 15 to 20 needles are utilized per session. During needle insertions to the chest or neck, special precautions are taken to avoid pneumothorax. When placing needles close to the spine, care is taken to avoid inserting needles into the subarachnoid space or the spinal cord. Each needle is connected with an alligator clamp to a stimulator, and each pair of needles is stimulated at 4 Hz for 60 seconds using a current that produces maximum tolerable stimulation. Needles frequently oscillate with induced muscle contraction. In our experience, manual stimulation is more painful and induces significant histamine release around the needle site; we also occasionally find the needle more difficult to remove after utilizing rotational stimulation. At completion of stimulation, the needles are removed and the patient is allowed to rest before dressing. The initial course of treatment consists of five treatments over a period of 2 weeks. At this time the patient is reevaluated. If no benefit has been obtained, the acupuncture is discontinued.

REFERENCES

Annual meeting report: acupuncture. *J Tenn Med Assoc* 1981; 75:202–204.

Lewith GT, Vincent C: On the evaluation of the clinical effect of acupuncture: a problem reassessed and the framework for future research. *J Altern Complement Med* 1996;2:91–100.

Melzack R: Myofascial trigger points: relation to acupuncture and mechanism of pain. *Arch Phys Med Rehabil* 1981;62:114–117.

Vincent CA, Richardson PH: The evaluation of therapeutic acupuncture: concepts and methods. *Pain* 1986;24:1–13.

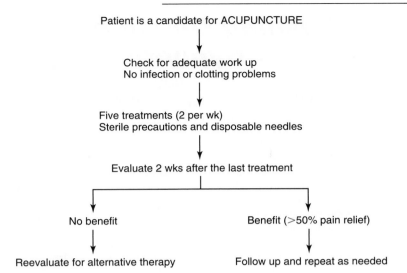

Patient is a candidate for ACUPUNCTURE

Check for adequate work up
No infection or clotting problems

Five treatments (2 per wk)
Sterile precautions and disposable needles

Evaluate 2 wks after the last treatment

No benefit

Reevaluate for alternative therapy

Benefit (>50% pain relief)

Follow up and repeat as needed

Weaning Opioid and Sedative Hypnotic Drugs

JAVIER CANON

A. Weaning the patients who are on significant doses of opioids and sedatives becomes necessary during the pharmacologic management of chronic pain in the following circumstances. When the drugs produce more side effects than benefit, medications are no longer needed because the patient's pain is relieved by other therapeutic modalities, the patient wants to get off of these medications, or the physician decides that the patient is noncompliant with the rules that apply to chronic opioid use.

Patients who exhibit true addictive behavior are candidates for drug detoxification. Detoxification from illicit drugs, according to The Controlled Substances Act, CSA, title II of the Comprehensive Drug Abuse Prevention and Control Act of 1970, should be performed by a specially licensed physician or a program.

Although not life-threatening (except in patients who have cardiovascular problems or who are pregnant) withdrawal from opioids can produce severe discomfort with hyperalgesia, dysphoria, anxiety, bone and muscle pain, spinal grip plexus hyperactivity, diarrhea, yawning, sweating, and rhinorrhea. Withdrawal from benzodiazepines can even precipitate convulsions.

B. The goal of the weaning process is to ensure safe discontinuance of the drugs without producing serious withdrawal symptoms. The patient should be motivated to participate in this program and should be fully aware of the process. Patients who have concurrent psychiatric conditions may be best managed with the participation of the psychiatrist. Generally, the weaning process is done on an outpatient basis, but occasionally hospitalization may be necessary because of the patient's medical condition.

C. The total daily opioid dose is converted into morphine equivalents. Twenty-five percent of the total daily dose is sufficient to prevent withdrawal, although most clinicians proceed at a slower pace. There are various weaning protocols. The patient's medication can be tapered using the opioid of choice over a period of weeks. The night-time dose is the last one to be discontinued to facilitate sleep. Methadone substitution is very effective, with minimal withdrawal symptoms and low cost. Buprenorphine can be used after methadone has been reduced to less than 30 mg per day. Buprenorphine has been used from 4 to 32 mg per day. Preparations containing buprenorphine and naloxone are also available. Clonidine is useful in suppressing the sympathetic nervous system–induced withdrawal symptoms although craving, lethargy, insomnia, restlessness, and muscle aches may not be well suppressed. The dose of clonidine used is weaned 0.3 to 1.2 mg per day while blood pressure is monitored.

D. Benzodiazepine and sedative hypnotics can produce physical dependence with a potential for severe life-threatening withdrawal syndrome. Patients who are taking very large doses of benzodiazepines may require inpatient weaning. Patients tolerate gradual tapering of the benzodiazepines, 10% to 20% per day. Benzodiazepines can be weaned using Diazepam, after calculating the equivalent daily dose and administering in divided doses four times a day and reducing the dose 10% each day. Benzodiazepines can also be weaned using equivalent daily doses of phenobarbital administered in divided doses. Antiepileptic medications such as gabapentin and carbamazepine in a small amount and valproic acid have been used, especially when patients are being weaned from benzodiazepines and opioids simultaneously.

REFERENCES

American Psychiatric Association: Practice guideline for the treatment of patients with substance use disorders: Alcohol, cocaine, opioids. *Am J Psychiatry* 1995;152(Suppl):11.

Fishbain DA: Detoxification of nonopiate drugs in the chronic pain setting and clonidine opiate detoxification. *Clin J Pain* 1997; 8:191–203.

Jaffe JH: Pharmacological treatment or opioid dependence: Current techniques and new findings. *Psychiatry Ann* 1995;25:369–375.

Smith DE, Wesson DR: Benzodiazepine and other sedative-hypnotics. In: Galanter M, Leber HD (eds) *Textbook of Substance Abuse Treatment*, 2nd ed. Arlington, VA, American Psychiatric Press.

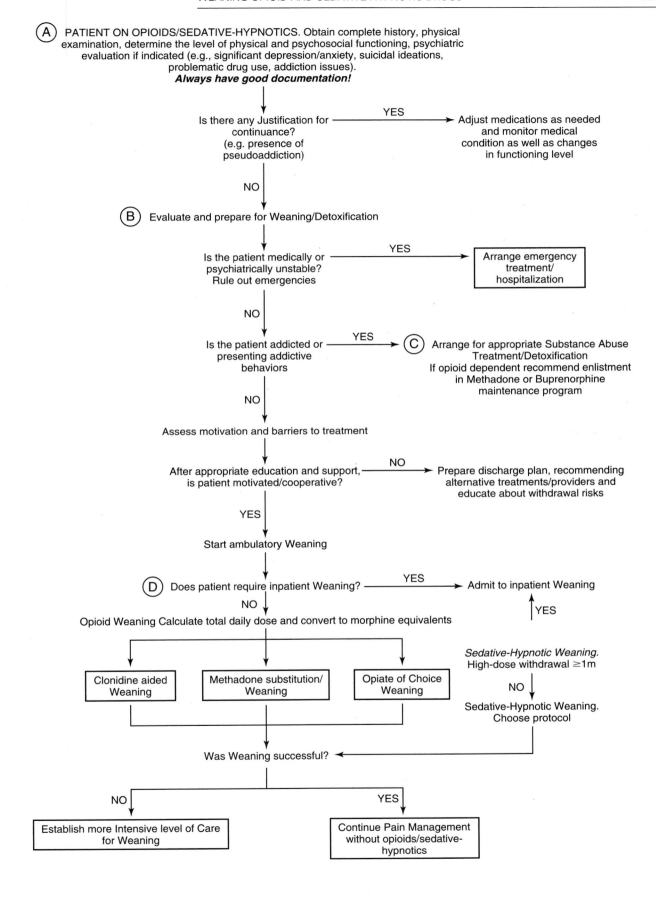

(A) PATIENT ON OPIOIDS/SEDATIVE-HYPNOTICS. Obtain complete history, physical examination, determine the level of physical and psychosocial functioning, psychiatric evaluation if indicated (e.g., significant depression/anxiety, suicidal ideations, problematic drug use, addiction issues).
Always have good documentation!

Is there any Justification for continuance?
(e.g. presence of pseudoaddiction) ——— YES ———▶ Adjust medications as needed and monitor medical condition as well as changes in functioning level

NO

(B) Evaluate and prepare for Weaning/Detoxification

Is the patient medically or psychiatrically unstable? Rule out emergencies ——— YES ———▶ Arrange emergency treatment/ hospitalization

NO

Is the patient addicted or presenting addictive behaviors ——— YES ———▶ (C) Arrange for appropriate Substance Abuse Treatment/Detoxification. If opioid dependent recommend enlistment in Methadone or Buprenorphine maintenance program

NO

Assess motivation and barriers to treatment

After appropriate education and support, is patient motivated/cooperative? ——— NO ———▶ Prepare discharge plan, recommending alternative treatments/providers and educate about withdrawal risks

YES

Start ambulatory Weaning

(D) Does patient require inpatient Weaning? ——— YES ———▶ Admit to inpatient Weaning

NO

Opioid Weaning Calculate total daily dose and convert to morphine equivalents

| Clonidine aided Weaning | Methadone substitution/ Weaning | Opiate of Choice Weaning |

Sedative-Hypnotic Weaning. High-dose withdrawal ≥1m

NO

Sedative-Hypnotic Weaning. Choose protocol

Was Weaning successful?

NO ———▶ Establish more Intensive level of Care for Weaning

YES ———▶ Continue Pain Management without opioids/sedative-hypnotics

APPENDICES

Appendix 1: Definitions of Common Pain Terms

Allodynia — Pain due to a stimulus that does not normally provoke pain

Analgesia — Absence of pain in response to stimulation that would normally be painful

Anesthesia dolorosa — Pain in an area or region that is anesthetic

Central pain — Pain initiated or caused by a primary lesion or dysfunction in the central nervous system

Deafferentation pain — Pain due to loss of sensory input into the central nervous system (CNS), as occurs with avulsion of the brachial plexus or other types of lesions of peripheral nerves or due to pathology of the CNS

Dysesthesia — Unpleasant abnormal sensation, whether spontaneous or evoked

Hyperalgesia — Increased response to a stimulus that is normally painful

Hyperesthesia — Increased sensitivity to stimulation, excluding the special senses

Hyperpathia — Painful syndrome characterized by an abnormally painful reaction to a stimulus, especially a repetitive stimulus, as well as an increased threshold

Hypoalgesia — Diminished pain in response to a normally painful stimulus

Hypoesthesia — Decreased sensitivity to stimulation, excluding the special senses

Neuralgia — Pain in the distribution of a nerve or nerves

Neuritis — Inflammation of a nerve or nerves

Neurogenic pain — Pain initiated or caused by a primary lesion, dysfunction, or transitory perturbation in the peripheral or central nervous system

Neuropathic pain — Pain initiated or caused by a primary lesion or dysfunction in the nervous system

Neuropathy — Disturbance of function or pathologic change in a nerve: in one nerve, mononeuropathy; in several nerves, mononeuropathy multiplex; if diffuse and bilateral, polyneuropathy

Nociceptor — Receptor preferentially sensitive to a noxious stimulus or to a stimulus that would become noxious if prolonged

Noxious stimulus — One that is damaging to normal tissues

Pain — Unpleasant sensory and emotional experience associated with actual or potential tissue damage, or described in terms of such damage

Radiculalgia — Pain along the distribution of one or more sensory nerve roots

Radiculopathy — Disturbance of function or pathologic change in one or more nerve roots

Radiculitis — Inflammation of one or more nerve roots (term does not apply unless inflammation is present)

Suffering — State of emotional distress associated with events that threaten the biologic and/or psychosocial integrity of the individual (suffering often accompanies severe pain but can occur in its absence; hence pain and suffering are phenomenologically distinct)

Trigger point — Hypersensitive area or site in muscle or connective tissue, usually associated with myofascial pain syndromes

Modified from Merskey H, Bogduk N (eds): *Classification of Chronic Pain,* 2nd ed. Seattle, IASP Task Force on Taxonomy, IASP Press, 1994;209–214.

Appendix 2: Pain Clinic Organization

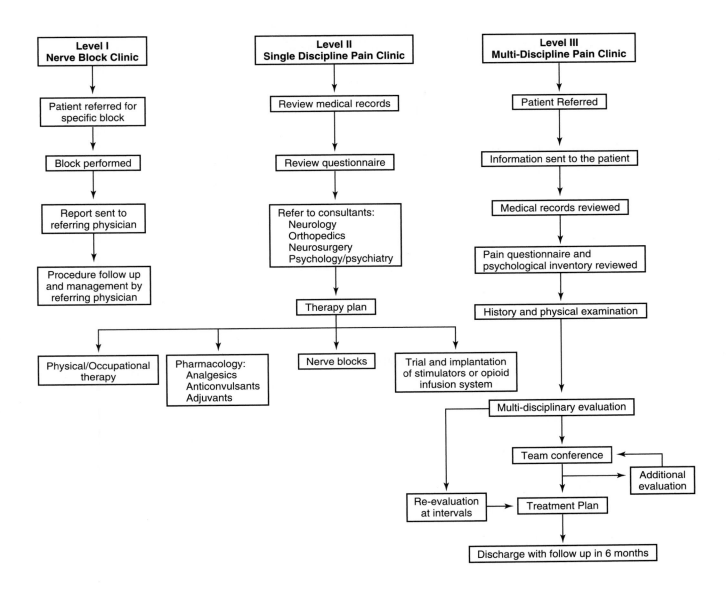

Appendix 3: Assessment Tools

PAIN INTENSITY SCALE: SINGLE-DIMENSION SELF-REPORT MEASURES

Numerical

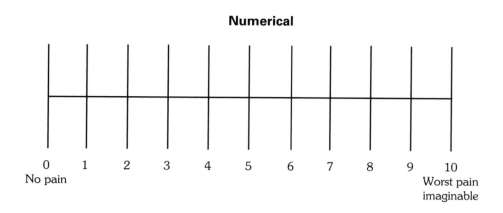

0   1   2   3   4   5   6   7   8   9   10

No pain   Worst pain imaginable

Categorical

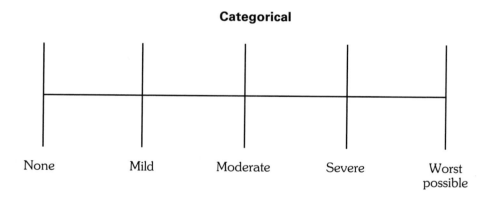

None   Mild   Moderate   Severe   Worst possible

Visual Analogue Scale

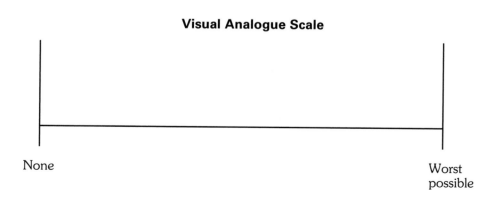

None   Worst possible

Pain Relief Scale

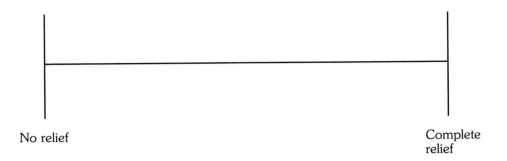

No relief   Complete
                                                 relief

McGILL PAIN QUESTIONNAIRE*

1. *WHERE IS YOUR PAIN?*

Please mark, on the drawings below, the areas where you feel pain. Put "E" if external or "I" if internal near the areas you mark. Put "EI" if both external and internal.

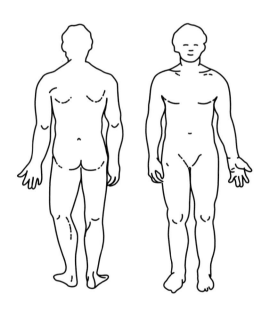

2. *WHAT DOES YOUR PAIN FEEL LIKE?*

Some of the words below describe your present pain. Circle *only* those words that best describe it. Leave out any category that is not suitable. Use only a single word in each appropriate category — the one that applies best.

Sensory: 1–8   *Evaluative:* 16
Affective: 9–15   *Miscellaneous:* 17–20

---

*From Melzack R: The McGill Pain Questionnaire: major properties and scoring methods. *Pain* 1975;1:277–299.

1	2	3	4
Flickering Quivering Pulsing Throbbing Beating Pounding	Jumping Flashing Shooting	Pricking Boring Drilling Stabbing Lancinating	Sharp Cutting Lacerating

5	6	7	8
Pinching Pressing Gnawing Cramping Crushing	Tugging Pulling Wrenching	Hot Burning Scalding Searing	Tingling Itchy Smarting Stinging

9	10	11	12
Dull Sore Hurting Aching Heavy	Tender Taut Rasping Splitting	Tiring Exhausting	Sickening Suffocating

13	14	15	16
Fearful Frightful Terrifying	Punishing Grueling Cruel Vicious Killing	Wretched Blinding	Annoying Troublesome Miserable Intense Unbearable

17	18	19	20
Spreading Radiating Penetrating Piercing	Tight Numb Drawing Squeezing Tearing	Cool Cold Freezing	Nagging Nauseating Agonizing Dreadful Torturing

3. HOW DOES YOUR PAIN CHANGE WITH TIME?

a. Which word or words would you use to describe the *pattern* of your pain?

1	2	3
Continuous Steady Constant	Rhythmic Periodic Intermittent	Brief Momentary Transient

b. What kind of things *relieve* your pain?
c. What kind of things *increase* your pain?

4. HOW STRONG IS YOUR PAIN?

People agree that the following five words represent pain of increasing intensity.

1	2	3	4	5
Mild	Discomforting	Distressing	Horrible	Excruciating

To answer each question below, write the number of the most appropriate word in the space beside the question.

1. Which word describes your pain right now? _____
2. Which word describes it at its worst? _____
3. Which word describes it when it is least? _____
4. Which word describes the worst toothache you ever had? _____
5. Which word describes the worst headache you ever had? _____
6. Which word describes the worst stomachache you ever had? _____

SHORT-FORM McGILL PAIN QUESTIONNAIRE

Patient's name: _____ Date: _____

	None	Mild	Moderate	Severe
1 Throbbing	0) _____	1) _____	2) _____	3) _____
2 Shooting	0) _____	1) _____	2) _____	3) _____
3 Stabbing	0) _____	1) _____	2) _____	3) _____
4 Sharp	0) _____	1) _____	2) _____	3) _____
5 Cramping	0) _____	1) _____	2) _____	3) _____
6 Gnawing	0) _____	1) _____	2) _____	3) _____
7 Hot, burning	0) _____	1) _____	2) _____	3) _____
8 Aching	0) _____	1) _____	2) _____	3) _____
9 Heavy	0) _____	1) _____	2) _____	3) _____
10 Tender	0) _____	1) _____	2) _____	3) _____
11 Splitting	0) _____	1) _____	2) _____	3) _____
12 Tiring-exhausting	0) _____	1) _____	2) _____	3) _____
13 Sickening	0) _____	1) _____	2) _____	3) _____
14 Fearful	0) _____	1) _____	2) _____	3) _____
15 Punishing-cruel	0) _____	1) _____	2) _____	3) _____

PPI

No Pain _____ Worst Possible Pain

0	No pain	_____
1	Mild	_____
2	Discomforting	_____
3	Distressing	_____
4	Horrible	_____
5	Excruciating	_____

Note: 1 to 11 represent the sensory dimension of pain, and 12 to 15 represent the affective dimension.
PPI = present pain intensity.
Modified from Melzack R: The short form McGill Pain Questionnaire. *Pain* 1987;30:191, with permission.

Appendix 4: Opioids

Drug	Approximate equianalgesic oral dose	Approximate equianalgesic parenteral dose	Recommended starting dose (adults more than 50 kg body weight)		Recommended starting dose (children and adults less than 50 kg body weight)*	
			Oral	Parenteral	Oral	Parenteral
Morphine[†]	30 mg (long term) 60 mg (single dose)	10 mg	30 mg q3-4h	5–10 mg q3-4h	0.3 mg/kg q3-4h	0.1 mg/kg q3-4h
Codeine[‡]	130–200 mg	75–100 mg	60 mg q3-4h	60 mg q2h (IM/SC)	1 mg/kg q3-4h	Not recommended
Hydromorphone[†]	7.5 mg	1.5 mg	6 mg q3-4h	1.5 mg q3-4h	0.06 mg/kg q3-4h	0.015 mg/kg q3-4h
Hydrocodone	30 mg	Not available	10 mg q3-4h	Not available	0.2 mg/kg q3-4h	Not available
Levorphanol	4 mg	2 mg	4 mg q6-8h	2 mg q6-8h	0.04 mg/kg q6-8h	0.02 mg/kg q6-8h
Meperidine	300 mg	75–100 mg	Not recommended	100 mg q3h	Not recommended	0.75 mg/kg q2-3h
Methadone	20 mg	10 mg	20 mg q6-8h	5–10 mg q6-8h	0.2 mg/kg q6-8h	0.1 mg/kg q6-8h
Oxycodone	20–30 mg	Not available	10 mg q3-4h	Not available	0.2 mg/kg q3-4h	Not available
Oxymorphone[†]	Not available	1 mg	Not available	1 mg q3-4h	Not recommended	Not recommended

Note: Published tables vary in the suggested doses that are equianalgesic to morphine. Clinical response is the response in the criterion that must be applied for each patient; titration to clinical response is necessary. Because there is not complete cross-tolerance among these drugs, it is usually necessary to use a lower than equianalgesic dose when changing drugs and to retitrate to response.

Caution: Recommended doses do not apply to patients with renal or hepatic insufficiency or other conditions affecting drug metabolism and kinetics.

*Caution: Doses listed for patients with body weight less than 50 kg cannot be used as initial starting doses in babies less than 6 months of age. Consult the *Clinical Practice Guideline for Acute Pain Management: Operative or Medical Procedures and Trauma* section on the management of pain in neonates for recommendations.

[†]For morphine, hydromorphone, and oxymorphone, rectal administration is an alternate route for patients unable to take oral medications, but equianalgesic doses may differ from oral and parenteral doses because of pharmacokinetic differences.

[‡]Caution: Codeine doses above 65 mg often are not appropriate because of diminishing incremental analgesia with increasing doses but continually increasing constipation and other side effects.

Caution: Doses of aspirin and acetaminophen in combination opioid/NSAID preparation must also be adjusted to the patient's body weight.

Adapted from Acute pain management guideline panel. In: *Acute Pain Management: Operative or Medical Procedures and Trauma. Clinical Practice Guideline.* AHCPR Publ. No. 92-0032. Rockville, MD, Agency for Health Care Policy and Research, Public Health Service, U.S. Department of Health and Human Services. February 1992.

Appendix 5: Opioid Side Effects and Treatment

EULECHE ALANMANOU

Nausea and Vomiting	Promethazine 1 mg/kg up to 25 mg IV or PO q6h (Black Box Warning for Pediatric Use) Ondansetron 0.1 mg/kg up to 4 mg IV or 8 mg PO q6h
Constipation	Stool softeners, cathartics
Pruritus	Antihistamines (diphenhydramine, 0.5–1mg/kg IV or PO up to 300 mg/day)

Sleep disturbance
  (persisting despite adequate analgesia)
	Low-dose tricyclics (imipramine, 0.2–0.4 mg/kg PO 1 hr before bedtime;
	  may increase by 50% every 2–3 days up to 1–3 mg/kg solidus/day)

Somnolence	Reduce opioid doses; consider regional techniques; psychostimulants
	  (dextroamphetamine or methylphenidate for adult A.M. and noon,
	  0.1–0.5 mg/kg up to 60 mg/day; for children > age 6 yr, 2-5 mg at A.M. and noon
	  increase by 0.1 mg/kg/dose up to 60 mg/day)

Respiratory depression: Mild	Apply oxygen; reduce opioid dose; stimulate; provide careful observation
Respiratory depression: Severe	Support ventilation; naloxone, 10 µg/kg–titrate slowly to effect

Appendix 6: Antidepressants

Drug	Analgesia	Norepinephrine Reuptake Block	Serotonin Reuptake Block	Anticholinergic	Orthostatic	Sedation	Cardiac Arrhythmia	Elimination Half-life of Parent Drug (hr)
Classic Tricyclics								
Amitriptyline	+++	++	++	+++	+++	+++	+++	9–46
Imipramine	+++	++	++	+++	+++	++	+++	6–28
Nortriptyline	+++	++	++	++	+	+	+++	18–48
Desipramine	++	+++	0	+	++	+	+++	12–28
Selective Serotonin Reuptake Inhibitors								
Paroxetine	+	0	+++	0	0	0	0	21
Citalopram	+	0	+++	0	0	0	0	24
Serotonin-Norepinephrine Reuptake Inhibitors								
Venlafaxine	?	++	+++	0	0	0	0	4

Modified from Max MB, Gilron IH: Antidepressants, muscle relaxants, and N-methyl-D-aspartate receptor antagonists. In: Loeser JD (ed) *Bonica's Management of Pain.* Philadelphia, Lippincott Williams & Wilkins, 2001:1716.

Appendix 7A: Acidic Antipyretic Analgesics (Antiinflammatory Antipyretic Analgesics, NSAIDs): Chemical Classes, Structures, Pharmacokinetic Data, and Therapeutic Dosage

Chemical/ Pharmacokinetic Subclasses	pKa (Binding to Plasma Proteins)	Time to Peak Plasma Conc.*	Elimination Half-life[†] (hr)	Oral Bioavailability (%)	Single Dose (Range); Max. Daily Dose
Low Potency/Fast Elimination					
Salicylates					
Aspirin*	3.5 (>80%)	~0.25[‡]	~20 min[‡]	20–70	0.05–0.1 g; ~6 g[†]
Salicylic acid	2.9 (<90%)	0.5–2[§]	2.5–7[¶]	80–100	0.5–1 g; 6 g
Arylpropionic acids					
Ibuprofen	4.4 (99%)	0.5–2	2–4	80–100	0.2–0.4 g; 3.2 g
High Potency/Fast Elimination					
Arylpropionic acids					
Ketoprofen	4.2 (99%)	0.5–2	1.1–4	~90	15–100 mg; 300 mg
Arylacetic acids					
Diclofenac	4 (99%)	0.5–24**	1–2	30–80[¶]	25–75 mg; 200 mg
Indomethacin	4.5 (99%)	0.5–2	2.6–11.2[††]	90–100	25–75 mg; 200 mg
Ketorolac	3.5 (99%)	0.5–1	5	~100	
Oxicams					
Lornoxicam	4.9 (99%)	0.5–2	4–10	~100	4–12 mg; 16 mg
Intermediate Potency/Intermediate Elimination					
Salicylates					
Diflunisal	3.8 (98–99%)	2–3	8–12	80–100	250–500 mg; 1 g
Arylpropionic acids					
Naproxen	4.15 (99%)	2–4	13–15[††]	~95	0.5–1 g; 2 g
High Potency/Slow Elimination					
Oxicams					
Piroxicam	5.1 (>99%)	3–5	14–160[††]	~100	20–40 mg; initially 40 mg
Tenoxicam	5.0 (>99%)	3–5	25–175[††]	~100	20–40 mg; initially 40 mg

*Time to reach maximum plasma concentration after oral administration.
[†]Terminal half-life of elimination.
[‡]Of aspirin, the prodrug of salicylic acid.
[§]Depending on galenic formulation.
[¶]Dose-dependent.
**Monolithic acid-resistant tablet or similar form.
[††]EHC = enterohepatic circulation.
Modified from Brune K: Non-opioid (antipyretic) analgesics. In: Giamberardino MA (ed) *Pain 2002—An Updated Review: Refresher Course Syllabus.* Seattle, IASP Press, 2002; and *2004 Physicians Desk Reference.*

Appendix 7B: Nonacidic Antipyretic Analgesics: Chemical Classes, Structures, Pharmacokinetic Data, and Therapeutic Dosage

Chemical/ Pharmacologic Class	Fraction Bound to Plasma Proteins	Time to Peak Plasma Conc.* (hr)	Elimination Half-life† (hr)	Oral Bioavailability (%)	Daily Dose (Single Dose) in Adults
Aniline Derivatives					
Acetaminophen (paracetamol)	5–50% dose-dependent	0.5–1.5	1.5–2.5	70–100	1–4 g (0.5–1 g)
Phenazone Derivatives (Pyrazolinone‡)					
Phenazone (antipyrine)	<10%	0.5–2	5–24	~100	1–6 g (0.5–2 g)
Propyphenazone (isopropylantipyrine)	~10%	0.5–1.5	1–2.5	~100	1–6 g (0.5–1 g)
Metamizole-Na (Dipyrone-Na)§					
4-MAP¶	<20%	—	—	—	1–6 g (0.5–2 g)
4-AP**	~50%	1–2	2–4	~100	—
Active metabolites	~50%	—	4–5.5	—	—
Selective COX Inhibitors††					
Celecoxib	>90%	2–4	9–15	~100	400 mg (40–200 mg)
Valdecoxib	98%	3	~8	~83	40 mg (10–20 mg)
Rofecoxib ᶦ	>80%	2–4	~12	~100	25 mg (12.5–25 mg)

*Time to reach maximum plasma concentration after oral administration.
†Terminal half-life of elimination, dependent on liver function with phenazone.
‡Terms such as pyrazole and, incorrectly, pyrzolone, are also in use.
§Noraminopyrinemethanosulfonate-Na.
¶4-MAP = 4-methylaminophenazone.
**4-AP = 4-aminophenazone.
††Other antipyretic analgesics (exception: acetaminophen) block both COX isoforms at therapeutic concentrations.
Modified from Brune K: Non-opioid (antipyretic) analgesics. In: Giamberardino MA (ed) *Pain 2002—An Updated Review: Refresher Course Syllabus.* Seattle, IASP Press, 2002; and *2004 Physicians Desk Reference.*

INDEX